Theory and Research for Academic Nurse Educators Application to Practice

Rose A. Utley, PhD, RN, CNE

Associate Professor
Missouri State University
Springfield, Missouri

JONES AND BARTLETT PUBLISHERS
Sudbury, Massachusetts
BOSTON   TORONTO   LONDON   SINGAPORE

World Headquarters
Jones and Bartlett Publishers
40 Tall Pine Drive
Sudbury, MA 01776
978-443-5000
info@jbpub.com
www.jbpub.com

Jones and Bartlett Publishers
Canada
6339 Ormindale Way
Mississauga, Ontario L5V 1J2
Canada

Jones and Bartlett Publishers
International
Barb House, Barb Mews
London W6 7PA
United Kingdom

Jones and Bartlett's books and products are available through most bookstores and online booksellers. To contact Jones and Bartlett Publishers directly, call 800-832-0034, fax 978-443-8000, or visit our website, www.jbpub.com.

Substantial discounts on bulk quantities of Jones and Bartlett's publications are available to corporations, professional associations, and other qualified organizations. For details and specific discount information, contact the special sales department at Jones and Bartlett via the above contact information or send an email to specialsales@jbpub.com.

The authors, editor, and publisher have made every effort to provide accurate information. However, they are not responsible for errors, omissions, or for any outcomes related to the use of the contents of this book and take no responsibility for the use of the products and procedures described. Treatments and side effects described in this book may not be applicable to all people; likewise, some people may require a dose or experience a side effect that is not described herein. Drugs and medical devices are discussed that may have limited availability controlled by the Food and Drug Administration (FDA) for use only in a research study or clinical trial. Research, clinical practice, and government regulations often change the accepted standard in this field. When consideration is being given to use of any drug in the clinical setting, the health care provider or reader is responsible for determining FDA status of the drug, reading the package insert, and reviewing prescribing information for the most up-to-date recommendations on dose, precautions, and contraindications, and determining the appropriate usage for the product. This is especially important in the case of drugs that are new or seldom used.

Production Credits
Publisher: Kevin Sullivan
Acquisitions Editor: Amy Sibley
Associate Editor: Patricia Donnelly
Editorial Assistant: Rachel Shuster
Production Editor: Amanda Clerkin
Marketing Manager: Rebecca Wasley
V.P., Manufacturing and Inventory Control: Therese Connell
Composition: Datastream Content Solutions, LLC
Cover Design: Kristin E. Parker
Cover Image: © Dmytro Hurnytskiy/ShutterStock, Inc.
Printing and Binding: Malloy, Inc.
Cover Printing: Malloy, Inc.

Library of Congress Cataloging-in-Publication Data
Utley, Rose.
    Theory and research for academic nurse educators : application to practice / Rose Utley.
        p. ; cm.
    Includes bibliographical references and index.
    ISBN-13: 978-0-7637-7413-4 (alk. paper)
    ISBN-10: 0-7637-7413-8 (alk. paper)
    1. Nursing—Study and teaching. I. Title.
    [DNLM: 1. Faculty, Nursing—standards. 2 Competency-Based Education—methods. 3. Nursing Education Research—methods. 4. Nursing Faculty Practice. 5. Professional Competence. WY 19 U91t 2011]
    RT71.U85 2011
    610.73071'1--dc22

                                                            2009033393

6048

Printed in the United States of America
14 13 12 11 10   10 9 8 7 6 5 4 3 2 1

Contents

Introduction

Nurse educators have been essential to the development of the nursing profession since the advent of formal nursing education programs. Today, academic nurse educators (ANEs) teach theory in the classroom, skills in the simulation laboratory, and clinical practice in a variety of specialty settings. ANEs teach in traditional face-to-face settings as well as in a variety of distance learning formats, at the undergraduate and graduate levels. Over the years, as nursing education programs have gradually become incorporated into institutions of higher education, the responsibilities of the ANE have expanded. This shift has led to greater involvement of nursing faculty in interdisciplinary collaborations and in the leadership functions within the institution.

Despite the prevalence and centrality of the ANE to the profession of nursing, the roles and responsibilities of nursing faculty had remained undefined for over a century. Then, in 2002, the Southern Regional Education Board (SREB) identified the primary roles of the ANE as teacher, scholar, and collaborator and identified competencies related to each role. Later, in 2005, an expert panel of nurse educators delineated 8 core competencies for ANEs, which served as the foundation for the development of *The Scope of Practice for Academic Nurse Educators* (NLN Certification Governance Committee, 2005). After the publication of the scope of practice document, a national certification examination for ANEs was developed. The Certified Nurse Educator (CNE) examination is now available to validate and recognize the ANE's distinct body of knowledge in the area of academic nursing practice.

This text is designed to explore theoretical and research knowledge that is foundational for practice as an ANE. Therefore, theory and research related to the core competencies delineated by the NLN *Scope of Practice for Academic Nurse Educators* serves as an organizing framework for the chapters of this book. Chapter 1 provides an overview of each competency and integrates the three role functions of teacher, scholar, and collaborator. Suggestions for application to practice are provided at the end of the chapter. Chapters 2 through 9 are devoted to theory and research related to each of the eight competencies. Within each of these chapters, the reader will find objectives, a list of key terms, a description and definition of the competency, discussion of theory and research related to the competency, resources, a bulleted summary, and references to facilitate further study. The application of theoretical and research knowledge to teaching practice is integrated throughout these chapters.

This book is written for nursing faculty ranging from experienced to inexperienced, certified or noncertified; and for graduate students who are enrolled in a nurse educator program. Nurses who are currently teaching in a nursing program will find the text provides a synthesis of knowledge that may be helpful in fulfilling responsibilities and expectations of academic practice and for preparing for national certification as a CNE. The experienced ANE who may already be nationally certified as a CNE will find that the text provides a useful overview of academic practice knowledge and resources for further self-study and exploration. For nursing faculty who teach in a graduate nurse educator program, the text will provide a useful reference for courses within the nurse educator curriculum. In addition, graduate students will find that the text complements the nurse educator curriculum by providing content related to teaching learning theories, assessment, evaluation, and curriculum design. Graduate students will also gain a comprehensive picture of teaching practice and competencies related to scholarship, leadership, and functioning in the educational environment. And finally, this book is for the ANE who simply seeks to better understand her or his scope of practice and the foundational knowledge used in the roles of teacher, scholar, and collaborator.

As mentioned earlier, theory and research related to each competency are discussed in each chapter. In this book, the term theory is used broadly to depict formalized theories related to each competency as well as models, frameworks, concepts, and/or principles. The term *research* refers to knowledge derived from quantitative and qualitative studies, meta-analysis, evaluation research, and systematic reviews of the literature. Because nursing has a history of using theoretical and research knowledge from nursing as well as other disciplines, the chapters reflect this broad knowledge base. The term *application to practice* is also used in the title of this book. In this case, application refers to how theoretical and research information can be used in practice. Using this definition, application involves a range of processes from simply internalizing the information cognitively or affectively, and perhaps teaching the information to others; to taking the information and using it as guide for taking deliberate action.

It is my hope that you will find this text helpful as you explore and continue your professional development as an ANE.

REFERENCES

Southern Regional Education Board, Council on Collegiate Education for Nursing. (2002). *Nurse educator competencies*. Atlanta, GA: Author.

NLN Certification Governance Committee. (2005). *The scope of practice for academic nurse educators*. New York: National League for Nursing.

Acknowledgments

A big thank you to the nursing faculty and administration at Missouri State University for their support and encouragement while writing this book. A special thank you to Dixie Burns who reviewed several chapters of this text and provided valuable feedback; and to Mary Beth Houser, Michele La Forest, Marilyn Morriss, Elizabeth Ozark, Carole Petty, and Carol Robson who provided much support and encouragement along the way. And finally to my dogs, Buster and Sam, who sat by my side for hours on end while I prepared this manuscript.

CHAPTER 1

Academic Nursing Practice—Roles and Core Competencies

OBJECTIVES

After completion of this chapter the reader will be able to

1. Define the teacher, scholar, and collaborator role components of the academic nurse educator (ANE).
2. Differentiate the eight core competencies of the ANE.
3. Identify core competencies related to the ANE roles of teacher, scholar, and collaborator.
4. Compare the four types of scholarship described in Boyer's model.
5. Describe how to use the core competencies in professional development and in ANE program development and evaluation.

KEY TERMS

Academic Nurse Educator (ANE)
Teacher role
Scholar role
Collaborator role
Core competencies
Certified Nurse Educator (CNE)

Boyer's model of scholarship
Scholarship of discovery
Scholarship of integration
Scholarship of application
Scholarship of teaching

INTRODUCTION

The core competencies of the academic nurse educator (ANE) reflect the essential knowledge, skills, values, and beliefs of nursing faculty. The competencies were originally developed by the National League for Nursing Task Group on Nurse Educator Competencies (2005) to reflect the role functions of teacher, scholar, and collaborator. Regardless of the type of specialty or type of didactic course the ANE teaches, the roles of teacher, scholar, and collaborator are reflected in educational practice.

However, the emphasis placed on these role functions depends on the ANE's work setting, educational preparation, teaching experience, and the specific needs of the nursing program. The exact mix of these roles will also vary with the academic mission and philosophy of the institution and with the type of educational program (i.e., undergraduate or graduate). For most ANEs the role component of teacher is primary, with the scholar and collaborator components integrated within the faculty role. In this chapter, an overview of the roles and competencies of the ANE are presented along with a model depicting the relationship between the ANE roles of teacher, scholar, and collaborator and the core competencies.

ROLES OF THE ACADEMIC NURSE EDUCATOR

Over the years, the role of nurses teaching in nursing education programs has evolved and expanded. Initially, much of the didactic content in nursing programs was taught by physicians, with the role of the nursing instructor focused on clinical supervision and enforcement of rules of conduct. Gradually, nurses began to publish and build an identifiable clinical knowledge base and assume more responsibility for classroom didactic instruction, as well as clinical supervision. As nursing education programs became affiliated within academic institutions, the role of teacher expanded to include an emphasis on scholarship and service to the nursing program, institution, profession, and community.

The Teacher Role

The role of teacher includes activities that directly enhance learning. The nursing process, which serves as a framework to guide nursing practice, can be readily applied to guide teaching. In the first part of the process, the ANE assesses the learner's needs, abilities, and learning styles using theories and assessment tools. Based on the learning needs of our students, the next step of the learning process involves diagnosis. In the learning process, diagnosis of problems correlates with establishing learning objectives. The learning objectives guide the next step of the process, which is planning. Planning involves developing and organizing the content and determining learning activities that will address the objectives. The implementation part of the process involves the use of research, and theory-based knowledge of teaching methods and strategies. In the final step of the learning process, a variety of formal and informal evaluation methods can be used. Verbal questioning, games, examinations, formal writing assignments, performance checklists, simulations, and clinical observations can be used to determine the type and degree of learning that has occurred. The evaluation findings can then be used to guide modifications in the learning experience.

Today, nurses function in a fast-paced, high technology environment, and performance expectations for new graduates have grown in complexity. These expectations require the ANE to skillfully integrate teaching and clinical practice knowledge. The ANE needs to be able to share his or her knowledge of clinical practice and enhance learner development and socialization using best practices in interpersonal skills, educational technology, and teaching strategies.

The Scholar Role

Teaching nursing is a scholarly endeavor. It demands awareness of and application of the latest clinical knowledge, as well as knowledge of teaching and evaluation processes. Boyer recognized that academic scholarship went beyond conducting and disseminating research. In his classic work, *Scholarship Reconsidered: Priorities of the Professoriate* (1990) he describes four types of scholarship in which faculty engage. First is the scholarship of discovery. When engaging in the scholarship of discovery, the ANE conducts research that leads to new knowledge. The scholarship of integration emphasizes the synthesis of knowledge from nursing as well as other disciplines. The use of knowledge in clinical and educational practice describes the scholarship of application. Finally, the scholarship of teaching recognizes the importance of the process of disseminating new knowledge to the learner (Box1-1). Further discussion of each type of scholarship is found later in this chapter under competency 7—"Engage in Scholarship" and in Chapter 8.

The Collaborator Role

The collaborator role is useful in all three realms of academia, including teaching, research, and service. In the realm of teaching, the ANE collaborates with faculty colleagues, administrators, and community agencies to deliver optimal learning experiences. Collaboration in teaching may involve establishing new program models such

---

BOX 1-1   Boyer's Four Types of Academic Scholarship

1. Scholarship of Discovery—conducting research and disseminating findings

2. Scholarship of Integration—synthesizing knowledge and research findings

3. Scholarship of Application—using knowledge in education and or clinical practice

4. Scholarship of Teaching—disseminating new knowledge to students

Data from Boyer, E. (1990). *Scholarship reconsidered: Priorities of the professoriate.* Princeton, NJ: The Carnegie Foundation for the Advancement of Teaching.

as service learning or community based education, or may result in formalization of specific strategies for teaching such as mentoring or the development of study groups. In the realm of research, the ANE may collaborate with colleagues from nursing or other disciplines to develop scholarly projects or research studies, or may collaborate with community agencies to obtain grant funding for educational or service related initiatives. Collaboration is also involved in the dissemination of new knowledge via publication or presentation of research findings.

CORE COMPETENCIES OF ACADEMIC NURSE EDUCATORS

Eight core competencies of academic nurse educators (Box 1-2) have been delineated by the National League for Nursing (NLN) and articulated into the Scope and Standards of Academic Nursing Practice (NLN, 2005). These competencies play an important function in curriculum design and development, and in the educator's professional development. Many graduate programs involved in preparing ANEs explicitly use the core competencies as a curriculum guide to assure that the ANE student is introduced to the knowledge and skills related to each competency. The competencies are also used as a blueprint for developing test items for the certified nurse educator (CNE) examination developed by the NLN. To assist the ANE in selecting continuing education offerings that meet their personal learning needs, edu-

---

BOX 1-2   Core Competencies of Academic Nurse Educators

1. Facilitate learning

2. Facilitate learner development and socialization

3. Use assessment and evaluation strategies

4. Participate in curriculum design and evaluation of program outcomes

5. Function as a change agent and leader

6. Pursue continuous quality improvement in the nurse educator role

7. Engage in scholarship

8. Function within the educational environment

Data from NLN Certification Governance Committee. (2005). *The scope of practice for academic nurse educators*. New York: NLN.

cation providers now identify which core competencies are addressed in the program brochures.

In addition to these uses, many academic nursing units have adopted the core competencies as a framework for development and evaluation of promotion and tenure portfolios. The bottom line is that the core competencies delineate the knowledge, skills, and values inherit in teaching nursing students. To be effective in teaching nursing students and to function fully in all aspects of the academic role, critical self-reflection is needed. The core competencies provide a comprehensive framework that can guide the ANE in self-reflection, self-evaluation, and identification of professional development learning needs.

Competency 1: Facilitate Learning

Of all of the eight competencies, "facilitate learning" covers the broadest array of educator knowledge and skills. This competency incorporates 14 task statements that serve to delineate the scope of facilitation of learning. The task statements cover the use of teaching strategies and technology in teaching, skills in all forms of communication, the ability to engage in cognitive processes such as critical thinking and self-reflection, the use of educational theories and role modeling, and assessing learner characteristics that can influence learning. This competency also recognizes the importance of the personal characteristics and behaviors of the teacher such as the ability to inspire, motivate, and establish respectful working relationships with students. In addition to having knowledge of the content area that is taught, the ANE also needs the ability to use appropriate teaching strategies and apply educational theories to the classroom. Skills in using educational technology and the application of evidence-based teaching practices that facilitate learning are also helpful.

An awareness of personal attributes of the student and instructor and how these facilitate or impede learning is also important. The ANE needs to be able to tailor teaching strategies to the content and context of the specific learning situation, and to the unique attributes of the learner such as age, gender, culture, and experience.

In addition to the knowledge areas previously identified, the ANE needs the ability to implement strategies and create effective learning environments, which requires specific skill sets. The instructor also needs the ability to implement diverse teaching strategies such as lecture, discussion, cooperative learning activities, demonstration, simulations, and case studies. Other skills include the ability to create learning opportunities and positive learning environments in the classroom, laboratory, and clinical practice settings. The teacher may create effective learning environments by using positive personal qualities such as caring, integrity, humor, and confidence to create learning environments that empower the learner. By modeling these attributes along with critical thinking, reflective thinking, and communication skills, the ANE is able to facilitate learning.

Competency 2: Facilitate Learner Development and Socialization

Facilitating learner development and socialization focuses on helping students develop as nurses and incorporate the values, knowledge, and skills they have learned into the role of the nurse. Unlike competency 1 in which initial learning of nursing knowledge and skills is emphasized, competency 2 is concerned with facilitating the assimilation of professional attitudes and behaviors, and development of personal and professional goals. The ANE facilitates the transitioning of the student nurse to novice nurse by recognizing learner attributes that may influence professional socialization. The ANE provides resources, and advises and counsels learners with diverse learning styles, educational, and cultural backgrounds. Assisting the student to develop self-reflection and peer evaluation skills is recognized as useful in promoting the student's critical thinking and self-determination.

The ANE also engages in role modeling to facilitate socialization and development of the learner. However, in competency 2, the emphasis shifts from role modeling skills such as critical thinking and communication, which are components of competency 1, to role modeling professional behaviors such as involvement in nursing organizations, serving as an advocate, and pursuing life-long learning opportunities.

Competency 3: Use Assessment and Evaluation Strategies

For the ANE, competency 3 entails skillfully using a variety of assessment and evaluation strategies that are evidence-based. Six task statements are identified for this competency, which reflect the selection and or development of assessment and evaluation strategies for all learning domains. The ANE uses information from the assessment and evaluation strategies to guide the teaching–learning process and to provide feedback to the learner.

Assessment and evaluation may be formative, occurring periodically during a course of study. However, evaluation also may be summative, occurring at the end of a course of study, thereby providing a measurement of achievement and mastery of the course objectives. The ANE needs knowledge and skills in using and interpreting a variety of formative and summative assessment and evaluation strategies when teaching face-to-face, online, or in clinical and laboratory practice. A final aspect of this competency involves using evidence-based literature to design and implement the use of assessment and evaluation tools, and procedures.

Competency 4: Participate in Curriculum Design and Evaluation of Program Outcomes

Another area of responsibility for the ANE involves designing, developing, and evaluating courses and programs of study. Programs of study, or curriculum, are composed of a set of courses each with distinct purposes, objectives, content, assignments, and experiences. When combined, the individual courses that comprise a program of study should provide the opportunity for the learner to meet program outcomes.

The NLN has identified eight task statements that identify key components in the curriculum design and evaluation process. The process involves the integration of curriculum and content knowledge with the application of education principles, theory, and research. This creates opportunities for learning. The ANE designs curriculum to meet the current healthcare needs of the community and society at large. In addition, the ANE designs a curriculum to be consistent with the mission and philosophy of the parent institution.

Curriculum revision is based on determining if program outcomes, student learning needs, and societal healthcare needs are being met. Appropriate change theory and strategies are used by the ANE during curriculum implementation and revisions. To assure that curriculum revisions are seamlessly implemented and program goals continue to be met, the ANE collaborates with outside agencies and maintains community and clinical partnerships that support the program's goals. A final aspect of this competency is assuring continuous program quality by developing and using program assessment models that enable the ANE to recognize and respond to emerging curriculum needs.

Competency 5: Function as a Change Agent and Leader

Many academic institutions define the roles of faculty as including teaching, research/ scholarship, and service responsibilities. Functioning as a change agent and leader describes a continuum of activities that cross into the academic roles of teaching, scholarship, and service, and relies heavily on collaboration. The number and type of tasks that the ANE demonstrates will vary depending on the ANE's experience, education, and the specific expectations of the educational institution. At the beginning of the continuum, the novice ANE may be focused on developing leadership skills, may participate in interdisciplinary efforts at local and regional levels, advocate for change, and promote innovative practices. As experience and leadership skills are acquired, the ANE may incorporate additional change agent and leadership tasks. These include implementing strategies for organizational change, and participating in interdisciplinary scholarly and professional service activities at the national or international levels. Additional advanced tasks include evaluating organizational effectiveness, and providing leadership in the nursing program, institution, profession, and or community.

In the teaching role, being a change agent and leader requires collaboration (with students, faculty peers, and clinical agencies) to provide and evaluate educational experiences. In the researcher/scholar role, the ANE may participate in interdisciplinary clinical or educational research, or promote or implement evidence-based educational practices within the nursing program or the institution. In the service component of the faculty role, the ANE participates in the governance and operation of the nursing program and institution as a whole. Many academic institutions also recognize the value of service to professional and community organizations, which can further enhance the ANE's functioning as a teacher and scholar. For example, serving as a manuscript reviewer may allow the ANE to function as a change agent and leader in the profession by determining the value of publishing certain manuscripts. The role of scholar is enhanced by evaluating the scholarly qualities of the manuscript and by being on the cutting edge of receiving new information. The role of teacher may be enhanced when the review process exposes the ANE to information or experiences that are helpful in fulfilling teaching responsibilities. Therefore, functioning as a change agent and leader may occur in various degrees in the realms of teaching, scholarship, and service.

Competency 6: Pursue Continuous Quality Improvement

The ANE requires knowledge and skills related to the content subject matter and knowledge and skills related to assessment, planning, implementation, and evaluation of the teaching process. In other words, the ANE needs knowledge and skills related to whatever content areas are taught, whether it involves clinical experiences in obstetrics or a didactic course in research. The ANE also needs knowledge and skills related to teaching processes, such as how to design and implement effective assessment, teaching, and evaluation strategies. While a nurse may teach without a high degree of knowledge in a specific content area, the learning experience of students may not be optimal. Likewise, a nurse who lacks knowledge and skills related to the teaching process may not be able to provide the most optimal learning experiences. Therefore, to be most effective, the ANE needs to be attentive to developing and maintaining knowledge and skills in subject matter and in the teaching–learning process.

Competency 6 recognizes the dual nature of the knowledge and skills required by the ANE. The competency recognizes that the knowledge and skills are continually evolving and expanding at a rapid pace. Healthcare procedures and treatments for existing disorders evolve and change. New disorders are discovered with new, expanded understanding of the pathophysiology that underlies the condition. Likewise, new teaching technologies and approaches, as well as new understandings of students and educational theories are continually emerging. To be most effective, the ANE needs to participate in activities that enhance content knowledge and skills, and teaching effectiveness. Feedback from students and peers, and self-reflection are used to determine areas for further professional development. Nursing faculty also may participate in activities that promote socialization into the ANE role such as faculty mentoring, and the development and implementation of educational policies and procedures that impact teaching practice.

Competency 7: Engage in Scholarship

Boyer (1990) offers a reconceptualization of the scope of academic scholarship that incorporates four elements of scholarship (see Box 1-1). In academic settings, scholarship is a broad term that many institutions have internalized to include Boyer's four elements: discovery, integration, application, and teaching. The emphasis placed on achievement in these areas depends on multiple factors, including the institution's mission and goals, the type of program (undergraduate or graduate), the faculty member's educational preparation, and the needs of the program.

The scholarship of discovery is the most widely recognized element of scholarship and is synonymous with conducting original research. The scholarship of discovery not only includes conducting original research but all of the activities associated with research such as grant writing, publishing, and presenting research findings. The scholarship of discovery is often a focus in universities that emphasize graduate education.

The second element of scholarship is referred to as the scholarship of integration. According to Boyer (1990), the scholar involved in integration "seeks to interpret, draw together, and bring new insight to bear on original research" (p.19). The ANE may practice integration through interdisciplinary review of data, interpreting data in a new way, and making connections between disciplines. Boyer acknowledges that the scholarship of integration can involve interpreting one's own research, as well as synthesizing and interpreting the data from studies by other researchers.

The third element of scholarship is a dynamic process that Boyer (1990) refers to as the scholarship of application. It is essentially a form of scholarly service in which "theory and practice vitally interact and one renews the other" (p. 23). As a practice discipline, the scholarship of application is highly valued in nursing. It involves more than merely using data from research studies. It involves applying research and contributing to the knowledge of the discipline. The scholarship of teaching is also a dynamic process in which the teacher studies the subject matter and engages in the teaching process, from assessment through evaluation. The scholarship of teaching "means not only transmitting knowledge, but transforming and extending it as well" (p. 24).

The exact mix of the four scholarship domains varies from institution to institution, from programs within an institution, and from faculty to faculty within a specific program. The philosophy and mission statements of doctoral and master level institutions will by necessity emphasize the scholarship of discovery and integration. The faculty will typically be engaged in grant writing, conducting research, interpreting findings, and publishing and presenting research as primary responsibilities. In comparison, institutions focusing on undergraduate education tend to emphasize the scholarship of teaching and application.

The emphasis placed on the four elements of scholarship also varies within programs, influenced by the ANE's educational preparation and rank. A focus on the scholarship of teaching and application is likely during the early years of one's teaching career or for faculty who do not have advanced educational preparation in research methodology. In comparison, doctorally prepared faculty teaching in graduate nursing programs will typically find greater emphasis on demonstrating the scholarship of discovery and integration.

Competency 8: Function Within the Educational Environment

In 1923, Yale University School of Nursing became the first nursing program to abandon the apprenticeship model of education, shifting from hospital-based instruction to an academic-based educational model (Yale University School of Nursing, 2008). With this shift, nursing instructors were expected to function within a broader faculty role to provide support and meet the goals inherent in the institution's mission and philosophy. Functioning within the educational environment subsumes networking and collaborating with faculty from other disciplines to meet the institution's goals. Therefore, competency 8 concerns the ANE's ability to function as an effective member and leader in the governance structure of the institution and nursing program. Inherent in this competency is the ANE's ability to use knowledge of current educational and professional trends to make informed decisions.

INTEGRATING EDUCATOR ROLES AND
CORE COMPETENCIES

To fully and effectively function as an educator in an academic setting requires integration of the roles of teacher, scholar, and collaborator. The fulfillment of these roles is expressed in the eight core competencies and the task statements that delineate each competency (Figure 1-1). The emphasis placed on each of the roles and the related competencies will vary from individual to individual and from institution to institution.

The role of teacher emphasizes core competencies 1 through 4, (i.e., facilitating learning, facilitating socialization and development, using assessment and evaluation strategies, and participation in curriculum design and program development). The collaborative role emphasizes competency 5, serving as a leader and change agent, and also integrates aspects of several other competencies including competency 2 (facilitate learner development and socialization) and competency 7 (engage in scholarship). The scholar role emphasizes competency 7 (engage in scholarship), and integrates aspects of competency 6 (pursue continuous quality improvement). The scholar role also integrates task statements from other competencies that emphasize the importance of using evidence-based practices. Finally, competency 8 (function within the educational environment), integrates aspects of all three roles, teacher, scholar, and collaborator.

APPLICATIONS TO EDUCATIONAL PRACTICE

The core competencies of ANEs provide a framework that can be useful in individual professional development and evaluation, and in the development and evaluation of graduate curriculum focused on preparing ANEs.

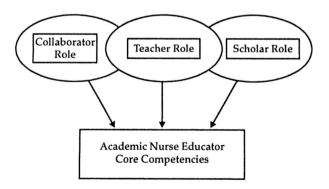

FIGURE 1-1   Integration of Academic Educator Roles and Core Competencies.

Using the Core Competencies for Professional Development

There are two aspects that are essential to using the core competencies for individual professional development. First is to assess one's knowledge and skill level in each of the core competencies. This can be done informally by reading the competencies and related tasks statements and engaging in self-reflection on your knowledge and skill level in each competency. Reflecting on questions such as, "How comfortable and confident do I feel with each competency and task described?" and "How often do I engage in selected tasks?" can be helpful.

A more formal self-assessment can also be performed using assessment tools. Kalb (2008) developed an online Nurse Educator Self-Evaluation Tool that provides the ANE with formalized and quantifiable feedback. The ANE is asked to rate his or her level of knowledge and skill in each of the 66 task statements using a 4-point Likert scale. Results can be tabulated and printed for future reference and can be used to identify areas for future development.

Formal self-assessment also can be accomplished by completing the Certified Nurse Educator Self-Assessment Exam, which is fashioned after the CNE test blueprint in terms of content coverage and question complexity. The self-assessment examination provides 65 multiple-choice questions, along with the opportunity to review rationales for each answer. Upon completion, a score report is provided to assess strengths and identify areas for further study.

After conducting a self-assessment, using one of the methods described, the second step is to identify personal learning needs and set personal learning goals. This text can serve as a helpful self-study review of theory and research related to each competency. In addition, students enrolled in graduate programs to prepare for the ANE role will find the text helpful for setting individual learning goals and meeting nurse educator course objectives. Suggestions for application to educational practice are integrated throughout the text along with resources and references to support further study.

Self-assessment of core competency knowledge also is helpful in providing guidance for selecting appropriate continuing education programs. Most nurse educator conferences and continuing education programs will identify the competencies that the offering addresses, making it easy to select educational programs that will meet the ANE's needs. Thus, after specific learning needs have been identified, this information can be used to select continuing education programs and conferences that emphasize the competency areas needed.

In addition to these applications, many nursing faculty are now seeing the core competencies integrated within job descriptions, and into criteria for tenure and promotion. The ANE seeking tenure or promotion can use the core competencies as a framework for validating performance as well as for guiding professional development. Mentoring programs for nursing faculty are also recognizing the value of using the core competencies to guide the development of less experienced faculty.

Using the Core Competencies in the Nurse Educator Curriculum

The competencies provide a natural framework for developing curriculum and course content in graduate programs. Most nurse educator programs include courses and content covering the teaching process, including how to implement specific teaching strategies, learning theories, and educational technology into the classroom. Many nurse educator programs also include a course on curriculum design and at least one education practicum in which the student can gain teaching experience and begin the process of socialization to the ANE role.

In addition to using the core competencies as a curricular framework, they can be used to guide the self-reflection of ANE students. Nurse educator practicum courses, especially those that allow the student to determine and evaluate personal learning objectives, can easily integrate the core competencies. Students can be asked to self-evaluate their knowledge and skills related to the core competencies, and document activities and experiences that address the competencies. Another option is to have the students develop a course or program portfolio. In the portfolio, the students document their knowledge, skills, and experiences related to the core competencies. Program portfolios are particularly useful for documenting the student's achievement of program outcomes.

CONCLUSION

The eight core competencies reflect the knowledge, skills, values, and beliefs that facilitate effective teaching, scholarship, and service to the institution, the community, and the profession. Acquiring knowledge and skills in each of the competencies reflects developmental progression of the ANE over time. Factors such as years of teaching experience, type of educational preparation, and type of teaching institution play a role in the level of competence demonstrated by the ANE and in the expectations for performance as a teacher, scholar, and collaborator. The competencies and corresponding task statements provide a useful tool for personal professional development of the ANE, as well as a framework for teaching nurse educator students about the role functions of the ANE.

SUMMARY

- The eight core competencies of the academic nurse educator (ANE) reflect knowledge, skills, and values inherent in the role of the ANE.
- The core competencies reflect the academic functions of teaching, scholarship, and service, with the ANE fulfilling the roles of teacher, scholar, and collaborator.
- The role of teacher includes activities that directly enhance learning.
- The scholar role incorporates Boyer's four types of scholarship (i.e., teaching, application, integration, and discovery).
- The scholarship of teaching involves disseminating knowledge to students.
- The scholarship of application involves using knowledge in clinical practice.
- The scholarship of integration involves synthesizing knowledge and research findings.
- The scholarship of discovery is the planning and implementation of research and dissemination of research findings.
- The role of a collaborator is useful in fulfilling teaching, scholarship, and service functions.
- The core competencies provide a comprehensive framework that can guide the educator in self-reflection, self-evaluation, and identification of professional development learning needs.
- Competency 1: Facilitate learning—covers the broadest array of educator knowledge and skills including assessing students' learning preferences, abilities, and needs; and implementing and modeling effective teaching and learning strategies.
- Competency 2: Facilitate learner development and socialization—focuses on helping students develop as nurses and incorporate the values, knowledge, and skills they have learned into the role of the nurse.
- Competency 3: Use assessment and evaluation strategies—entails skillful use of a variety of assessment and evaluation strategies that are evidence-based and/or theoretically sound.
- Competency 4: Participate in curriculum design and evaluation of program outcomes—requires familiarity with the institution and program mission, philosophy, professional standards, and practice expectations.
- Competency 5: Function as a change agent and leader—involves advocating for change, providing leadership within the program, institution, nursing profession, and the community.

- Competency 6: Pursue continuous quality improvement—is concerned with assessing one's performance as an ANE and taking actions to develop and maintain competence.
- Competency 7: Engage in scholarship—involves designing and implementing scholarly activities and using, integrating, and disseminating knowledge derived from scholarship activities.
- Competency 8: Function within the educational environment—involves integrating knowledge of history and trends, and social factors to develop collaborative relationships, advocate for nursing, and provide leadership within the organization.
- Each of the core competencies relate to one or more academic role functions (teaching, scholarship, and/or service).
- The competencies and task statements can be used a framework for self-assessment and as a guide for professional development activities.
- The core competencies provide a natural framework for developing curriculum and course content in graduate nurse educator programs.

RECOMMENDED RESOURCES

National League for Nursing, Faculty Resources: Available at http://www.nln.org/facultydevelopment/facultyresources.htm.
National League for Nursing, Excellence and Innovation in Nursing Education: Selected resources are available at http://www.nln.org/excellence/excellence resources.htm.
National League for Nursing, Task Group on Nurse Educator Competencies has published the core competencies of academic nurse educators with task statements. The document is available from http://www.nln.org/facultydevelopment/pdf/corecompetencies.pdf.

REFERENCES

1. Boyer, E. (1990). *Scholarship reconsidered: Priorities of the professoriate.* Princeton, NJ: The Carnegie Foundation for the Advancement of Teaching.
2. Kalb, K. (2008). Core competencies of nurse educators: Inspiring excellence in nurse educator practice. *Nursing Education Perspectives, 29*(4), 217–219.
3. National League for Nursing, Certification Governance Committee. (2005). *The scope of practice for academic nurse educators.* New York: National League for Nursing.

4. National League for Nursing, Task Group on Nurse Educator Competencies. (2005). *Core competencies of nurse educators with task statements*. Retrieved September 10, 2008 from http://www.nln.org/facultydevelopment/pdf/corecompetencies.pdf

5. Yale University School of Nursing. (2008, May). *About YSN*. Retrieved November 15, 2008 at http://nursing.yale.edu/About/.

CHAPTER 2

Facilitate Learning—Competency 1

OBJECTIVES

1. Compare major educational theories and learning principles used to facilitate learning.
2. Explore theory and research related to the learner, teacher, content, teaching strategies, and the learning environment.
3. Identify research-based teaching strategies and best practices for teaching in the face-to-face classroom, practice laboratory, clinical practicum, and distance learning environments.
4. Explore critical thinking, self-reflection, learner motivation strategies, and processes that facilitate learning.

KEY TERMS

Andragogy
Advance organizer
Behaviorism
Brain dominance
Bruner's cognitive growth theory
Cognitivism
Collaborative teaching
Concept mapping
Constructivism
Connectivism
Critical thinking
Dunn and Dunn Learning Style Model
Emotional intelligence
Generational theories
Gestalt psychology
Gardner's Theory of Multiple Intelligences
Grasha's teaching styles
Humanism
Information processing
Keirsey's four temperaments
Kolb's learning cycle

Kolb's learning styles
Mosston's Spectrum of Teaching Styles
Myers-Briggs personality types
Novice to Expert Theory
Parse's Human Becoming
    Teaching–Learning Model
Pedagogy
Piaget's Theory of Cognitive Development
Principles of learning
Problem-based learning
R2D2 model
Reflective journaling
Reusable learning objects
Schemata
Seven Principles of Good Practice in
    Education
Social Learning Theory
Socratic questioning
Self-Determination Theory
Transformational learning
VAK Learning Styles

DEFINITION AND DESCRIPTION OF COMPETENCY _____

Facilitation of learning represents a range of diverse factors that the academic nurse educator (ANE) needs to consider when teaching. The competency includes 14 task statements that involve knowledge, skills, and values inherent in the teaching process (National League for Nursing [NLN], Task Group on Nurse Educator Competencies, 2005). These task statements describe two types of knowledge needed by the ANE; content or subject matter knowledge, and knowledge of pedagogy, or the art and science of teaching. The subject matter knowledge needed by the ANE varies depending on the courses taught and whether teaching at the graduate or undergraduate level. For example, teaching nursing research requires specific content knowledge in research designs, methods, and analysis strategies; however, the depth, complexity, and scope of instruction will differ for undergraduate and graduate students. The importance of subject matter or content knowledge is recognized in task statement 13, "Maintains the professional practice knowledge base needed to help learners prepare for contemporary nursing practice" (NLN, Task Group on Nurse Educator Competencies, 2005, p. 1).

The second type of knowledge needed by the ANE relates to knowledge of the science and art of teaching, or pedagogy. Examples include knowledge of educational theory and research, teaching strategies, and educational technology; and the art of selective application of science and theory to the learning process. The ANE applies the familiar steps of the nursing process: assessing, diagnosing, planning, implementing, and evaluating to the learner and the learning situation. Thus, attributes of the learner such as learning styles and teaching preferences are assessed and learning needs are determined. The ANE also uses knowledge of the learning situation derived from observation and assessment to determine how learning can best be achieved. This helps create an optimal learning environment.

Next, the teaching plan is implemented and learning is evaluated. Implementation of the teaching plan requires skill in communicating information, organizing presentations, and engaging the student using a variety of strategies. To facilitate learning, the ANE also uses knowledge of "the self" to establish collegial relationships and to motivate and inspire learners. The ANE is able to construct a positive learning environment by skillfully communicating interest, respect, and caring, and by modeling critical thinking and reflective practices.

The final component reflected in the task statements involves the values underlying the teaching process. Each ANE conducts their teaching practice based on personal values and beliefs about teaching and learning. In other words, the ANE operates from assumptions and beliefs about the relationships between the teacher, the learner, and the environment. These values and beliefs influence the type and amount of interaction and communication that is provided to facilitate learning. Even the personal attributes revealed during the teaching process, such as caring, respect, and enthusiasm stem from values and beliefs.

OVERVIEW OF CONCEPTS

In this section, foundational knowledge related to major educational theories is reviewed, followed by research and theories related to the learner, the teacher, the content, teaching strategies, and the learning environment. The ANE will find that each educational theory reflects a unique perspective based on differing assumptions, values, and beliefs about teaching, learning, and the learning process. The ANE who is knowledgeable about the various theoretical perspectives will have a repertoire of approaches to draw on when teaching. As a result, the ANE will be equipped to adjust the teaching styles, methods, and strategies and modify the environment and learning content as needed.

Figure 2-1 is a model that depicts factors that facilitate learning. At the center of the model are the key players in the learning process; the teacher and the student. Both have unique personal attributes, learning style preferences, and teaching style preferences that influence the learning process. To enhance the learning process, the

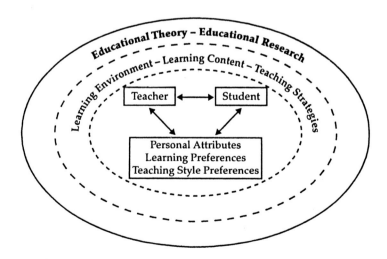

FIGURE 2-1   Factors That Facilitate Learning

ANE skillfully uses self-knowledge of personal attributes and preferences as well as knowledge of the students' attributes and preferences. Through self-reflection, the ANE recognizes how personal attributes and teaching styles affect student learning. Based on sound theoretical principles, the ANE assesses what the student brings to the situation and differentiates between those attributes that facilitate and impede learning. The ANE gains an understanding of the student's attributes such as learning styles, motivation, and learning abilities, and is able to select strategies and processes to enhance the achievement of learning outcomes.

The ANE also uses knowledge and skills to create an optimal learning environment, to design the content, and implement selected teaching strategies. The ANE is able to facilitate learning by being familiar with these components and the dynamic interactions between them, and taking appropriate actions. Each of the core concepts of student, teacher, environment, content, and teaching strategies depicted in the model is surrounded by a field of educational theory and research, which are major sources of educational knowledge, values, and skills used in teaching practice. Using theoretical and research knowledge, the ANE is aware of how aspects of the core components can be strengthened, molded, or modified to enhance student learning.

The factors that facilitate the learning model, depicted in Figure 2-1, serves as an organizing framework for the content of this chapter. Each component will be discussed, beginning with the theoretical knowledge from the outer sphere of the model followed by the core concepts of student, teacher, environment, content, and teaching strategies represented in the inner spheres. To complete the model, the findings from selected research studies and literature reviews will be integrated throughout.

EDUCATIONAL THEORIES AND PERSPECTIVES _____

The earliest theories used to guide teaching approaches and strategies were actually psychological theories of human behavior. These major educational perspectives include behaviorism, cognitivism, social cognitivism, humanism, and constructivism. Each of these perspectives has added a new dimension to our understanding of learners and the learning process. Principles of learning derived from these theories that are useful for guiding the ANE's teaching practice will be highlighted at the end of this section.

Behaviorism

Behaviorism represents a school of thought formulated by the works of Watson, B.F. Skinner, Thorndike, Guthrie, and others. What characterizes these authors' works are their underlying assumptions about the process of learning. To behaviorists learning is seen as a change in behavior, and the environment is key in shaping that behavior. New behaviors are acquired through the process of conditioning in which the learner connects certain responses with certain stimuli (Huitt & Hummel, 1997).

Skinner developed the theory of operant conditioning, or the idea that we behave the way we do because the behavior had certain consequences in the past. The concept of positive and negative reinforcement describes the use of stimuli to increase a behavior. In teaching, a positive reinforcer could be anything the learner will work toward to obtain, such as a reward, praise, or a good grade. A negative reinforcer involves the removal of a negative stimulus, which will increase the likelihood of the behavior occurring again in the future. Schunk (2008) describes a case in which the instructor gives the student independent study time for completing an assignment. If the student uses the time wisely and then receives praise for the good work done, the desired response of using the time wisely is reinforced. In the same situation, the likelihood of a positive behavior can be increased by using negative reinforcement. In negative reinforcement, when the student uses the independent study time wisely, the instructor could reward the good outcome by not providing an additional assignment. In this case, the negative reinforcer is the potential extra assignment. The desired response of using the independent study time wisely was reinforced by removing the negative reinforcer from the situation.

Another related concept in behaviorism is punishment, which in the behaviorist context refers to either presenting a negative reinforcer or removing a positive reinforcer (Schunk, 2008). Punishment can be instituted when the student does not engage in the desired response. For example, in the previous situation in which the instructor gave the student independent study time to complete a task, if the student wasted time and did not adequately complete the task, a negative reinforcer would be to assign additional homework. An example of removal of a positive reinforcer would be to stop providing independent study time.

In applying reinforcement or punishment to a situation, the reinforcing or punishing stimulus needs to be administered close in time to the event so that the student makes the connection between the behavior and the reinforcer or punishment. The principle of contiguity (how close in time two events must be for a connection to be made) and reinforcement (any means of increasing the likelihood that an event will be repeated), are central to explaining the process of conditioning (Schunk, 2008). Based on these principles, it becomes important for the teacher to present the material in small segments, assess for the achievement of the learning outcome, and give immediate feedback to the learner. Immediate feedback allows learners to make a connection between their behavior, the positive or negative reinforcer received, and the desired response (Schunk, 2008).

Although behaviorism is no longer a dominant educational perspective for adult learners, the concepts of positive and negative reinforcement are still useful today, and the application of the principles of behaviorism have supported several other common approaches. For example, generating behavioral objectives, establishing learning contracts, and programmed instruction have roots in behaviorism. Behavioral objectives are clear statements of the intended student learning outcomes of instruction. Thus, students are given a clear description of how they will know if they have achieved the objective.

Another teaching approach that is based in behaviorism is the use of contingency or learning contracts. These are defined as an agreement between the student and teacher that specifies the amount and type of work that will need to be done to accomplish a specific grade (reinforcement). Some faculty have used contingency contracts for specific assignments, especially long-term or complex assignments. Others have used contracts for determining course grades. In either case, a contingency contract helps learners enhance performance by giving them a goal to work toward and by breaking the task into smaller series of steps, which helps them gage their progress (Schunk, 2008, p. 71).

Finally, the use of programmed instruction modules, which were especially popular in the 1960s and 1970s, are also based in behaviorism. Programmed instruction involves designing instructional materials so the student is moved through the material in small steps called frames. At the conclusion of each frame, the student is asked questions about the content in the form of short-answer, fill-in the blank, true/false, or multiple choice questions. If the student responds correctly, the student continues to move forward to explore more content at their own pace. However, if the student responds incorrectly, the student is directed to restudy specific material in the module and is retested using slightly different questions. Because programmed instruction allows the student to work at his or her own pace, it can be used for students who have demonstrated a deficiency in knowledge and need additional study, or for students wanting enrichment in a certain topic. Today, many student workbooks contain exercises and activities that utilize the concept of programmed instruction.

Cognitivism

Cognitivism is comprised of a group of theoretical perspectives encompassing the works of Brunner, Ausubel, Gagné, Vygotsky, gestalt psychologists, and others (McInerney, 2005). Cognitive theories were generated in response to behaviorism, which was seen as offering a narrow and incomplete explanation for learning. As the name implies, cognitivism emphasizes the person's cognitive or thinking processes. Learning is considered "an internal process that involves higher-order mental activities such as memory, perception, thinking, problem-solving, reasoning, and concept formation" (Hand, 2005, p. 57). Compared with the behaviorist perspective, constructivism views the learner as more active in the learning process. Constructivists see learning as the result of the individual using thinking processes to acquire or assimilate new knowledge. Assimilation involves the interaction between new information and the learner's current cognitive structures to form a new understanding of the information (Hand, p. 57).

Cognitivism has been distinguished as two separate schools of thought, the cognitivist and the social cognitivist. The cognitivist view emphasizes understanding the thinking or cognitive processes of the individual. Ausubel's advance organizer, gestalt psychology, Gagné's information processing, and Mayer's multimedia principles are examples of theoretical perspectives based in cognitivism. The social cognitivist perspective, represented by Vygotsky's social development theory, values the role of social processes in learning in addition to cognition. What these theories within the cognitivism umbrella all have in common is the view of learning as more than a change in behavior, but as specific mental processes used by the learner. Cognitivism considers how the mind and memory work to promote learning and is concerned with mental processes such as thinking, memory, knowing, and problem solving.

Cognitivism views learning as schema, or symbolic mental constructions that provide a foundation for organizing and building knowledge. Therefore, cognitivism views learning not as a change in behavior, but as a change in the learner's schemata. According to cognitivism, changes may be observed in the learner, but they are ultimately an indication of change in cognition. Thus, a major difference between behaviorist and cognitivist perspectives is the locus of control for learning. For behaviorists, the locus of control lies with the environment via conditioning and reinforcement. For cognitivists, the locus of control is within the learner's mental processes, and the mental schema or organization of that knowledge. In the following section, a brief overview of selected cognitivist theories is presented.

Bruner's Cognitive Growth Theory

An American developmental psychologist, Jerome Bruner, proposed a theory of cognitive growth to describe the learning process (Bruner, 1964). He believed that a central process of learning involved categorizing information that is perceived. Learners of all ages interpret the world in terms of comparison, noting similarities and differences, and eventually categorize information based on those similarities and differences. Brunner noticed that a child's actions or responses to stimuli were mediated by cognitive processes, such as thoughts and beliefs. He also noticed that children represented information using three modes: enactive, iconic, and symbolic representation. Enactive representation concerns muscle memory or how past events are demonstrated through motor response (Bruner, 1964, p. 2). Iconic representation involves selective organization of images by spatial, temporal, or other dimensions. The learner recognizes that images "stand for" or represent actual objects or events in the same way that a photograph represents the actual object or event (p. 2). The third mode of representation involves the use of symbols such as language to represent the actual objects. Learners using symbolic representation are able to appreciate that words represent an object or event, but are not the actual object or event (p. 2). According to Bruner, children adopt these representations sequentially.

Bruner also believed that children could be taught the same concepts adults learn, but at a less complex level (Schunk, 2008). Thus, as a person's cognitive abilities mature, the same topics can be presented again with greater complexity. Today, ANEs see this principle expressed in the leveling of program objectives and in building upon concepts throughout the nursing curriculum.

Bruner also believed that when new information is presented to learners, the way information is structured and organized can facilitate or detract from learning (Hand, 2005). He proposed that individuals learn by discovery, which is an active and deliberate process of obtaining knowledge by inductive reasoning from specific observations to general concepts. Today, types of discovery or inductive learning that commonly occur in schools include: experiments, independent or group projects, role playing, and computerized simulations of patient care situations. The ANE can use aspects of Bruner's theory by using discovery-based learning methods, as well as by facilitating development of the learner's schemata through analyzing and categorizing acquired knowledge.

Ausubel's Advance Organizer

Ausubel (1968) proposed the use of an advance organizer to help the learner recognize relevant information and see the connections between previous learning and the current topic. When using an advance organizer, the instructor needs to identify explicit connections between past content and how the current topic relates to what is already known. The rationale is that if the learner makes a connection between the new information and previous knowledge, the learning experience will become more meaningful and learning will be facilitated.

In contrast to the inductive reasoning approach used in Bruner's discovery learning, Ausubel's concept of advance organizer relies on deductive processes in which the learner gains perspective on how the subject matter relates to broader concepts and past learning. An advance organizer contains information the student already knows and an overview of the components of what will be learned, in a more abstract form. However, an advance organizer is more than a review of what was and what will be covered, and it is not the same as presenting the lesson objectives. Those are helpful approaches; however, they do not contain the attributes of an advance organizer. Advance organizers use familiar terms and concepts to link what the students already know to the new information that will be presented, therefore an advance organizer is more abstract than an overview.

Schunk (2008) differentiates between two types of organizers—expository and comparative. Expository organizers assist the learner in linking new information to old and assist the learner in seeing the value of the new learning. Using expository organizers may include offering concept definitions and generalizations about the concept. When using a comparative organizer, new information is introduced and connected to the learner's past knowledge, which serves as a structure on which new knowledge can be built. Analogies make effective comparative organizers provided the analogy is made of a concept or situation that is common knowledge to the audience. A common example of a comparative type of advance organizer for teaching about the circulatory system is to relate the circulatory system to a transportation system or to plumbing system concepts of pressure, flow, and constriction. According to Schunk, "Comparative organizers introduce new material by drawing analogies with familiar material. [They serve to] activate and link networks in long-term memory" (p. 284).

Research supports the effectiveness of advance organizers in a variety of contexts. Several meta-analyses on advance organizers (Luiten, Ames & Ackerson, 1980; Stone, 1983) and a systematic review of over 20 experimental studies by Corkill (1992) found positive effects on learning with the proper use of advance organizers.

Gestalt Psychology

The gestalt psychology movement began in Germany, founded by the works of Max Wertheimer, Kurt Koffka, and Wolfgang Kohler, in the early 1900s. *Gestalt* is a German word that has no literal translation in English; however, it is related to the mental form or configuration that is perceived (Gestalt Center of Gainesville, 2009). Gestaltists are therefore concerned with the person's perceptions of things. Schunk (2008) explains that when a person perceives an object, they see the entire figure or object against a background. It is the entire configuration of the object that is meaningful, not the individual parts that make up the object. For example, a tree is not a random arrangement of leaves and branches but an organized whole, and the whole tree cannot be perceived by focusing on the parts. Therefore, gestalt psychology emphasizes the ability to see the whole, to see the entire system and complete structures, rather than a reductionistic approach of looking at parts of a phenomenon in an attempt to understand the whole. The phrase "the whole is greater than the sum of its parts" reflects the gestaltist's emphasis on the perception of the whole and the appreciation of pattern recognition for envisioning the whole. What the phrase implies is that something of the whole is lost when the learner focuses on individual parts.

When gestalt concepts are transferred to the education domain, a sharp contrast with behaviorism is evident. Behaviorism emphasizes a mechanistic view in which the parts are important and can be connected to make a whole. From the gestalt perspective, something of the whole is lost whenever the focus is on the parts, as in the example of perceiving a tree by focusing on the leaves of the tree. Gestaltists' concentrate on the way the mind tends to discover patterns in things and how this contributes to the process of learning and obtaining insight. Perception is emphasized rather than the individual's response to specific stimuli. Gestaltists acknowledge that learners respond to the learning situation by selectively perceiving and responding to certain aspects of the situation. The aspects that the learner perceives are influenced by internal dynamics such as attitude, motivation, personal needs, and external dynamics of the learning situation. Gestalt psychology helps explain why learners attend to certain aspects of a learning situation and screen out other aspects.

Several principles derived from gestalt psychology are useful for educators to consider. First, perception is influenced by unique attributes of the individual and as a result, perception is selective. This means learners may differ in their perception of the same situation. According to gestalt psychology, our perceptions are organized by a variety of principles such as proximity, similarity, common direction, simplicity, and closure (Schunk, 2008, p. 143–144). The principle of proximity concerns the closeness of two objects in a person's perception. The closer they are in space or time the more likely they will be viewed as related. Schunk points out that proximity operates in speech recognition and learning foreign languages, as well with items placed in visual proximity to each other. According to the similarity principle, when items are viewed as similar in color, size, or shape they are perceived as belonging together. When items appear to flow in a similar direction and form a pattern, they are perceived as a figure. The principle of simplicity purports that people tend to organize their perceptual field in simple ordered ways to see the whole. The principle of closure refers to the person's ability to fill in missing formation to create a complete and meaningful picture. The ANE can apply these gestalt-based principles to the design and presentation of instructional materials.

Information Processing Model

Information processing theory focuses on how the individual remembers information. Gagné (1985) describes four stages the brain works through to process information

(Figure 2-2). The first stage, attention, is foundational to all the other stages. Attention involves the physiological process of receiving stimuli or sensory information and generating neural impulses. Second is the processing stage in which the neural impulses are sent to the brain to a sensory register that filters the relevant from the irrelevant. The third stage involves memory storage and specific strategies used to remember and move sensory information from short-term to long-term storage. Sensory information is encoded and stored temporarily in short-term memory. For information to reach long-term memory, the learner engages in deliberate strategies to facilitate storage such as associating the information with something already existing in the learner's schemata or cognitive structure. If the learner wants to keep the information in long-term storage, the information must be organized and given meaning. Research supports that learners remember information more readily when meaning is given to the information (Gagné, Wager, Golas, & Keller, 2005). The fourth stage is referred to as the action stage in which the individual responds to or takes action based on information from long-term memory.

Several learning principles have been derived from the information processing perspective. The need for learner arousal or attention so that the information can be selectively perceived and filtered from irrelevant information is paramount. Arousal can be achieved by changing the pace of instruction, and/or switching to a different teaching modality, or using a novel approach to introduce the topic.

The principle of chunking, or organizing information into smaller familiar groupings is also derived from the information-processing model. In a classic paper,

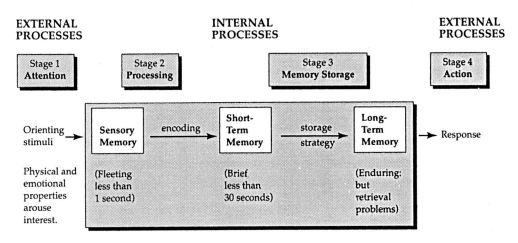

FIGURE 2-2 Information Processing Model of Memory
Source: Data from Bastable S. (2008). Nurse as educator. Principles of teaching and learning for nursing practice. (3rd ed.) Sudbury, MA: Jones and Bartlett, p. 62.

The Magical Number Seven, Plus or Minus Two: Some Limits on our Capacity for Processing Information, Miller (1956) discusses the optimal capacity of our short-term memory to recall lists and sequences of information longer than seven (plus or minus two). When dealing with information that exceeds the seven plus or minus two rule, items can be divided into smaller learning units to facilitate retention. The creation of mnemonics can aid in remembering longer strings of information.

Information processing emphasizes several principles that are useful for the ANE. First, present the foundational facts before higher levels of knowledge. Second, engage students in reasoning with higher-level concepts after they have learned the prerequisite information. Third, use teaching steps that match the internal order in which the brain processes information. The ANE can use key concepts of information processing by using strategies that promote long-term storage of information. Using the principles of arousal and chunking of information when presenting content can assist students in achieving long-term storage of information.

Social Cognitivism

Vygotsky's Social Development Theory represents a branch of cognitivism called social cognitivism. Vygotsky's theory emphasizes the cognitive aspects of learning such as content and teaching methods along with interpersonal aspects such as the context in which content is expressed (Long & Coldren, 2006, p. 238). Although the theory recognizes that learner control is central in construction of new knowledge, the teacher may collaborate with the learner to facilitate the student's construction of meaning. The interpersonal context of learning and the dynamic relationship between the student and instructor are important factors in facilitating learning from the social constructivist view. Thus, effective instruction is based largely on whether the teacher is knowledgeable of the content, knows and uses appropriate methods to teach the content, and is able to create a positive learning environment.

According to Vygotsky's theory, it is important for the instructor to share and make "explicit and external those thinking processes so that the learner may internalize them" (Long & Coldren, 2006, p. 241). This provides the student with scaffolding or schemata that can be used to learn the material.

Constructivism

Constructivism represents a perspective of learning, a broad theoretical framework that views learning as constructed by the individual by building upon previous learning. The name constructivism implies that the learner must generate the knowledge structure or schema; however, the student may acquire the knowledge through active learning strategies or through passive strategies such as reading and lectures. The constructivism view of learning contrasts with behaviorism, which views learning as a passive transmission of information from one individual to another. From the constructivism perspective, the teaching method is not the determining factor; instead, the active processes that the learner uses during the learning process are central. Thus, a key factor in construction of knowledge is that it involves more than merely receiving information.

Constructivist theory suggests that learners take an active role in learning and actually construct knowledge out of their own experiences. This concept represented a dramatic departure from the prevailing learning theories that viewed the learner and learning process as more passive. Major influences in the development of constructivism included the writings of John Dewey and developmental theorist Jean Piaget. Dewey's classic work, *How We Think*, (1910/1997) emphasized the importance of thinking and the processes by which we construct meaning. The idea of creating accurate meaning of a concept or an event is vital. Dewey says, "Through vagueness of meaning we misunderstand other people, things, and ourselves; through its ambiguity we distort and pervert" (p. 129–130).

One way people create meaning is through defining terms used in our language. Dewey delineated three types of definitions—denotative, expository, and scientific (1910/1997, p. 132). Denotative meanings are determined through information gathered by the learner's senses or direct experience. It is through the learner's direct experiences and through identification of aspects of the concept that understanding of the concept is achieved. Expository meanings are derived through associations with established denotative meanings. Dewey explained that learners have a given store of denotative meanings that can be used to create or clarify the understanding of new terms. For example, a person who is familiar with the concept of a cat but has no concept of a tiger can enhance their understanding of what a tiger is by having the teacher build upon the denotative definition and understanding of a cat. To do this, the teacher would compare attributes of the cat such as size, general body shape, and presence of claws, to those of the tiger. The description of the tiger helps the learner create an understanding of the previously unfamiliar concept. Making comparisons and associations is a common strategy the ANE can use to build on previous knowledge.

The third type of definition Dewey identified is the scientific, which uses rules or criteria for identifying and classify items (1910/1997, p. 133). Dewey differentiated popular definitions such as those found in a dictionary, from scientific definitions in several ways. "Popular definitions select certain fairly obvious traits as keys to classification. Scientific definitions select conditions of causation, production, and generation as their characteristic material" (1910/1997, p. 133).

Dewey also recognized that reflective thinking is a key process by which learners construct knowledge, create new meanings, and learn. He defined reflective thinking as "Active, persistent, and careful consideration of any belief or supposed form of knowledge . . . the grounds that support it, and the conclusion to which it tends" (Dewey, 1910/1997, p. 6). Inherent in the process of reflective thinking and learning is the "willingness to endure a condition of mental unrest and disturbance" (p. 13). The process of reflective thinking involves what Dewey calls a "double movement" in which the learner moves between inductive and deductive thinking. The learner engaging in reflection begins by considering the details of the specific event or condition using inductive thinking. Then, the learner moves to a discovery of a deeper understanding of how details are connected to form a comprehensive whole, which can be viewed from a broader perspective. This broader perspective can then be applied to specific conditions (using deductive thinking) and tested. Thus, inductive reasoning involves generating or discovering knowledge that may be generalizable to other situations. Deductive thinking involves thinking in the opposite direction; that is, taking a generalization and applying and testing the generalization to other instances. Dewey's in-depth analysis expanded the cognitivists' emphasis on mental processes, to consider how we use those processes to create meaning and new understanding. The ANE can foster contructivism in learning by encouraging active learning and reflective strategies that make the content meaningful to the learner.

Piaget's Theory of Cognitive Development

In addition to Dewey's influences, Piaget's work also played a role in the development of the constructivist learning perspective. In the field of nursing, Piaget's Theory of Cognitive Development has been tremendously influential, outlining the sensorimotor, preoperational, concrete operational, and formal operational stages of cognitive development (Piaget, 1972; 2003). Although the speed at which a person develops and moves through these stages is highly variable, the sequential nature of progression is not (p. 2). Inherent in the developmental processes described in Piaget's theory is the concept that individuals construct new knowledge from their experiences using the processes of assimilation and accommodation. Assimilation is a process in which information from the outer world is incorporated into the learner's inner world. When a learner assimilates knowledge, the information fits within the learner's current understanding and the learner is able to include or build the new experience into an already existing cognitive framework. When new information doesn't fit the learner's existing understanding, a process of accommodation occurs. Accommodation involves reframing one's mental representation to allow the new information to fit within existing cognitive structures.

Humanism

Humanism emerged in the 1960s as a paradigm that assumed that people act with intentionality based on their values and needs. From the humanism perspective, a person's primary purpose is personal development or self-actualization. In humanism, the educator functions as a facilitator of learning in an environment that is student-centered and personalized.

Perhaps the most well known proponents of humanism are Carl Rogers and Abraham Maslow. Psychologist Carl Rogers (1961) proposed the idea of client-centered therapy that is concerned with the motivations for behavior. In client-centered therapy, the seeking of love, affection, attention, nurturance, and positive self-regard (self-esteem, self-worth, and a positive self-image) are viewed as key factors. These concepts, when translated to the field of education, support a perspective in which educators value and utilize approaches and interactions that maintain or enhance a student's sense of positive regard.

Rogers viewed learning as a continuum that ranged from memorizing nonmeaningful information such as random sequences of numbers or words in an experimental memory study, to experiential or personally meaningful learning (Rogers & Freiberg, 1994). According to Roger's perspective, teaching at the experiential end of the continuum requires student-centered classrooms in which teachers and students can express themselves (Rogers, 1980; 1983; Rogers & Freiberg, 1994).

Another humanistic psychologist, Abraham Maslow, developed a well-known theory of motivation, commonly referred to as the Hierarchy of Human Needs (Maslow, 1968). Similar to the values inherent in Roger's client-centered therapy and experiential learning, Maslow's hierarchy depicts human motivation progressing from personal physical needs, through more subjective affective-based needs, and culminating in the motivation for growth. The hierarchy of needs provides a useful framework for assessing learner motivation and identifying unmet needs that may inhibit learning. The hierarchy includes (1) physiological; (2) safety; (3) love, affection and belonging; (4) self-esteem; and (5) self-actualization needs. The first four needs are considered deprivation needs. When one of these needs is not satisfied, the person is motivated by the deficiency of that need. Generally, each deprivation need must be met in sequence before successive needs can be realized. Self-esteem and self-actualization represent enduring growth or being needs. These growth needs can also serve to motivate learners, provided they perceive the learning to be something that will serve their growth and development, and they are able to focus on those higher-level needs.

When applying the humanistic perspective to learning, the ANE is concerned with the student's motivation, personal growth, and development. Personal interactions with students that enhance their sense of positive regard are valued.

Andragogy: Adult Learning Theory

The term andragogy, or the art and science of teaching adults, was introduced in the United States in the 1970s by Malcolm Knowles. Prior to that time, the educational system in the United States focused on the art and science of teaching children, called pedagogy. Pedagogy describes a system of education in which the teacher has complete responsibility and control over all aspects of learning, including content, teaching strategies, and evaluation. Andragogy recognizes that adults have different learning needs than children. Because of the background and experiences adults bring to the learning environment, they benefit from different teaching approaches than those used for children. Andragogical teaching and learning is problem centered rather than content centered and focuses on the relevance and usefulness of knowledge (Galbraith & Fouch, 2007). Andragogy recognizes that unlike children for whom school attendance is compulsory, when it comes to learning, adult learners are more influenced by career path choices, personal interests, and the social-cultural environment.

When the term andragogy was first introduced, the idea that learning operated under different assumptions for children and adults (thus requiring the use of different principles and approaches) was revolutionary. A persistent misconception about andragogy is that it refers to teaching persons of a specific biological, social, legal, or chronological age group. Knowles preferred to define an adult from a psychosocial perspective as someone who performs roles in society that demonstrate personal responsibility such as employee, spouse, or citizen (Knowles, 1984). Becoming an adult is viewed by Knowles as a process that is achieved by degrees, as the individual accepts increasing responsibility for their life and becomes self-directed.

Andragogy learning theory is based on six assumptions that delineate adults from children in terms of learning (Knowles, Holton, & Swanson, 2005). These assumptions include:

1. Need to Know. Adult learners need to know why, what, and how. The adult learner wants to know the value, and usefulness of what is being taught.
2. Learner Self-Concept. The adult learner's self-concept is autonomous and self-directing. The adult learner may experience conflict with his or her self-concept and previous school experience, in which learning was more teacher dependent.

3. Role of Previous Learning. The adult's life experiences and formal education play a significant role. According to Knowles *et al.* (2005) previous learning experiences result in greater diversity in groups of adult learners. Thus, teachers need to individualize learning approaches for adults.

4. Readiness to Learn. The need to acquire knowledge and skills required for a new role (i.e., career, marriage, or parenthood) enhances the adult's readiness to learn.

5. Orientation to Learning. Adults are more focused on problem-centered learning rather than subject-centered learning. If learning content is problem-centered, it will be meaningful.

6. Motivation. Adults tend to be more motivated to learn by intrinsic, internal pressures such as the desire for personal satisfaction and increased self-esteem, than by external circumstances (Knowles *et al.*, 2005).

Andragogy also operates from a set of core principles based on these assumptions about the nature and characteristics of adult learners. One principle is that adult learners are characterized by autonomy and self-directed behaviors (Galbraith & Fouch, 2007). In applying this principle, the role of the ANE becomes less controlling and more facilitative. The second principle values the adult's life experiences as important to learning. Conducting a needs assessment will help ensure that the learning experiences provided will meet the unique needs of the learners and conveys to the learners that their experiences are valued. A teaching approach in which the instructor encourages students to share and discuss personal experiences related to the subject matters also validates the importance of the student's previous knowledge base. The principle of valuing of life experiences recognizes that adults are motivated or demotivated by their experiences, and that adults operate from a foundation of life experiences that need to be recognized and built upon. A third principle is that learning needs to be relevant. For the teacher this means the usefulness of the information needs to be explicit. Learning goals and objectives need to be stated in terms that depict the relevance of the material to the student's lives. The assumptions and principles of andragogy can be used to develop learning materials and activities, and can help to tailor the learning approaches to the needs of adult learners.

Social Learning Theory

Bandura's Social Learning Theory represents a hybrid of the behaviorist and cognitivist perspectives. According to Bandura (1977), Social Learning Theory explains human behavior as a "continuous reciprocal interaction between cognitive, behavioral, and environmental determinants" (p. vii). Rather than seeing the person as passive in the learning process, (as in the behaviorism perspective), Bandura describes the learner and the environment as in a reciprocal relationship in which each influences the other. Social Learning Theory values the influence of the environment on learning and sees learning as a social process in which the individual can learn vicariously or deliberately by watching others' interactions and behaviors (Figure 2-3). In contrast to the humanistic perspective, which views the internal motivation of the learner as central, Bandura questioned the use of motivational theories as a primary explanation for human behavior (1977, p. 1–2).

The concept of modeling or learning through observation is essential to social learning theory. For an individual to learn by observation requires the cognitive processes of attention, memory, and the influence of motivation. However, Bandura (1977) points out that people do not enact everything that is modeled. Learners are "more likely to adopt a modeled behavior if it results in outcomes they value. . . ." (p. 28). When an observer sees a behavior of another person (i.e., role model), the observer processes the event into memory; then, uses the memory to reproduce the behavior. If positive reinforcement for the behavior was observed, the behavior is likely

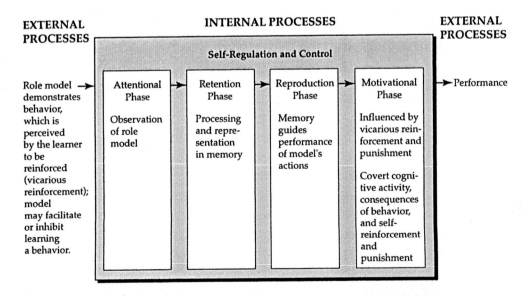

FIGURE 2-3   Model of Bandura's Social Learning Theory
Source: Data from Bastable S. (2008). Nurse as educator. Principles of teaching and learning for nursing practice. (3rd ed.) Sudbury, MA: Jones and Bartlett, p. 62.

to be repeated by the observer. Factors besides positive reinforcement such as the characteristics and status of the role model can also influence the likelihood that the learner will repeat a behavior.

According to Bandura's Social Learning Theory, people learn from passive as well as deliberate observation of another's behavior (Bandura, 1977). The implications for learning in the clinical setting via Social Learning Theory are numerous. Although exposure of the student to only perfect and positive behaviors may be desirable, students will no doubt observe behaviors in the clinical arena that should not be emulated. In these situations, Bandura sees the person's psychological dynamics as influencing the reproduction of the behavior (Bandura, 2001). Processes such as self-efficacy or one's sense of personal ability, one's sense of self-determination, and the ability to engage in self-evaluation and reflection are viewed as influential in the social learning process. The ANE can use critical and reflective thinking strategies to assist the learner in identifying the negative consequences of the behavior and evaluate what was observed. Awareness of the negative consequences of the behavior may serve to discourage the learner from repeating the behavior.

Emerging Learning Theories

In this section, two newer perspectives in learning theory will be discussed. The first is Parse's Human Becoming Teaching–Learning Process based on the Theory of Human Becoming, followed by Siemens's Connectivism theory that explores the learner's relationship with information in our technology rich environment.

Human Becoming Teaching–Learning Process

Parse, a nurse theorist and scholar, developed a perspective on the teaching–learning process that stems from her Theory of Human Becoming (Letcher & Yancey, 2004; Parse, 2004). According to Parse, "the human becoming paradigm offers a different view of what it means to be human, thus, a different view of teaching–learning as a human endeavor" (2004, p. 34). In the human becoming paradigm, the person is viewed as a holistic, unitary being, which is indivisible and ever-changing. Parse defines teaching–learning as "a never-ending journey of giving-receiving in coming to know" (2004, p. 34). Learning is viewed as "a cocreated journey" versus the traditional teaching-learning paradigm in which "teaching is telling" and "learning is destination" (Parse, 2004, p. 34). The human becoming paradigm of teach–learning is described as having a focus on the teacher–learner rather than on the teacher and teacher-designed learning opportunities. The traditional teaching–learning paradigm is developmental, linear, predictable, outcome driven, and teacher-focused compared with the cocreative, ever-changing, human becoming paradigm (Parse, 2004, p. 34).

A qualitative study by Letcher and Yancey (2004) used Parse's teaching–learning theory as a framework for reflective journaling. Nursing students from two different nursing programs used Parse's framework as guide for clinical journal entry topics. Five teaching–learning processes from Parse's theory were used as a framework for journal entries. The processes included "living with ambiguity, appreciating the mystery, inventing the possibilities, witnessing the unfolding, and honoring the wisdom" (Letcher & Yancey, 2004, p. 36). The students from both programs indicated that the journaling process resulted in unanticipated personal growth. The researchers found that the students' journal entries displayed progressive insights and depth of understanding. By the end of the 9-week session, many students were describing their clinical reflections using rich metaphors versus descriptive text (Letcher & Yancey, 2004, p. 40).

Connectivism

Connectivism was first proposed by Siemens in 2005, as a modern-day theory that reflects learning in today's digital age. According to Siemens, "Connectivism is the integration of principles explored by chaos, network, complexity, and self-organization theories" (2005, para. 23). Siemens acknowledges that when knowledge is abundant, as it is in today's world, it is imperative that the individual be able to evaluate the knowledge quickly. "New information is continually being acquired. The ability to draw distinctions between important and unimportant information is vital" (para. 24). To do that requires skills such as the ability to synthesize information, recognize connections, and recognize patterns within the information (para. 4).

Siemens differentiates connectivism from other theories based on five aspects believed to be common to all educational theories (2008, p. 11). The first aspect is concerned with how learning occurs. In connectivism, learning is "distributed within a network" and occurs through social and technological interaction. Learning involves recognizing and interpreting patterns. Second, the factors that influence learning include the "diversity of the network and the strength of network ties" (2008, p. 11). The third component, the role of memory, is described as "Adaptive patterns, representative of current state, existing in networks" (2008, p. 11). Transfer of learning occurs by "connecting to (adding) nodes" (2008, p. 11). Finally, Siemens sees each theoretical perspective as relevant for certain types of learning. He views behaviorism as suited to task learning, cognitivism to reasoning and critical thinking, and constructivism to less well-defined social and interactive concepts. Connectivism is suited to "complex learning, characterized by a rapid changing core, (and) diverse knowledge sources" (Siemens, 2008, p. 11).

In addition to delineating connectivism based on these aspects, Siemens synthesized new roles for educators by drawing on the metaphors developed by Brown, Fisher, and Bonk. Brown (2005) made an analogy between educator and master artist/architect to describe the role of the educator in today's digital world. He explains the analogy by describing an art studio in which students create their art in an open forum, in full view of fellow artists and the master artist or teacher. In the studio, the master artist is able to observe the activities of all students and provide comments and guidance (Siemens, 2008, p. 15). The art studio operates similarly to blogs and wikis that are constructed and used in teaching. Blogs and wikis are constructed by students in the open, where their products are subject to commentary and scrutiny of peers and teachers as they are constructed. Other metaphors for educators were developed by Fisher (as cited in Siemens, 2008) and Bonk (2007). Fisher proposed the role of the teacher as "network administrator." He viewed the network administrator as focusing on helping students create and evaluate new learning networks and make connections between existing networks (Siemens, 2008, p. 16). Bonk (2007) developed the analogy of educator as concierge, seeing the role of educator as one of "directing learners to resources or learning opportunities that they may not be aware of" (Siemens, 2008, p. 16).

Siemens added the final role of "educator as curator"—defining the curator as one who "creates spaces in which knowledge can be created, explored, and connected" (Siemens, 2008, p. 17). Educators as curators are also seen as experts within their field, who are capable of guiding and encouraging the student's exploration. Curators "create learning resources that expose learners to the critical ideas, concepts, and papers within a field" (Siemens, 2008, p. 17).

Siemens also outlined principles of connectivism to provide additional understanding of this new perspective (Box 2-1). The first four principles provide an understanding of learning as both process and substance. As a process, "learning is no longer an internal, individualistic activity" (Siemens, 2005, p. 9). As substance, learning relies on diversity and may exist outside of the individual. Principles 5 and 6, depict aspects of the individual that are important in learning, such as diversity of opinions and capacity to know more. Principle 7 identifies the goal or desired outcome of learning as accurate, up-to-date knowledge. The last principle recognizes that decision-making is indicative of what Siemens refers to as "sensitive dependence on initial conditions," which means that "if the underlying conditions used to make decisions change, the decision itself is no longer as correct as it was at the time it was made" (Siemens, 2005, p. 5). Thus, for learners, there is a need to continually reevaluate the importance of the information and adjust decisions accordingly. More

---

BOX 2-1   Principles of Connectivism

Learning involves:

1. Development and preservation of connections between information sources

2. Seeing connections between sources of information

3. Decision-making processes

4. The use of technology

Connectivism values:

5. Diverse opinions

6. Capacity to know more

7. Accuracy and currency of information

8. Decision-making based on the changing nature of information

Data from Siemens, G. (2005). Connectivism: A learning theory for the digital age. *International Journal of Instructional Technology and Distance Learning, 2*(1), 20.

---

details about this emerging theory can be found at the Web site listed in the resource section.

Principles of Learning

Each educational theory looks at the learning situation from a unique perspective. Each emphasizes different attributes important to learning and provides guidance for teaching. The ANE who is familiar with a range of theoretical perspectives and the key principles of educational theories will be more flexible, adaptable, and deliberate in selecting approaches that facilitate learning. Principles of learning represent the core values, beliefs, and practices that underlie the major educational theories. Principles of learning can be used to help the ANE develop and guide his or her teaching practice.

Although each theoretical perspective has a unique focus and assumptions, principles have been derived from these that can be useful regardless of one's particular perspective. Just as it is important to use a variety of teaching styles and strategies, flexibility in the use of principles can enhance teaching and facilitate learning. Slavin (2006) identified 16 evidence-based principles that are useful to facilitate learning (Table 2-1). Some of these principles are learner focused, others are instructor focused, and some are a combination of both. The learner bears primary responsibility

TABLE 2-1	Principles of Learning	
Principle	**Examples**	**Theoretical Basis**
1. Focusing	Focus is on visual, auditory or kinesthetic clues or tasks	Behaviorism Cognitivism
2. Repetition	Rereading notes, text book, studying flash cards, programmed instruction	Behaviorism Information processing
3. Learner control	Self-paced learning assignments, group projects, problem-based learning	Constructivism Humanism
4. Active participation	Class discussion, small group activities	Constructivism Humanism
5. Learning styles	Preferences for visual, auditory, kinesthetic modes, individual or group activities, structured vs unstructured activities	Cognitivism
6. Organization	Learner physically and or cognitively organizes information by asking questions, highlighting readings, note taking strategies, or teaching the content to peers	Cognitivism Constructivism
7. Association	Learner clarifies the relationship of new information to old. Instructor builds on previous knowledge or uses advance organizer	Cognitivism Information processing Advance organizer
8. Imitation	Return demonstration, learning through observation	Social Learning Theory
9. Motivation	Comments and questions that peek student's curiosity, pointing out the benefits of learning the content Student sets personal learning goals	Humanism
10. Spacing	Presenting content in brief segments to allow learner to absorb information	Cognitivism Information processing
11. Recency	Reviewing information before a test	Cognitivism Information processing

(continues)

TABLE 2-1	Principles of Learning *(continued)*	
Principle	**Examples**	**Theoretical Basis**
12. Primacy	Presenting the most critical information first in a series	Cognitivism
13. Arousal	Appealing to an emotional aspect, use of a novel teaching strategy, a change in pattern	Cognitivism Gestaltism
14. Feedback	Verbal and written comments Peer evaluation activities	Humanism Constructivism
15. Application	Problem-solving activities, case studies, clinical practice	Cognitivism Constructivism
16. Personal history	Assessing and building upon previous learning experiences using questioning, surveys	Social Cognitivism Humanism

Some data from Slavin, R. E. (2006). *Educational psychology: Theory and practice*. New York. Pearson; and Babcock, D., & Miller, M. (1994). *Client education: Theory and practice*. St. Louis: Mosby.

for implementing the learner-focused principles into the learning situation. However, the instructor who is aware of the importance of student-focused principles can guide and facilitate the student in applying them to the learning situation.

The principles of focusing and repetition reflect the behaviorism and cognitivism perspectives. Focusing refers to the need to attend to the information that is to be learned, to mentally focus on the content. Learners find it is easier to attend when the teaching style matches their own style, such as in the use of visual, auditory, or kinesthetic styles. Others need certain types of environmental conditions to aid in the focusing process such as a firm or a soft chair, beverages and snacks, and music or silence. The principle "repetition enhances learning" is concerned with forming a connection between a stimuli and response, and is a helpful cognitive strategy for encoding information into long-term memory.

The principles of learner control, active participation, and feedback (written and verbal), stem from constructivist and humanistic theory. According to Babcock & Miller (1994), learners who feel in control of their learning situation are "more likely to choose methods and approaches that work for them" (p. 45). The principle of active participation refers to mentally engaging with the content and the active teaching strategies being utilized. Discussion, critical thinking, and problem-solving strategies actively engage the learner. The principle of feedback is an instructor-focused principle. The instructor uses written or verbal feedback, or in cases in which peer evaluation is used, the instructor will guide the students through the process and provide specific criteria for the students to use when providing feedback.

Seven principles outlined by Slavin (2006) are derived predominately from cognitivism, including principles of learning styles, organization, association, spacing, recency, primacy, and arousal. The principle that individual learning styles vary is consistent with every learning style theory. Individuals have preferences and strengths in terms of receiving and processing information, in terms of studying, and in the types of learning activities and environments preferred. The meaning of the principle of organization is two-fold. On one level it refers to the organization of content in an appropriate manner. For example, organizing the content from simple to complex when teaching complex topics; or using sequential organization when teaching procedures or critical thinking strategies. Perhaps more importantly, organization also refers to strategies the learner uses to mentally organize information such as note taking, and asking questions. The principle of association refers to relating new information to previous learning, building upon a foundation of knowledge, and creating a structure in which the new information is connected to the previous knowledge. According to Babcock and Miller (1994), establishing an association makes the new information meaningful for the learner. Information that is meaningful is more likely to be remembered. The principle of spacing refers to the learner's ability to process small segments of new information easier than larger amounts of information presented all at one time. Presenting new content in small segments allows the learner time to mentally process the new information, before introducing new content.

The principles of recency and primacy relate to the timing of when content is covered. Recency refers to the ability to more easily recall information that has been recently covered. This principle explains why cramming for an exam is effective for some students, at least in the short term. Learners also tend to learn the first few items in a grouping best, which reflects the cognitivist concept of primacy. Implications for teaching are to present the most critical information early in a learning unit and cover material in small segments.

According to cognitive theorists, arousal also influences retention. Arousal can be achieved by using novelty to introduce the topic, changing the pattern of the presentation by vocal inflection, humor, asking a question to raise an issue, or doing something that stimulates the senses or the emotions and creates a tension in the learner. Application of learning to a variety of life situations through case study, problem-solving, and clinical practicums will help the learner integrate and generalize the knowledge to clinical practice.

Imitation is a principle linked to social learning theory. The process of imitation accounts for learning new skills and behaviors that reflect underlying attitudes, values, and beliefs. The humanist perspective places the principle of motivation as central to the learning process. The reason motivation works may relate to activation of several other principles. Motivation may enhance the learner's ability to focus. Thus, the more motivated the person is to learn the content, the easier it may be for the person to remember. When learners are motivated to learn, it also may be related to the sense of arousal that is generated by the topic and the anticipation the learner feels about learning the content.

The last two principles Slavin (2006) identifies are application and personal history, which reflect influences from the cognitivist and constructivist perspectives. By applying new learning to a variety of different contexts, the learner is creating a cognitive structure in which the new learning becomes meaningful. According to Babcock and Miller (1994), application of new learning helps the learner generalize knowledge and determine other situations in which the learning could be appropriately applied (p. 47). The social cognitivist perspective is reflected in the valuing of personal history in the learning experience. The person's biological, psychological, sociological, and cultural experiences are seen as influencing multiple aspects of learning including mental processes, motivations, self-esteem, attitudes, and more. Each principle of learning describes aspects that can be utilized by the ANE to shape positive learning experiences and facilitate learning.

Seven Principles of Good Practice in Education

The *Seven Principles of Good Practice in Education* were developed from a synthesis of over 20 years of educational research (Chickering & Gamson, 1987). These principles, along with strategies for implementation, are outlined in Table 2-2. Although these principles were initially developed to guide traditional face-to-face classrooms, the principles have a timeless quality that makes them easily applied to other learning environments. In fact, several authors have used these principles as a guide for developing online teaching practices (Graham, Cagiltay, Lim, Craner, & Duffy, 2001; Palloff & Pratt, 2003).

TABLE 2-2   Implementation of Principles of Good Practice in Undergraduate Education

Principles of Good Practice	Strategies for Implementation
1. Encourage student-faculty contact.	• Meet students individually early in the course. • Establish and inform students of communication expectations. • Establish turnaround time for returning assignments.
2. Encourage cooperation between students.	• Incorporate group activities and assignments. • Provide discussion assignments that involve student cooperation.
3. Encourage active learning.	• Have students explore an issue or real problem in the community and share findings with the entire class. • Participate in service-learning projects.
4. Give prompt feedback.	• Establish clear expectations for the timing and nature of written and verbal feedback. • Provide informational and acknowledgement feedback as needed.
5. Emphasize time on task.	• Space assignment deadlines evenly throughout the course.
6. Communicate high expectations.	• Include assignments that are challenging. • Commend students for high quality work.
7. Respect diverse talents and ways of learning.	• Suggest varied ways of learning content. • Use teaching approaches that address multiple learning styles. • Offer choices in assignments when possible. • Encourage creativity in student projects and presentations.

Data from Chickering, A. & Gamson, Z. (1987). Seven principles for good practice in undergraduate education. *AAHE Bulletin, 39*(7), 3–7.

THEORY AND RESEARCH RELATED TO LEARNER ATTRIBUTES

There is a vast amount of theoretical and research-based knowledge relevant to the core competency, facilitate learning. This section will address selected theories and research that relate to the learner (or student) as depicted in the facilitation of learning diagram presented at the beginning of the chapter (see Figure 2-1).

Assessment of students for factors that influence learning should be conducted early in the teaching process. Using information from the assessment of students allows the ANE to make informed decisions regarding the most appropriate learning activities and approaches to implement. Student assessment involves determination of learning styles and preferences; learning strengths and weaknesses; knowledge and experience; the influence of social, cultural, and cohort attributes; and environmental characteristics. A major factor that affects learning is the student's learning style. In this section, various learning style perspectives are discussed and strategies for capitalizing on these styles are presented.

Learning Styles

Learning style refers to inner characteristics and preferences that reflect the way learners think and learn. These inner characteristics and preferences are not stagnant but are influenced by age and experience, and may change with time. Awareness of learning styles allows the learner and the teacher to engage in ways that enhance receptivity and learning, and allows both the teacher and learner to use approaches and strategies that speak to the diverse needs of the learner.

Learning style theories can be categorized based on: (1) learner attributes; (2) ways of processing information; (3) ways of interacting with the physical, social, or cultural environment; and (4) as integrative, in which aspects of several theories are synthesized. In Table 2-3, examples of learning style theories within each category are compared in terms of general focus and assumptions. Awareness of student attributes is helpful when teaching one-on-one, such as in the clinical setting, or when teaching groups of students in the classroom. For example, the ANE can tailor the approaches and language used during one-to-one teaching interactions to challenge, guide, and encourage learning. In large classroom settings, the ANE will likely find students with a wide range of diverse learning styles, preferences, backgrounds, and motivations. Therefore, it may not be practical or effective to use a single strategy that appeals to only one type of learner. For teaching groups of students, the use of diverse strategies throughout the teaching session that appeal to a range of student learning

TABLE 2-3	Comparison of Learning Style Theories			
Categories	**Learner Attributes**	**Ways of Processing**	**Ways of Interacting**	**Integrative**
Examples of theories	• Myers-Briggs Personality Types • Keirsey's Four Temperaments	• Multiple intelligences • Visual, auditory, kinesthetic styles • Brain dominance	• Kolb's Learning Styles • Emotional intelligence theory	• Generational Cohort Theories • Dunn and Dunn Learning Styles Model
General focus	Inner attributes of the learner, i.e., personality characteristics	Cognitive preferences: preferred ways of learning and processing information	Interaction between internal characteristics and learning processes	Integrates multiple perspectives of internal and external influence
Assumptions	Learners have dominant traits that influence the learning process. Each type has unique attributes.	Learning is facilitated when the dominant processing mode is used.		Learning is facilitated when multiple personal and environmental factors are considered.

styles are recommended. Therefore, the ANE will benefit from knowing about a range of learning styles and being able to select strategies that will engage students who prefer those styles. In the following section, each learning style theory is discussed and selected theory-based teaching-learning strategies for the learning style are presented.

Learning Styles Based on Learner Attributes

Learning styles focusing on learner attributes are concerned with the inner characteristics of the person such as personality and temperament. In this section, the Myers-Briggs Personality Theory and Keirsey's Four Temperaments Theory and their applications to teaching and learning are discussed.

Myers-Briggs Personality Theory

Influenced by the work of Carl Jung, Myers and Briggs developed a personality inventory that identifies an individual's preference in each of four dichotomous personality attributes. These dichotomous attributes include (1) introvert–extrovert, (2) sensing–intuitive, (3) thinking–feeling, and (4) perceiving–judging (Myers & Briggs Foundation, MBTI Basics, n.d.). In 1942, Myers and Briggs began testing the type indicators on a small group of friends and relatives. Testing progressed to include larger and more diverse samples, including a sample of 10,000 student nurses (Myers & Briggs Foundation, MBTI Basics, n.d.). As a result of many years of testing, the Myers-Briggs Type Inventory (MBTI) has been revised several times, resulting in a well-validated tool.

The MBTI determines the learner's dominance or preference in each of the four personality traits. The introversion–extroversion trait refers to where the learner prefers to focus. Preference for the outer world of people and events is called extroversion (E) and preference for the inner world of thoughts, ideas, and reflection, is referred to as introversion (I). The dominance of either introversion or extroversion is what Myers and Briggs refers to as the person's "favorite world." For introverts the favorite world involves preferring to focus inwardly and for extroverts the preference is for focusing on the outer world. The introversion–extroversion attribute also identifies where the learner obtains his or her key source of energy. Introverts will be more energized and engaged in solitary activities involving inner dialog, reflection, and analysis of problems, whereas the extrovert will be more energized by exchanging ideas and interacting with others. The ANE can address the introversion–extroversion preferences by incorporating a mix of reflective and solitary learning activities that will appeal to introverts, as well as small group or collaborative activities that will appeal to extroverts.

The sensing–intuiting dichotomy represents "the way people prefer to take in information, and ways they become aware of things, people, events, or ideas" (Western Nevada College, 2001; para. 1). The preference to focus on the information itself is referred to as sensing (S), and the preference to interpret the information is called intuition (N). Individuals who are dominant in sensing pay close attention to physical reality and to the information gathered with the senses. They are concerned with what is real vs. abstract and like to see the practical use of things they are learning. Intuitors like to work with symbols and abstract theories, even if they do not know how they will use them. The ANE can appeal to each preference by offering learning opportunities that allow sensing learners to focus on concrete, factual information by providing opportunities for intuitive learners to interpret information using case studies, reflective activities, and reaction papers.

The third component of Myers-Briggs typology deals with how individuals make decisions, how they evaluate information and draw conclusions. Those classified as thinking (T) value the logical consistency of the information, whereas those in the feeling (F) category consider the particular conditions and people when making decisions. According to the Myers & Briggs Foundation (MBTI Basics, n.d.), people may use thinking for some decisions and feeling for others; however, there usually is a dominate preference. Those operating from the thinking category value being objective and unbiased in their decision making, whereas those in the feeling category base decisions on subjective data. They are concerned with what is best for the people involved and what will produce the most harmonious resolution. The ANE can encourage the student's growth and learning by asking questions that call for the student to consider both the thinking and feeling aspects when making decisions and reaching conclusions.

The fourth set of preferences—judging–perceiving—revolves around what Myers and Briggs call structure (Myers & Briggs Foundation, MBTI Basics, n.d). Structure refers to the type of life style and work habits people prefer. Those who prefer high structure in the form of planned and organized activities fall within the judging (J) domain, whereas those who prefer less structure and seek to stay open to receiving new information are classified as perceivers (P). Judgers prefer to have things decided and appear to others as task oriented. Perceivers prefer a flexible and spontaneous way of life, and seek to understand and adapt to the world rather than organize it. The judging–perceiving preference may also be thought of as the person's orientation to the outer world. The ANE can address these preferences by providing a mix of highly structured and less structured activities and assignments throughout the course of study.

According to the Myers-Briggs Type Inventory (MBTI), a person is dominant in one of each of the four preferences, resulting in a range of 16 personality types. Each preference identifies a range of normal human behaviors and characteristics. Thus, one characteristic is not better or worse than another, but simply different. Recognition of one's type can enable the teacher and student to engage in activities that are supportive, facilitative, and intellectually challenging. For further information on the Myers-Briggs personality typology and the science behind the MBTI, see the Center for Application of Psychological Types Web site listed in the resources section.

Keirsey's Four Temperaments

Building upon the Myers-Briggs typology, Keirsey (1998) outlined a concise framework of four temperaments, referred to as the artisan, guardian, idealist, and rationalist. Keirsey defines temperament as, "a configuration of observable personality traits, such as habits of communication, patterns of action, and sets of characteristic attitudes, values, and talents" (Keirsey.com, 2008, para. 1). The temperaments stem from the interaction of two aspects of human behavior: our communication and actions, in other words, what we say and what we do (The Four Temperaments Overview, 2008, para. 2). Keirsey (1998) describes our communication patterns as being either abstract or concrete. Concrete communicators talk about the reality of day-to-day life, whereas abstract communicators talk about ideas, values, and beliefs. In terms of how people go about their daily business, Keirsey also describes two opposite perspectives, the utilitarian, and the cooperative. The utilitarian acts in a manner that is practical, efficient, and focused on results. The cooperative doer, on the other hand, focuses on the need to do the right thing and considers the effectiveness of the actions as secondary. The four temperament types, characteristics, and teaching strategies are outlined in Table 2-4. Note that each type differs in terms of communication and action preferences.

Regardless of the framework used to determine one's learning style, there are several advantages to knowing the personality or temperament types of the teacher as well as the student. First, students whose style is different from the teacher's may have difficulty adjusting to the classroom environment and to the teaching methods used. Recognition of incongruous learning styles is the first step toward taking action that may help the student and or teacher make adjustments. Second, educators who are aware of the potential individual variations among students in the classroom will be armed with options and strategies that can be used to meeting the student's diverse needs.

Learning Styles Based on Ways of Processing

Each learner has one or more preferred ways of receiving and processing information. Several processing-based models have been developed to describe learner's strengths in terms of learning. These processing models generally focus on innate preferences

TABLE 2-4 Four Temperament Types: Needs, Skills, & Teaching Strategies			
Temperament	**Core Needs**	**Skills**	**Learning Activities/ Teaching Strategies**
GUARDIAN Sensing/Judging (40%-45% of population)	• Group membership • Belonging • Responsibility • Duty	• Logistics • Organizing • Planning • Facilitating • Inspecting • Supporting	• Traditional well organized lectures • Activities that are planned and can be prepared for in advance
ARTISAN Sensing/Perceiving (30%-35% of population)	• Freedom & action • Ability to make an impact • Prefers excitement & variation	• Tactics • Composing • Producing • Motivating • Operating • Executing • Performing	• Hands-on activities • Giving demonstrations • Presentations • Performing skits • Projects that are quick paced
IDEALIST Intuitive/Feeling (15%-20% of population)	• Identity & self-actualization • Meaning & significance	• Diplomacy • Clarifying • Unifying • Individualizing • Inspiring • Mediating	• Activities involving words • Communication of ideas • Group discussions • Role-playing • Small group projects
RATIONALIST Intuitive/Thinking (5%-10% of population)	• Knowledge • Competence • Willpower & mastery	• Strategy • Engineering • Conceptualizing • Theorizing • Coordinatin • Designing	• Activities that are challenging • Activities that generate new understanding • Problem-solving and discovery vs. activities where they demonstrate what they already know

Adapted with permission from D. Hilliard. Western Nevada College. (2001). Learning Styles and Personality Types. From http://www.wnc.edu.

for certain sensory processing channels and on types of intelligences. In this section the visual, auditory, and kinesthetic learning styles, multiple intelligences, and brain dominance theories are explored.

Visual, Auditory, and Kinesthetic Learning Styles

A well-known and easy-to-use processing classification is the visual, auditory, and kinesthetic, or VAK model. Visual, auditory, and kinesthetic refers to the learner's preferred mode of receiving and processing new learning experiences. Despite the popularity of the VAK model, its exact origin is not clear. One group of authors links the origin to the work of Smith in the 1980s (Sharp, Byrne, & Bowker, 2007). However, others link the origin to Bandler and Grinder who founded neuro-linguistic programming (NLP). According to Dunbar-Wells (2003), NLP is based on the idea that we use five information-gathering processes to make sense of our world: visual, auditory, kinesthetic, gustatory (taste), and olfactory (smell). The first three, visual, auditory, and kinesthetic, were found to be used most commonly for acquiring information about our world. From this foundation, the linkage to teaching and learning evolved. Congruence between the teacher and learner in terms of their modes of information gathering and processing has been identified as important (Dunbar-Wells, 2003). Today, the VAK concepts have become widely known and applied to teaching adults and children in diverse settings.

The VAK perspective proposes that visual learners learn best by seeing and reading. Auditory learners transfer information through hearing and speaking, whereas the kinesthetic learner learns by touching and doing. Most learners display a mix of preferences, with one way of receiving and processing information being more dominant than the others. These preferred ways of receiving information have direct implications for the design and implementation of the teaching session. It is believed that the learner's style preference changes over time because of age and life experiences. For example, compared with adults, young children have weaker reading and language skills and short attention spans, and thus tend be kinesthetic dominant learners by default. However, as learners develop language and writing skills that enable them to process verbal and written information, learning preferences may shift to visual or auditory modes. If you wish to explore your VAK learning style, check the Web site listed in the resource section or conduct a search for learning style assessment tools.

Gardner's Theory of Multiple Intelligences

Gardner's Theory of Multiple Intelligences represents another perspective on the preferred ways of receiving and processing information. Gardner popularized the theory of multiple intelligences in his book *Frames of Mind* (1983; 2004). Based on a synthesis of hundreds of studies from multiple disciplines, Gardner originally proposed that learners had seven intelligences, each oriented to a specific type of information such as: linguistic, spatial, kinesthetic, musical, logical-mathematical, interpersonal, and intrapersonal (Gardner, 1999; Gardner & Moran, 2006). Later, Gardner revised the theory, integrating inter- and intrapersonal categories into one category labeled "personal" and adding a category titled "naturalistic" (Table 2-5). Most individuals will have one dominant intelligence, and the other intelligences will range from strong to weak preferences. Gardner proposes that when teaching individuals, learning can be facilitated by recognizing the learner's dominant and preferred intelligences and providing teaching approaches that speak to those intelligences when possible. When teaching groups of students who will collectively have a range of preferred modes of intelligences, learning can be facilitated by providing learning opportunities that address several different intelligences.

The multiple intelligences model can be used in a variety of ways to teach virtually any subject. Hooper & Hurry (2000) recommend using multiple intelligences as a framework for offering students a choice of activities. This approach allows for student-directed learning and self-discovery of strengths related to each intelligence. A second approach is to develop intelligence-specific approaches for teaching a topic. Rather than rigidly adhering to using all of the intelligences when teaching, or randomly selecting intelligences to emphasize, Hooper and Hurry recommend incorporating selected intelligences as appropriate for the students at that point in time.

Hooper and Hurry (2000) found that using one of the flexible approaches to teaching, as described earlier, had three distinct effects on learning. First, it increased awareness in students and faculty about the processes used in learning and allowed the teacher to reach more students than with using only traditional approaches (p. 27–28). Second, by acknowledging the different ways people learn, the use of multiple intelligences places more emphasis on individual learning processes and provides more emphasis on student-centered learning and responsibility (p. 29). The third benefit of using multiple intelligences is in facilitating active learning (p. 29). Active learning using strategies based on multiple intelligences tends to engage learners and provide successful learning experiences that serve to motivate the learners (p. 30).

Armstrong (1994) claims that the key to using the intelligences is to create learning objectives that address the essential features of an intelligence, as described in Table 2-5. Asking questions related to how an intelligence can be used to present and learn the content will allow the teacher to use many intelligences to teach a topic (Armstrong, 1994, p. 3). Some topics will lend themselves more readily to certain

TABLE 2-5 Teaching Approaches for Gardner's Theory of Multiple Intelligences		
Types of Intelligences	**Questions for Developing Learning Activities (Armstrong)**	**Teaching Approaches**
Linguistic or word smart	• "How can I teach this topic using spoken and or written words?" (p. 3)	• Use the spoken or written word in lecture, readings, in-class assignments.
Spatial	• "How can I use visual aids, color, art, metaphor, or visual organizers to teach this topic?" (p. 3)	• Use pictures, diagrams, color, and visualization.
Bodily kinesthetic	• "How can I involve the whole body or hands on experiences when teaching this topic?" (p. 3)	• Have physical models, equipment, or displays available for students to touch and manipulate. • Engage in classroom activities in which movement or hands-on experiences can be incorporated.
Musical	• "How can I use music, rhythm, or environmental sounds to teach this topic?" (p. 3)	• Incorporate or emphasize innate rhythms, music, or sounds relevant to the content or encourage the learner to create these to learn the material.
Logical-mathematical	• "How can I incorporate numbers, calculations, logic, classification, or critical thinking into the learning situation?" (p. 3)	• Use categorization schemes, classifications, numerical information, ask learner questions about their rationale and critical thinking.
Personal	• "How can I involve students in interaction, sharing, or group activity when teaching this topic?" • "How can I evoke personal feelings, memories, or give students choices when teaching this topic?" (p. 3).	• Engage students in sharing, cooperative learning, real-world field experiences, or large-group simulations. • Incorporate in-class or out-of-class assignments that provide personal experience. • Use stories and experiences that elicit feelings or memories about the learning session.
Naturalistic	Not addressed by Armstrong	• Employ activities involving empathy and categorization of natural events and situations.

Data from Gardner, H. (2004). *Frames of mind: The theory of multiple intelligences.* (10th Anniversary edition). New York: Basic Books; and Armstrong, T. (1994). Multiple intelligences: Seven ways to approach curriculum. *Educational Leadership, 52*(3), 27.

intelligences; however, asking the question "How can I use aspects of linguistic, logical, spatial, musical, kinesthetic, personal, or naturalistic intelligence to teach this topic?" will help uncover additional intelligences that can be used to reach students.

Brain Dominance Theories

Theories of brain dominance draw on Jung's perspective of brain functioning. In particular, Benziger's theory of brain dominance views the brain as containing four specialized areas called "modes" that are responsible for different brain functions. According to Benziger, research into brain typology has found that "each person holds what is known as a 'natural lead' or 'natural preference,' meaning that one segment of their brain actually works 'better' than the other sections" (Benziger, The Basics, 2000, para. 3). The four brain function typologies (left and right basal and left and right frontal) and corresponding teaching–learning strategies are outlined in Table 2-6. The Benziger Thinking Styles Assessment (BTSA) is used to discover the natural lead, or preferred mode of the learner.

Another important concept related to Benziger's brain dominance theory is the notion of "falsification of type." According to Benziger, "Though all minds hold their own natural style of thinking, many of us may be using a different segment of our brains in order to operate in our society, workplace, and family environment" (The Basics, 2000, para. 5). This is known as "falsification of type," which according to Benziger can be detrimental to the individual's productivity and health. Falsification of type is one of three interdependent factors that determine how skillfully a person thinks. The other two factors include the person's brain mode preference, and the person's competence.

TABLE 2-6   Brain Dominance Typology and Teaching/Learning Strategies

Brain Dominance Modes	Teaching–Learning Strategies
Basal Left	• "Sequenced, well organized materials" (para. 4) • Learner is energized by logical, proceduralized assignments
Basal Right	• Activities that involve discerning congruity and incongruity
Frontal Left	• Activities that require prioritization and evaluation
Frontal Right	• Activities that involve imagination and visualization

Data from Benziger, K. (2000). *Thriving in mind: Managing preferences to maximize effectiveness*. Retrieved from http://www.benziger.org/articles/pdf/tim_maximizing_preferences, (para. 4–7).

Benziger suggests some general strategies when learners are forced to use their nonnatural mode of thinking, thereby engaging in falsification of type. One strategy is to encourage the learner to be proactive in managing learning situations by scheduling nonpreferred activities during peak energy times or by sandwiching nonpreferred activities between preferred activities. This strategy would be helpful when advising students to register for courses that will demand intense use of the learner's nonpreferred mode or recommending that the student study or do homework involving the nonpreferred mode during his or her peak energy times. Another strategy is to enlist the aide of a mentor. This could be a peer or nonpeer mentor who has expertise in the topic, or someone who functions well in the learner's nonpreferred mode, referred to as a "modal mentor."

Learning Styles Based on Ways of Interacting

Interaction-based learning style theories share the commonality of describing and explaining the nature of the learner's interaction with the learning experience. These theories focus on how the individual's mental processes interact with the content, teaching strategies, and learning environment. Kolb's learning style theory and emotional intelligence theory are two perspectives in this category that will be discussed along with strategies appropriate for each learning style. For the ANE, the value in these theories is in the increased understanding of the learner and an enhanced ability to work with learners who have diverse styles.

Kolb's Experiential Learning Model and Learning Styles

Kolb's (1984) model of experiential learning describes a process of engagement and interaction with the learning situation and provides educators with a useful model for creating learning experiences. According to Kolb, "Learning is a holistic process of adaptation to the world" (1984, p. 31). It involves the "integrated functioning of the total organism—thinking, feeling, perceiving, and behaving" (p. 31). Learning is created through transformation of experience and is best viewed in terms of a process versus an outcome (1984, p. 38).

According to Kolb (1984), if learners are to be effective in learning they need skills and abilities in four areas: (1) concrete experience, (2) reflective observation, (3) abstract conceptualization, and (4) active experimentation. Concrete experience abilities involve direct experiences of sensing and feeling. Learners need to be able to involve themselves freely and openly in the learning experience. Reflective observation abilities refers to learners being able to reflect on their experiences from different perspectives and create personal meaning from their observations. Learners also need to be able to think abstractly and create concepts that integrate their observations into sound theories. The abstract conceptualization process involves solitary thinking, such as analyzing case studies and reading assignments. Active experimentation involves physical and or mental engagement with the learning situation. Kolb proposes that in optimal learning situations, the learner will move through all four processes.

Kolb (1984) also describes four learning styles and teaching strategies that are derived from the processes depicted in his experiential learning model. The converger learning style relies on abstract conceptualization and active experimentation. Learners using the converger style learn through practical application of ideas to real world situations. They are able to use deductive reasoning in problem solving and decision-making. The converger is described as preferring to "deal with technical tasks and problems rather than social and interpersonal issues" (p. 77). The diverger learning style draws on concrete experience and reflective observation and displays characteristics opposite to those of the converger. Divergers do well with brainstorming and interactive learning activities. They are often described as creative learners because they tend to reflect on many diverse strategies for learning and problem solving. Those with the assimilator learning style use reflective observation and abstract conceptualization. They do well with inductive reasoning and creating theoretical models. Like the converger, the assimilator is less focused on people and more focused on ideas and concepts (p. 78). Kolb describes accommodators as learning by using concrete experience and active experimentation. Accomodators thrive in learning environments that involve hands-on activities and working with others, such as the skills laboratory and clinical practice. The four learning styles derived from Kolb's experiential learning model are summarized in Table 2-7 along with suggested strategies the ANE can implement to address each style.

Emotional Intelligence

Another interaction-based learning style is emotional intelligence. Emotional intelligence (EI) has been described as "a set of noncognitive abilities that influence the individual's capacity to succeed in life" (Salovey & Mayer, 1990, p. 92). In conjunction with a person's innate IQ level, EI works to enable the person to function successfully in society. Definitions of emotional intelligence have evolved over time. Salovey and Mayer (1990) initially defined emotional intelligence as "The ability to monitor one's own and others' feelings, to discriminate among them, and to use this information to guide one's thinking and action" (p. 189). More recently, the definition was expanded to include four separate yet interconnected abilities: the ability to perceive, use, understand, and manage one's emotions (Mayer & Salovey, 1997 & Mayer, Salovey, &

TABLE 2-7 Kolb's Learning Styles and Teaching Strategies

Learning Style	Learner Characteristics	Teaching Strategies
Converger	• Able to find practical uses for ideas • Able to solve problems and make decisions • Prefers to deal with technical tasks and problems rather than with social and interpersonal issues • Abstract conceptualization and active experimentation are dominant learning abilities.	• Participate in simulations • Laboratory assignments • Experiment with new ideas • Problem-solving scenarios • Practice skills
Diverger	• Able to view concrete situations from diverse perspectives • Concrete experience and reflective observation are dominant learning abilities.	• Activities involving gathering information • Brainstorming • Working in groups • Activities involving listening with an open mind • Receiving personalized feedback
Assimilator	• Less focused on people and more interested in ideas and abstract concepts • Able to synthesize diverse sources of information • Abstract conceptualization and reflective observation are dominant learning abilities.	• Readings • Lectures • Activities involving exploring analytical models • Solitary thinking activities • Reflective writing activities
Accommodator	• Often act on intuitive feelings • Prefers to work with others to get assignments done • Relies on people for information rather than on their own technical analysis • Concrete experience and active experimentation are dominant learning abilities.	• Learn from hands on experience • Group activities and projects • Clinical and practicum experiences • Test out different approaches to completing a project.

Some data from Kolb, D.A. (1984). *Experiential learning: Experience as the source of learning and development.* Englewood Cliffs, NJ: Prentice-Hall (p.141).

Caruso, 2004). Goleman, author of *Emotional Intelligence* (2005), defines emotional intelligence quite succinctly as "the ability to recognize and regulate emotions in self and others" (2001, p. 14).

Although Goleman notes that there is no single test for EI that yields an EI score, the abilities inherent in EI fall into five domains (Box 2-2), which can be helpful in explaining interpersonal differences and interactions (2005, p. 44). The first domain of EI involves the ability to monitor one's own emotions and be self-aware, which Goleman states is necessary for developing personal insight and self-understanding (p. 43). The second domain of EI, referred to as "managing emotions," depends on the person's ability to recognize their own emotions. Managing emotions involves demonstrating emotional resiliency, the ability to dissipate negative emotions and reduce lingering negative emotions. Goleman also describes the skill involved in using emotions to motivate oneself. This ability involves controlling emotions that would interfere with goal achievement and being able to get into a state in which creativity and productivity are heightened.

Unlike the first three domains of EI, which focused on the internal aspects of the self, the final two domains are concerned with other people. Domain 4 involves recognizing emotions in others. This domain reflects a crucial interpersonal skill in recognizing subtle clues that indicate what others need (Goleman, 2005, p. 43). In nursing, patients commonly experience stressful events; therefore, the ability of the nurse to recognize a patient's emotional response and empathize is important. The fifth domain of EI is what Goleman refers to as the ability to handle relationships (p. 43). To a large degree, this involves managing emotions in others by offering, praise, support, comfort, encouragement, and providing guidance and leadership,

BOX 2-2   Emotional Intelligence Domains

1. Self-awareness of emotions
2. Managing emotions
3. Using emotions to motivate self
4. Recognizing emotions in others
5. Handling relationships

Data from Goleman, D. (2005). *Emotional intelligence* (10th Anniversary Edition, p. 43). NY: Bantam Books.

when needed. As with any other multidimensional attribute, individuals will vary in their strengths and abilities in each of the domains of EI. Knowing about the domains of EI is helpful in teaching practice because it enables the educator to understand more thoroughly the clinical interactions of individual students. Knowing about the domains of EI is also essential for recognizing EI skills that have not been sufficiently developed. EI can be enhanced through self-reflection and deliberate practice. When difficulty in one of the EI domains is noted, the ANE can encourage affective-based learning activities that focus on the deficient domain. Activities such as scenario-based discussion, sharing in postclinical conferences, and reflective journaling can be useful strategies.

In a rebuttal to Waterhouse's (2006) criticism of EI as lacking sufficient scientific study, Cherniss, Extein, Goleman, & Weissberg (2006) state that "EI is a young theory, still in an early stage of development and hypothesis testing" (p. 239). However, Cherniss *et al.* concluded that there was sufficient evidence indicating the domains of EI are different from attributes of general intelligence as measured by IQ (p. 240). They cite seven supporting studies on IQ and EI, and two studies and a meta-analysis exploring EI and personality traits. Another criticism by Waterhouse related to a lack of evidence that EI contributes to real-world success. Cherniss and colleagues refuted that claim, citing 12 studies conducted between 2000 and 2005 that found positive relationships between EI domain scores and leadership, customer satisfaction, and work performance. They concluded, "EI matters greatly in selecting, promoting, and developing leaders" (p. 242).

According to Goleman (1998), EI influences our ability to learn and apply practical skills. Freshwater and Stickley noted that, "Every nursing intervention is affected by the master aptitude of emotional intelligence" (2004, p. 93). EI incorporates elements of motivation, self-awareness, empathy, self-regulation, and relationship skills, all of which have direct application to nursing. Much of nursing practice relies on the nurse's ability to sense what others are feeling, assist people in dealing with those feelings, and recognize how personal feelings can affect interactions and relationships. In a systematic review of the literature, Akerjordet & Severinsson (2007) concluded, "personal growth and development in the area of emotional intelligence are central to professional competence" (p. 1405). Emphasis on reflective educational strategies may be helpful in facilitating development of emotional intelligence (Goleman, 2001).

Integration of concepts and practices that help the learner develop EI is essential to the development of nurses who are well rounded in both the art and science of nursing. Strategies the ANE can use to support the development of EI include a variety of experiential learning activities. Examples of experiential learning activities in-

clude reflective discussion and writing, practicing listening skills, self-inquiry, narrative, and the use of video recordings for observation and feedback (Freshwater &
Stickley, 2004, p. 96). The ANE can facilitate holistic learning by valuing cognitive as
well as affective-based knowledge and skills that includes EI.

Learning Styles Based on Integrative Concepts

Integrative learning style theories reflect a synthesis of perspectives and concepts that
describe and explain the learner and their learning preferences. Theories within the
integrative category are broader in scope than individual learning style and learning
process theories alone. Generational or cohort theories, the Dunn & Dunn Model of
Learning, and the Felder-Silverman Learning Style Model are examples of integrative theories that will be discussed in this section.

Generational Theories

Generational or cohort theories describe the influence of multiple sociocultural dimensions on the learner. Cohort theories are based on the premise that individuals
born and raised during certain time periods share common history, values, and culture. These shared commonalities influence the learning preferences, and the
strengths and challenges that learners bring to the classroom. Over the decades,
teachers and researchers have described, explored, and compared various learning cohorts, and have used this information to guide the use of teaching approaches (Table
2-8). Several classification systems for generational learners have been outlined.
Howe & Strauss (2000) provide a nonoverlapping classification system that recognizes baby boomers as born between 1943 & 1960, generation X as born between
1961 and 1981, and millennials (generation Y) as born between 1982 to the present.
The classification system developed by Oblinger & Oblinger (2005), includes a category called the mature generation (those born between 1900 and 1946) and a one-
year overlap between other categories. Regardless of the classification system used,
the vast majority of ANEs today are in the baby boomer generation, whereas the student body is primarily a mix of generation X and Y (Skiba & Barton, 2006).

Referring to the generational characteristics of learners became prominent when
the largest cohort, the baby boomers, emerged. Boomers comprise the post-World
War II babies born roughly between the 1940s and 1964. Although the majority of
nursing students encountered in today's classrooms will share characteristics and values of generation X and Y, educators may still encounter baby boomers returning to
college for advance degrees or certification. Understanding the values and dispositions that boomers bring to the learning environment can allow the educator to be

TABLE 2-8   Comparison of Generational Learners

Generation	Boomers	Gen X	Gen Y
Characteristics	• Dependable • Hard working • Value doing good work	• Independent • Pragmatic • Able to multitask	• Tolerant of diversity • Heavy multi-taskers • May bore easily
Learning patterns	• Primarily exposed to teacher-lead, teacher-focused approaches	• Prefer more self-directed activities • Able to work in teams	• Technology is integral • Group oriented • Need active engagement
Implications for teaching	• Traditional lecture • Not comfortable with technology	• Use teaching time wisely • Emphasize application of information	• Provide frequent and prompt feedback • May challenge teacher s authority

Data from Arhin, A., & Cormier, E. (2007). Using deconstruction to educate generation Y nursing students. *Journal of Nursing Education, 46*(12), 562–567; Billings, D. (2004). Teaching learners from varied generations. *The Journal of Continuing Education in Nursing, 35*(3), 104–105; and Skiba, D., & Barton, A. (2006). Adapting your teaching to accommodate the net generation of learners. *Online Journal of Issues in Nursing, 11*(2), 6.

proactive in addressing the needs and concerns of this group. Billings (2004) describes boomers as more dependent on the educator, as they grew up with traditional teacher-lead and teacher-focused approaches. Baby boomers value doing a good job and they respond to positive feedback and recognition for their efforts. However, compared with later generations who are more technologically savvy, they do not expect frequent feedback and immediate responses from instructors. Harris adds to the description, stating boomers are dependable, accustomed to working long hours, and demonstrate commitment to their jobs (2005, p. 44).

Students classified as generation X have dominated the classrooms for several decades and will continue to be a significant presence as they continue their education and seek second degrees or graduate degrees. Generation X learners, born between the 1960s and 1980, have been described as concrete thinkers who are independent, pragmatic, outcome focused, able to solve problems, and engage in multi-tasking (Walker *et al.*, 2006, p. 371). Although not as technologically savvy as their successors, generation X students are able to easily develop the skills needed to use technology. Raised in a period of relative economic prosperity, by predominantly baby boomer parents, generation X learners are less accustomed to economic hardship than their predecessors, and may express a sense of entitlement in their work and school affairs (Harris, 2005, p. 49). They also value a balanced lifestyle, tend to challenge the status quo, and question authority more than the other cohorts (Walker *et al.*, 2006, p. 371). Generation X learners can be self-directed in their learning and can work in teams. They appreciate clearly presented information that can be applied to the real world (Billings, 2004, p. 104). Teaching approaches for generation X students are outlined in Table 2-8.

College students born after 1981 are referred to as generation Y, nexters, or millennials. They share the commonality of being raised by fathers and mothers who worked outside the home. They also experienced having surrogate parents in the form of extended family, babysitters, day care, peers, and television (Arhin & Cormier, 2007). They have been raised with technology, are accustomed to multitasking, and are group oriented. For educators this means the generation Y student is accustomed to immediate feedback, may have a shorter attention span, and may require more active engagement to counteract boredom (Arhin & Cormier, 2007).

Generation Y learners have been described as the most culturally diverse cohort of learners. They are respectful of authority but will not hesitate to challenge authority, if needed. They are more technologically literate than any other group and have a strong preference for visual media (Walker *et al.*, 2006, p. 272). Other characteristics include being future oriented and altruistic. Because they have been exposed to diversity through technology, media, and travel, they have tolerance for diversity (Arhin & Johnson-Mallard, 2003; Clausing, Kurtz, Pendeville, & Walt, 2003).

Researchers Arhin and Cormier (2007) describe the application of a philosophy of deconstruction, which is the practice of reading, criticism, and analytical inquiry, to teaching generation Y students. They discuss three pedagogies that meld with and invigorate generation Y learners. First is using transformative pedagogy—a process of interactive dialog, debate, and cross-examination to achieve empowerment and a better understanding of concepts. These approaches build on the student's need for active engagement and group orientation. A second approach uses narrative pedagogy, which involves sharing the lived experiences of the student and or teacher. The teacher may use case studies, discussion of real clinical cases, role-playing, and simulation. Students may journal or write a clinical log that integrates real clinical experiences. These strategies provide a high level of engagement and active participation needed by generation Y learners. The third strategy is the incorporation of techno-literacy–based activities such as digital communications and hypertext, to link to successive Web sites. Techno-literacy–based strategies utilize communication forms commonly used by generation Y, allowing the learner to critically analyze and deconstruct the information obtained.

Today many nursing classrooms are a composed of a mix of generation X and Y students. In teaching these groups, it is important to use strategies that recognize common attributes such as preferring nonauthoritarian approaches, being independent and resourceful, preferring immediate response and feedback, and being dependent on peers (Ahrin, & Johnson-Mallard, 2003). Accommodating these learners does not always require major modifications. Ahrin and Johnson-Mallard describe the reconfiguring of an existing assignment for juniors in an undergraduate clinical course. The assignment constisted of individual students presenting a case study to the class. Rather than prescribing the format of the presentations the assignment was modified to encourage a variety of approaches. The authors found that the modified assignment embodied several of the strategies that Caudron (1997) recommended for teaching generation X and Y such as, (1) making learning experiential, (2) allowing students to control their learning, and (3) having students construct knowledge from their own experiences (p. 122).

Very little research has been conducted to explore generational differences in online learning for nursing students. A study by Walker *et al.* (2006) compared generation X and Y BSN nursing students' teaching preferences using a 30-item survey. The only significant difference noted was that generation X students ($n = 25$) reported more struggle with reading comprehension compared with the generation Y students ($n = 103$). Both groups indicated a preference for lecture over Web-based course or group work, which may be related to a general preference for face-to-face classes.

In a larger study Billings, Skiba, & Connors (2005), surveyed 230 graduate and 328 undergraduate students from six schools of nursing about educational practices, the use of technology, student support, and learning outcomes (p. 128). Differences noted between undergraduate and graduate students related to faculty and student interactions and time factors (p. 130). The undergraduate students rated the faculty-student interactions higher than the graduate students, which could reflect undergraduate's concurrent interactions with faculty in face-to-face clinical courses (p. 130). As for time factor differences, the graduate students reported spending more time on task, more time on the course Web site, and more time studying than the undergraduate students (p. 130). The authors noted that the graduate students were older, more passive learners, who tended to associate course credit hours with seat time.

Dunn and Dunn Learning Styles Model

The Dunn and Dunn Learning Styles Model incorporates aspects of cognitive and brain dominance theories to provide a comprehensive integrated view of learner preferences (Morse, Oberer, Dobbins, & Mitchell, 1998, p. 27). According to Dunn and

Dunn (1993), learning style is a "biological and developmental set of personal characteristics that makes the identical instruction effective for some students and ineffective for others" (p. 5). They further define learning styles as "the way individuals concentrate on, internalize, and remember new and difficult academic information and skills" (Dunn & Griggs, 1998, p. 11).

The Dunn and Dunn Learning Styles Model includes preferences in five areas: the physical environment, and emotional, sociological, physiological, and psychological variables. Each of these preference areas contains from three to six elements that describe specific preference areas. For example, the category of physical environment includes preferences in sound, light, temperature, and design. Regarding sound preferences, some students may prefer studying and reading in a quiet environment, others do better listening to specific music. Students may also have lighting and temperature preferences that facilitate learning such as dim lighting or bright lighting and cool versus warm temperatures. Design refers to the types of seating a student prefers when studying. Some students are able to concentrate easier when using formal seating such as a table and hard chair, whereas other students may find concentration easier in a soft cushioned chair.

The emotional dimension of the model includes four preference areas: motivation, persistence, responsibility, and structure. A student's motivation to learn the subject can range from high to low and is influenced by multiple factors such as past exposure to the topic, perceived relevance, and difficulty. Persistence refers to the student's ability stay focused and to complete a project before moving to another task. Responsibility refers to the student's preference for conformity or nonconformity. The learner's preference for structure relates to the individuals "internal versus external needs for structure" (Van Wynen, 1998, p. 45).

The sociological dimension of the model concerns the number of people the learner prefers to interact with during the learning process and the type of preferred interaction with the teacher. Some students may prefer studying alone or working on class projects individually, whereas others prefer interacting with one other student, or in various small group configurations. In terms of the type of interaction with the teacher, preferences can range from authoritative to the more facilitative. The sociological dimensions also include the individual's preference for a routine schedule or for variety. Some students find learning easier if a routine is adhered to, whereas others may become disinterested if learning experiences follow a predictable routine.

The main component of the psychological or cognitive dimension incorporates brain dominance theory (Dunn & Griggs, 1998). Those who process predominantly with the left hemisphere are analytical learners and those who process information with the right hemisphere are global learners. Analytical learners tend to be detail oriented and prefer information that is logically organized and sequentially presented.

They need to explore and understand the parts first, for the most effective learning to occur. Global learners, on the other hand, are predominantly right-brain processors who need to see the big picture first, or understand the overall concept before they can focus on the details (Dunn, 1992). Both analytical and global processors tend to have distinct preferences in each of the other dimensions (See Table 2-9).

Aspects of perceptual preferences such as the visual, auditory, and kinesthetic learning styles are included within the physiological dimension. Another aspect of the physiological dimension is time, referring to the time of day in which the learner is best able to focus, concentrate, and retain information. In addition to these physiological preferences, some learners may prefer intake of some type of food or beverage while studying, others prefer no food or beverages until studying is completed. Some need to move about while processing new information, others need to be motionless.

Individuals are not equally affected by all of the learning style elements. Dunn and Dunn (1998) conclude that most learners are affected by between 6 and 14 combinations of elements. To determine the learner's preferences and strengths in each of these dimensions (emotional, physical, environmental, emotional, sociological, and

TABLE 2-9 Comparison of Global and Analytic Learners		
Type of Stimuli	Global Learner Preferences (Subjective/Intuitive)	Analytic Learner Preferences (Objective/Detached)
Environmental	• Background music, TV, or conversation • Subdued lighting • Relaxing, comfortable seating while studying	• Quiet setting with few interruptions • Bright lights • Desk and chair while studying
Emotional	• Need a high degree of interest in the subject to be motivated to learn • Prefer working on several tasks at one time	• Tend to be persistent and complete one task before starting another • Prefer to control the structure of learning tasks
Sociological	• Prefers group work	• Can work alone or with others
Physiological	• Prefers foods and beverages and frequent breaks while studying	• Prefers no intake while studying or working on a project • Works on task without frequent breaks

Data from Dunn, R., & Griggs, S. A. (Eds.). (1998). *Learning styles and the nursing profession.* New York: NLN Press, (pp. 30 & 45).

psychological), Dunn, Dunn, and Price (1989) developed and tested a 100-item learning style inventory. Since then, the Dunn and Dunn Learning Style Model has been studied extensively. In a meta-analysis of 36 studies of over 3000 learners, researchers found that students whose learning styles were accommodated achieved 75% of a standard deviation higher than those whose learning styles were not accommodated (Dunn *et al.*, 1995, p. 353). These gains were greater for adults than for children and adolescents and were greater for those with strong learning preferences, as opposed to those with weaker or mixed preferences (p. 358). A meta-analysis of 76 studies by Lovelace (2005), found strong support that "matching student's learning-style preferences with complementary instruction improved academic achievement and student attitudes toward learning" (p. 176). Lovelace concluded that "the Dunn and Dunn model had a robust and moderate to large effect size that was practically and educationally significant" (p. 176). The ANE's awareness of the dimensions in the Dunn and Dunn model, coupled with the ability to implement strategies that will accommodate various preferences, can have a significant effect on learning.

Felder-Silverman Learning Style Model

The Felder-Silverman Learning Style Model is an integrative model that synthesizes concepts from several theories to offer a unique perspective on learning styles. In 1988, Felder and Silverman published a model that integrated key ideas found in the VAK, brain dominance, and Myers-Briggs theories. Their model describes learning preferences in terms of four dichotomous factors: (1) active and reflective learners, (2) sensing and intuitive learners, (3) visual and verbal learners, and (4) sequential and global learners. The key ideas introduced in the Felder and Silverman model include the term sequential learner, which refers to those who gain understanding in progressive, stepwise fashion; and the term global learner, which refers to people who suddenly gain insight and understanding and tend to learn in large jumps rather than in smaller increments. The Index of Learning Styles (ILS) is an online instrument that is used to assess the learner's preferences in each of the four areas.

In a statistical analysis of the Felder-Silverman Learning Style Dimensions, Graf, Viola, Leo, & Kinshuk (2007) validated the four dimensions of the model. The first dimension looks at the active and reflective ways of processing information. Active learners learn best by doing and applying; and they do well with group learning activities. Reflective learners need to think about the material and prefer to work individually. The second dimension is similar to Myers-Briggs concept of sensing and intuition. Individuals classified as "sensing" prefer concrete, objective learning material and established ways of receiving information. However, intuitive learners prefer abstract material, new ways of learning, and tend to be less detail oriented than the sensing type of learner. The third dimension is the visual and verbal learner, which refers to receiving information by auditory or written means. Finally, the sequential/global dimension is characterized by how the learner processes information in terms of connections. Sequential learners prefer making connections from the parts to the whole and tend to be detail oriented. On the other hand, the global learner easily processes information presented nonsequentially, can grasp how information is connected to other areas and thus is able to see the big picture.

Faculty who wish to use the ILS may refer their students to the ILS Web site listed in the resource section. The tool is available online, at no cost to individuals who wish to determine their own learning style profile and for educators who wish to use it for teaching, advising, or research.

Self-Regulation Theory

Self-regulation theory combines concepts from social learning theory and social cognitivism to emphasize the learner's self-efficacy in the learning process. Bandura's Social Learning Theory emphasizes the role of the learner as agent. Agency has been defined by Martin (2004) as the capability of the learner to make choices, take action (p. 135), be self-reflective, and determine the specific behaviors to be modeled. The learner's internal feedback mechanisms determine and regulate the selection of behaviors the individual will model (Bandura, 2001). Social Cognitive Theory acknowledges that students with a high degree of self-regulation will evaluate factors in the learning situation to determine specific actions needed to achieve desired outcomes. Mccann & Turner (2004) note that "the interaction among behavioral, personal, and environmental processes forms the basis for the varied approaches that students take to tackle their academic work" (p. 1696). Self-regulation requires learner agency and has been deemed important in the inclination to practice life-long learning (Murphy, 2005; O'Shea, 2003) and the development of clinical reasoning skills (Kuiper, 2005; Kuiper & Pesut, 2004).

A study by Mullen (2007) explored the self-regulation practices of students in an accelerated second-degree BSN program. Using quantitative data from students in the second and third trimester of the program, they compared student responses on various subscales of self-regulation strategies. Both groups of students used cognitive, resource management, and self-regulation strategies such as organization, rehearsal, elaboration, time management, and control of the study environment (p. 410). The third trimester students scored higher in all subscales than the first trimester students except for scoring slightly lower in the critical thinking subscale. Findings also revealed that students who studied independently for a greater number of hours used significantly more self-regulatory strategies (p. 410). These findings have several implications for the ANE. The findings can be used to support assessment of the self-regulation strategies currently used by students and in teaching students about additional strategies. Knowledge of the importance of self-regulatory learning practices for the student's academic success can be integrated into orientation programs for students. Finally, the ANE can enhance the student's use of cognitive self-regulatory practices by modeling these approaches and explaining the use of these approaches to students (p. 411).

The volitional component of self-regulation is concerned with the students' ability to make choices and regulate their learning activities (Mccann & Turner, 2004). According to Mccann and Turner, "When it comes to achieving learning goals, academically successful students not only have a repertoire of effective strategies for learning, they also take control of their learning" (p. 1696). The use of volitional strategies affects the student's ability to persevere through difficult tasks and distractions, to stay on task, and stay motivated. Volitional strategies also serve as a protective mechanism for feelings of discouragement, overwhelment, and self-doubt in the face of temporary performance failures. Mccann and Turner (2004) suggest ways the ANE can encourage the student to develop volitional control and thus improve self-regulation of learning (Box 2-3).

BOX 2-3 Strategies for Enhancing Student's Volitional Control

1. Initiate diagnostic testing such as the Academic Volitional Strategy Inventory

2. Instruct students about effective strategies to counter distractions and lack of motivation

3. Discuss situations the students may encounter that could be distracting and strategies to use to say on task

4. Encourage the student to think of the positive result that will be achieved from successful completion of an assignment or task

5. Have the student consider how not doing well on the assignment would affect them

6. Suggest the use of self-rewards when the task has been completed

7. Incorporate group projects that enable student to see how others stay on task and deal with distractions and lack of motivation

8. Conduct in-class activities that require the students to think aloud about the assigned task

9. Help identify resources that can be used to complete the task

Data from Mccann, E., & Turner, J. (2004). Increasing student learning through volitional control. *Teachers College Record, 106*(9), 1695–1714.

Self-regulation theory suggests that the development of clinical reasoning skills depends on development of both cognitive and metacognitive skills. Kuiper and Pesat (2004) concur, citing cognitive skills such as critical thinking and metacognitive skills such as reflective thinking, as contributing to the development of clinical reasoning. Many teaching strategies that enhance critical thinking have been developed and tested. The task of educators is to determine the best strategies given the unique attributes of the learner, the nature of the content, and the learning setting.

THEORY AND RESEARCH RELATED TO TEACHER ATTRIBUTES

In all of the major educational theories, the instructor has a role in the learning process. However, the role varies in terms of control of the learning situation and the type of interaction with the learner. In the behaviorist perspective, the instructor controls the learning by manipulating rewards and punishments. In the cognitivist perspective, the instructor is active in the organization and presentation of the content and is concerned with promoting higher cognitive functions of critical thinking. The constructivist teacher is less controlling and allows the learner to process and construct their own learning. In this section, several perspectives for describing teaching styles are explored along with teacher skills in self-reflection and role modeling.

Teaching Styles

Just as learners have individual learning styles; teachers also have individual teaching styles that reflect various theoretical perspectives. However, teaching styles incorporate more than just the teacher's learning styles. Teaching styles generally mirror the teacher's values, beliefs, and his or her preferred ways of processing information. In other words, teachers tend to teach the way they are comfortable learning. Thus, identification of one's learning style is a starting point for understanding one's teaching style. Like learning styles, teaching styles stem from the teacher's perspective, personal strengths, and preferences.

Several of the NLN task statements speak to the importance of teaching style in facilitating learning. Specifically, task statement # 3 calls for the teacher to "recognize multicultural, gender, and experiential influences on teaching and learning" (NLN, Task Group on Nurse Educator Competencies 2005, p. 1) and task statement # 11 involves using "personal attributes that facilitate learning" such as "caring, confidence, patience, integrity, and flexibility" (p. 1). As with learning styles, each individual has a preference for specific teaching styles, which is influenced by personal attributes and experiences. Just as learners embrace different learning styles to accommodate different situations, teachers can adapt, change, and learn different teaching styles to achieve different learning goals.

Building on the learning styles discussed previously, specific teaching style taxonomies proposed by Grasha and Mosston will be explored in this section. The deliberate use of these teaching styles will require the ANE to engage in self-reflection on teaching practices, approaches, and philosophies commonly used.

Grasha's Teaching Styles

According to Grasha (1996), "Teaching styles, learning styles, and classroom processes are interdependent. . . . Each has direct implications for the appearance of the other two" (p. 233). Grasha (1996, 2003) describes five types of teaching styles including the expert, formal authority, personal model, facilitator, and delegator (Table 2-10). Each teaching style is characterized by specific teacher attributes and teaching methods that are most commonly used. Grasha acknowledges that the selection of a specific teaching style and effective use of corresponding teaching strategies depend on the student's learning styles and ability to engage in the types of tasks common to a particular style (1996, p. 233). For example, students who are more dependent and competitive tend to respond well to the expert and formal authority teaching styles, which offer a high degree of structure, emphasis on grades and examinations, and teacher-centered class sessions (1996, p. 234). However, students who are independent learners and enjoy collaborative activities, tend to respond well to the facilitator teaching style, which uses discussion, problem-based learning, and case studies. These two examples represent the extremes of teacher-centered and student-centered approaches.

Researchers have recently explored the relationship between teaching styles and learning styles, seeking scientific validation of these theoretical relationships (Giles, Ryan, Belliveau, De Freitas, & Casey, 2006). Students who were enrolled in four sections of an introductory statistics course ($n = 143$) received two units of instruction from the same instructor, one using a student-center approach and one using a teacher-centered approach. The student's ratings of each class in terms of teacher knowledge and ability to hold their interested were not significantly different for the teacher or the student-centered approach (Giles *et al.*, 2006). However, the teacher-centered class session was rated significantly higher in overall effectiveness and use of examples, and students reported increased confidence in their ability to successfully complete a quiz (p. 220). The majority of students also scored higher on quizzes that tested the teacher-centered content. On the surface, this seems to support the effectiveness of the teacher-centered approach. However, the authors analyzed the

TABLE 2-10 Characteristics of Grasha's Teaching Styles

Teaching Style	Description	Characteristics of Teaching
Expert	• Knowledgeable • Challenges students	• Emphasizes content knowledge • Concerned with providing information to ensure student meets learning outcomes
Formal authority	• Senior teacher status • Sets standards and expectations	• Provides classroom structure and feedback • Develops detailed syllabi to explain learning goals, standards, and expectations
Personal model	• Teaches by personal example • Values learning by direct observation	• Demonstrates and models desired behaviors • Guides and directs student's performance
Facilitator	• Concerned with student's needs, goals, and academic development	• Asks questions rather than providing answers • Works with students in a consulting fashion • Explores and suggests alternatives
Delegator	• Values student autonomy	• Serves as a resource to students • Encourages student problem solving and independence

Data from Grasha, A. F. (1996). *Teaching with style*. Pittsburgh, PA: Alliance Publishers, (p. 154).

student's quiz results in terms of their previous grade in their last math course. They found that students whose previous grade was above 90% scored significantly lower on the content presented using a teacher-centered approach and scored significantly higher on the content presented using the student-centered approach. Students whose grade in their last math course was lower than 90% scored significantly higher on the content presented using the teacher-center approach and scored lower on the content presented using the student-centered approach. Thus stronger students may do better by exploring the subject matter using creative, interactive approaches that tend to be more student-centered (p. 220).

Mosston's Spectrum of Teaching Styles

In 1966, Mosston delineated the Spectrum of Teaching Styles to depict the student/teacher involvement in the teaching and learning of psychomotor skill-based content. Mosston, a physical education teacher, believed that although teachers have their own individual styles of instruction, effective teaching needs to be dictated by more than style preference. Educators should select teaching styles based on logical and sound rationale. The Spectrum of Teaching Styles is conceptualized as a continuum of control and decision-making, with absolute instructor control at one end, and student self-teaching at the other end. Mosston and Ashworth (1990; 2002) delineated a total of 11 styles that vary in instructor and student control and decision-making (Table 2-11). At one end of the spectrum is the command style characterized by instructor control of content, methods, time on task, and all aspects of instruction and evaluation. The command style is followed by the practice, reciprocal, self-check, inclusion, guided discovery, convergent, divergent, learner-designed, and learner initiated styles, and ends with the self-teaching style. Each style has unique attributes, goals, and purposes, making each style appropriate for certain conditions.

A central premise of the Spectrum of Teaching Styles is that each style is designed to address specific types of objectives and that each style has value. Based on this premise, several styles may be used to teach a specific skill set. For determining which style is the best fit, Mosston and Ashworth (1990) suggests a simple process. First, determine the objectives and the observable outcomes of each activity within a lesson. Reflect on what you want the learners to accomplish. What is the task? What types of behaviors do you want the learner to develop? Next, determine the conditions that will govern the learner's task performance. Will the learner need to perform the task under specific environmental conditions such as time limits and distractions? Finally, determine the level of performance or standard of achievement that will be required for the task. Will the student need to perform with out hesitancy? Without error? Using behavioral objectives that describe the task, conditions, and criteria, will facilitate the process of matching the objective with a teaching style.

Self-Reflection

The terms reflection and self-reflection continually emerge in the literature as ways of gaining self-understanding and ultimately improving teaching practice and facilitating learning. The main functions of self-reflection in terms of teaching are to validate and make sense of the teaching-learning experience and gain insights and clarity about what has been learned. The concept of reflection places value on the idea that

TABLE 2-11	Mosston's Teaching Styles and Teacher Characteristics
Teaching Style	**Description**
Command	• Teacher is decision maker • Focus is on learning the task accurately & within a short period of time
Practice	• Teacher prescribes the tasks • Learner practices individually and receives guided feedback from the teacher
Reciprocal	• Students work in pairs: one performs, the other provides feedback • Uses criteria designed by the teacher
Self-check	• Students assess their own performance against criteria
Inclusion	• Teacher plans practice however, student monitors own work
Guided discovery	• Students solve teacher identified problems with teacher assistance
Convergent	• Teacher makes subject matter decisions, learner uses cognitive skills to discover answers
Divergent	• Students solve problems without assistance from the teacher
Learner designed	• Teacher determines content • Student plans the program of study
Learner initiated	• Student plans own program • Teacher advises
Self-teaching	• Student takes full responsibility for the learning process

Data from Mosston, M., & Ashworth, S. (2002). *Teaching physical education.* Columbus, OH: Charles Merrill Publishing; and Mosston, M., & Ashworth, S. (1990). *The spectrum of teaching styles. From command to discovery.* White Plains, NY: Longman, Inc.

experience alone does not lead to learning. The concept of reflection is also consistent with Kolb's theory of learning, which views reflection on the learning experience as a necessary component of the learning process.

Loughran (1996) defines reflection as "a personal process of thinking, refining, reframing, and developing actions" (p. 51). He emphasizes that a key aspect of reflection is the ability to see a problem or situation from different viewpoints. Furthermore, this process of framing and reframing occurs within one of three forms of reflection. Reflection may be anticipatory, contemporaneous, or retrospective in nature, indicating the time perspective from which the person is reflecting. Anticipatory reflection is focused on a future event or situation—a "what if" type of scenario in which the person thinks about possibilities and potential consequences of specific actions. Contemporaneous reflection is focused on the present time and involves viewing the situation from different perspectives, whereas retrospective reflection involves looking back on an actual event or situation. Depending on which type of reflection the individual is engaged in, the individual's "skills, experience, confidence, and expertise at these times may lead to different understandings of the same situation" (p. 47).

Reflective Practices

In the book *The Courage to Teach: A Guide for Reflection and Self-Renewal*, the authors, Livsey and Palmer, provide insightful rationale for engaging in self-reflection with colleagues. They note that:

> Teaching like any truly human activity, emerges from one's inwardness . . . As I teach, I project the conditions of my soul onto my students, my subject, and our way of being together . . . teaching holds a mirror to the soul. If I am willing took in that mirror. . . . I have the chance to gain self-knowledge—and knowing myself is as crucial to good teaching as knowing my students and my subject (1999, p. 1).

Livsey and Palmer (1999) describe a systematic process of self-reflection that begins with creating a physical, intellectual, emotional, and spiritual space for self-exploration. The type of physical space needed for conducting self-reflection should be private, relatively free of distractions and potential interruptions, and provide comfortable seating that is conducive to sharing. To create an intellectual space for group self-reflection, the facilitator considers the topic of self-reflection and tries to anticipate the needs of individual members in terms of discussion. For example, would discussion in one large group or in several small groups work best? One strategy for initial reflection and discussion that Livsey and Palmer suggest is to have the members write comment cards about a topic and their point of view. Then collect, shuffle, and redistribute the unsigned cards to the group. Each group member then can read the comment card and add their perspective. The anonymity of the comment cards can create an intellectual environment conducive to reflection and sharing.

Livsey and Palmer (1999) point out that creating an emotional space for this type of self-reflection is essential. Establishing ground rules and expectations for confidentiality, listening, speaking, and respecting others' feelings can help ensure that all individuals who wish to speak can he heard in a nonjudgmental atmosphere. One suggestion for addressing confidentiality is to assure "double confidentiality," meaning nothing said in the group leaves the room, and individuals will not be approached after the meeting for further discussion unless they indicate a wiliness to do so (p. 10). These guidelines help establish a trusting and safe emotional space for reflective learning.

Creating a spiritual space involves allowing each individual to actually reflect on the discussion and discover his or her own insights and answers (Livsey & Palmer, 1999). Advice and solutions should be offered only when a person asks. Often the tendency is to give advice and try to fix the person's problem. However well meaning this may be, it can tend to shut down further sharing. The authors provide additional questions and activities in their book that can guide faculty who wish to pursue group self-reflection.

In addition to the processes identified by Livsey and Palmer, other authors have identified approaches for reflective practice. Mezirow (1991) delineated three aspects of reflection that involve assessing the content, the process, and the premises (p. 104). Reflection involves analyzing the assumptions underlying the situation and problem solving, whereas critiquing the premises refers to posing potential problems that may be inherent in an everyday situation. Another approach is presented by Kuit, Reay, & Freeman (2001). They discuss several methods that can be used to reflect on teaching (Box 2-4). The DATA method describes four stages in the reflective process: describe, analyze, theorize, and act. Brookfield's critical thinking method involves identifying a triggering event, defining the problem underlying the event, exploring alternative ways to deal with the event, and identifying any insights gained or lessons learned.

BOX 2-4   Methods of Reflection Used in Teaching

- DATA Method—(Describe, Analyze, Theorize and Act)

- Brookfield's Critical Thinking—(Appraise event, define problem, explore alternatives and insights)

- Kolb's Experiential Learning Process

- Action Research

- Critical Incident Method

- Concept Mapping

- Storytelling

Data from Kuit, J. A., Reay, G., & Freeman, R. (2001). Experiences of reflective teaching. *Active Learning in Higher Education, 2,* 128–142.

Kolb's Experiential Learning Model can also be used to guide self-reflection. Kuit *et al.* (2001) suggest that the teacher decide on the situation that will be the subject of reflection and keep a written record of the event as it occurs, then use the written account to work through Kolb's phases of learning. In Kolb's phase of concrete experience, the teacher describes the teaching experience. In the reflective observation phase, the experience is analyzed in terms of what happened, why it happened, and what was expected to happen (1984, p. 132). Abstract conceptualization involves extracting meaning from the experience and determining what was learned. Active experimentation involves taking the lesions learned and applying them to the next learning encounter.

Another model for engaging in reflection involves the use of action research methods. Action research refers to the process of studying a teaching situation with a focus on improving the situation in the future and identifying how the practice informs theory. The processes of planning, taking action, observing the action, and reflecting involves determining the meaning of the experience, determining what was learned, and interpreting the meaning of the experience in theoretical terms.

The critical incident method uses a line of questioning to explore a significant teaching event. As with action research, the critical incident approach engages other people in the reflection process. First, the incident is described to a group of selected individuals. Then, group members are asked to explain why the incident was critical and identify assumptions made by the teacher. These factors are discussed in a group setting and new assumptions are derived that can be tested in subsequent teaching sessions.

The process of concept mapping also can be used by the ANE as a solitary reflection activity, or concept mapping can provide a structure for group reflection. In concept mapping, the topic of the reflection is written in a prominent location, usually at the top of a sheet of paper. Then other concepts related to the situation are placed on the paper and linked with arrows to indicate how they are connected to the situation. Then, the linkages are identified by verbs that describe the relationship. The map can then be analyzed by looking for missing concepts, relationships, and contradictions.

The story telling method outlined by Kuit *et al.* (2001) is often done informally with colleagues or can be done more formally to aid reflection. In formal storytelling, the teacher recounts the situation to a partner. They discuss the situation and identify assumptions. The assumptions are then compared to what actually happened and new assumptions are generated.

In summary, self-reflection emphasizes that learning is a personal, internal process of meaning making. Kolb's Learning Theory, Mezirow's Transformative Theory, and the approaches outlined by Kuit *et al.* (2001), provide a foundation for self-reflection in education. In addition, research supports the effectiveness of self-reflection in facilitating learning. The ANE can use self-reflection to improve teaching effectiveness and as a teaching strategy to facilitate deeper student learning.

Role Modeling

Teachers also facilitate learning by modeling clinical and professional behaviors and cognitive skills to their students. Bandura's (1977) Social Learning Theory outlines four processes that are involved in learning through role modeling (Table 2-12). The attention process is the prerequisite that determines whether a behavior will be adopted by the observer. Attention involves observing a behavior or situation and accepting or rejecting the importance of the activity being observed, depending on the fit with the observer's underlying values. Retention in role modeling is concerned with activating the learner's internal memory processes. The teacher can assist the student's retention by asking the student to identify key aspects of what was observed, describe what was observed, or create a concept map of what was observed (Armstrong, 2008). The next process is motor reproduction. During this process the learner recreates or demonstrates the observed behavior and evaluates his or her own performance of the behavior or skill. According to Bandura (1977), key factors in determining repetition of the behavior beyond the initial performance are the offering of praise (or other positive feedback) or the absence of negative consequences.

The motivation process is the final process of learning using role modeling. During the motivation process, the learner internalizes whether the behavior or skill was valuable and whether or not the behavior or skill will likely be repeated. Often the learner will test the situation to determine if positive responses will be forthcoming. According to Armstrong (2008), if the outcome continues to be positive, it serves to motivate the student to repeat the behavior.

Armstrong (2008) also discusses application of role modeling processes to real clinical situations. She cautions that for effective teaching to take place, role modeling needs to incorporate more than merely observing behaviors. Role modeling involves a continuum of learning from observation to participation. "It requires explanation, discussion, and feedback to allow the student to gain from the experience" (p. 601). Armstrong also points out that effective "role modeling relies heavily on the characteristics and consequences of the model's actions" (p. 601). Therefore, the learner's repetition of behaviors is a selective and active process. The ANE can facilitate role modeling of positive behaviors by addressing attention, retention, motor production, and motivational aspects and by talking about the positive and negative consequences of the behavior.

TABLE 2-12 Process of Learning Using Role Modeling		
Processes of Role Modeling	**Teacher Actions/ Characteristics**	**Learner Actions/ Characteristics**
Attention	• Requires consideration of the learner's expectations, values, and beliefs prior to modeling • Teacher models the behavior or skill • Teacher displays confidence, positive leadership, and communication skills • Teacher who is likable and respected is more likely to be modeled	• More likely to attend to the modeled behavior if it is perceived as not violating learner's moral principles or endangering their self-esteem
Retention	• Asks learner to describe what was observed • Asks learner to identify key aspects of what was observed	• Learner recalls what was observed (verbally, in writing, or using concept mapping) • Recalling activates cognitive retention processes
Motor reproduction	• Provides praise and positive feedback on learner's performance • Provides feedback using precise labels and imagery	• Performs the observed behavior or skill using information from the attention and retention processes
Motivation	• Provides positive responses to testing behaviors to motivate learner • Verbally reinforces the value or usefulness of the behavior or skill in future nursing practice	• Learner "tests" to determine if positive or negative (motivating or inhibiting) responses will be obtained in future learning situations

Data from Armstrong, N. (2008). Role modeling in the clinical workplace. *British Journal of Midwifery, 16*(9), 596–603; and Bandura, A. (1977). *Social learning theory.* NY: General Learning Press.

THEORY AND RESEARCH RELATED TO CONTENT

Factors to consider related to content or subject matter include the content domain (e.g., cognitive, affective, or psychomotor), and the design factors such as content structure, organization, and content delivery methods. This section will explore Bloom's original taxonomy of learning, the revised taxonomy, principles of instructional design, and content delivery methods that facilitate learning.

Content Domains: Cognitive, Affective, and Psychomotor

As participants in a caring, practice-based profession, ANEs rely heavily on the ability to develop the student's cognitive, affective, and psychomotor learning. Cognition refers to mental processes used to acquire and apply knowledge. The cognitive domain of learning refers to knowledge acquisition and utilization. Nursing education values and builds on a diverse array of cognitive knowledge, including knowledge of biological sciences, mathematics, English, informatics, social sciences, and humanities. The first cognitive taxonomy published in 1956 by Benjamin Bloom has become widely adopted as a classification system for developing learning objectives, and is commonly referred to as "Bloom's taxonomy." Later, Bloom's taxonomy was revised to reflect new understandings of cognitive learning (Anderson *et al.*, 2001). Today, both taxonomies are widely used in education to identify, level, and evaluate the achievement of learning outcomes.

Bloom's original cognitive taxonomy was followed in 1964 by the publication of volume II, which addressed the affective taxonomy (Krathwohl, Bloom, & Masia). The affective domain is concerned with feelings, values, underlying motives, and attitudes, and therefore is directly relevant to the caring and professional behaviors of nurses. As with the cognitive taxonomy, the affective taxonomy identifies a hierarchical progression of affective development. The affective levels and corresponding verbs can be use to develop learning objectives that can be leveled and used as a basis for evaluation of achievement.

The third volume in the taxonomy series proposed by Bloom and colleagues was intended to cover the psychomotor domain. Although this text did not come to fruition, other authors have developed psychomotor taxonomies (Dave, 1970; Harrow, 1972; Simpson, 1972). In nursing, the psychomotor domain involves the blending of cognitive and affective knowledge and skills in the performance of physical tasks that involve a degree of neuromuscular coordination. Similar to the other taxonomies, the psychomotor taxonomies provide progressive, hierarchical structures for developing and evaluating learning outcomes. Details of the cognitive, affective, and psychomotor taxonomies and their use in educational assessment and evaluation are discussed in Chapter 4. Because of the unique nature of nursing practice, each domain adds an essential dimension to nursing education.

Content Structure, Organization, and Delivery Methods

The use of technology to structure, organize, and deliver learning content has advanced rapidly over the past several decades. Teaching methods are no longer limited to scrolling transparencies, colored markers, chalk, blackboards, and filmstrips.

Nussbaum-Beach (2008) note that, "The speedy evolution of technology has often outpaced our ability to use it to transform teaching and learning in real and meaningful ways" (p. 14). To enhance the ANE's ability to effectively use technology to teach, scholars in education have articulated principles and identified best practices in technology-based education. In this section, empirically based principles and best practices to guide the use of technology and media in the creation and organization of learning content are highlighted.

Principles Guiding E-Learning Content

An overriding guiding principle for facilitation of online learning, as well as virtually every learning context, is what Kim (2008) calls e^3 learning. E^3 learning refers to ensuring that learning is effective, efficient, and engaging. In the book *e-Learning and the Science of Instruction*, Clark and Mayer (2008) present specific principles for effective online instructional design and review the underlying research supporting the concepts of effective, efficient, and engaging instruction (Table 2-13).

The Modality Principle

When both text and graphics are presented simultaneously on a slide, the learner needs to process both the text and the graphics through the visual channel, which can result in visual overload. The modality principle refers to reducing the load on the visual channel so that the learner is able to attend to and process the information. The modality principle supports presenting words as speech rather than as onscreen text whenever there are competing visual images. According the Clark and Mayer (2008), there is "strong and consistent support for using [verbal] narration rather than on screen text to describe graphics" (p. 100).

The Redundancy Principle

Repetition of information, especially complex information, is generally considered beneficial to learning. The redundancy principle supports explaining visuals with words in audio or text, but not both. In other words, do not display the printed text of the audio narration on the same slide as the graphic that is being explained. In this case, the text is considered redundant to the other media (Clark & Mayer, 2008, p. 117). However, there are situations in which it may be advisable to violate the redundancy principle and present both audio narration with simultaneous onscreen text of the narration. According to Clark and Mayer the use of onscreen text to describe or explain a graphic should be considered in cases in which students have language difficulties or when the use of graphics is limited.

TABLE 2-13 Evidence-Based Principles for Designing e-learning Presentations

Principle	Implementation
Modality principle	• Avoid providing the same information in two different visual modalities (text and graphics) simultaneously (p. 99)

Redundancy principle	• Avoid explaining a graphic with both audio and text
	• Consider including both on-screen text and narration only in the following situations:
	  – there is no pictorial presentation
	  – there is sufficient time to process the pictorial presentation
	  – when greater cognitive effort is required to process audio narration than printed text, such as non-native speakers or learning disabled (p. 125)

Contiguity principle	• When labeling parts of a table or graphic, align the label close to the part and use arrows to connect the label to the part
Segmenting principle	• Break a lesson into small parts
Pre-training principle	• Define key concepts and relationships between concepts prior to teaching the content
Multimedia principle	• Place on-screen words near the corresponding part of the graphic
Coherence principle	• Avoid adding material that does not support the instructional goal (p. 133)

Clark, R., & Mayer, R. (2008). *E-learning and the science of instruction: Proven guidelines for consumers and designers of multimedia learning* (2nd Ed). San Francisco, CA: Pfeiffer.

Clark and Mayer (2008) explain that the modality and redundancy principles are based on cognitive theory and are concerned with how visual and auditory information are processed. Learners are only able to process one type of visual information at a time. In this case, when simultaneously presenting a graphic such as a video, animation, or still shot along with onscreen text, two pieces of visual information are being presented simultaneously, the graphic and the text. The learner is able to focus only on one visual source at a time and as a result, the other visual source tends to get less attention. Furthermore, the combination of audio narration and on-screen text presented simultaneously provides a source of extraneous cognitive processing. Unfortunately, this is not beneficial to learning because the learners will tend to pay more attention to comparing the text and audio messages, thus ignoring the graphic.

The redundancy effect can be summarized by the statement "adding redundant onscreen text to narrated graphics tends to hurt learning" (Clark & Mayer, 2008, p. 124). Various researchers have tested the accuracy of the redundancy effect by comparing groups of students who receive redundant and nonredundant instructional material. Studies by Kalyuga, Chandler, and Sweller (1999, 2000, 2004), found that the nonredundant groups performed better on problem solving tests than the redundant groups, producing effect sizes ranging from .8 to 1.

The Contiguity Principle

The contiguity principle refers to aligning word labels, either written or spoken, to the corresponding part of a graphic (Clark & Mayer, 2008, p. 77). When printed words are used to label parts of a graphic, such as a table, spreadsheet, diagram, or photo, the word labels should be placed near the appropriate area of the graphic. To improve the correspondence of the label and graphic, Clark and Mayer suggest using an arrow to connect the text to the specific area of the graphic. If there is too much text to fit on the screen, a technique called a mouseover or rollover can be used (2008, p. 80). Using the rollover technique creates a popup text box when the learner's cursor rolls over a specific section of the screen. Many Web site menus use this technique to reveal a more detailed index of content available within each menu item. The text boxes appear and disappear as the cursor moves about the screen. In applying the contiguity principle, rollovers would be placed in close proximity to the graphic content being referred to and connected to the graphic with an arrow, if needed. When providing narration of something depicted on an animation or a video, the narration should be timed to correspond to the actions being described.

There are several benefits of using the contiguity principle when designing instructional materials. Clark and Mayer explain that when words and pictures are presented in a contiguous manner, the learner does not have use "scarce cognitive resources to match them up" (2008, p. 89). A lack of contiguity between the labels and the graphic creates the need for extraneous processing of information that is unrelated to the learning objective. However, when words and pictures are connected in time and space the learner is able to make meaningful connections between them.

Clark and Mayer (2008) cite a large body of research that supports the effectiveness of the contiguity principle on learning (Chandler & Sweller, 1991; Mayer, 1989; Mayer, Steinhoff, Bower, & Mars, 1995; Moreno & Mayer, 1999; Paas & Van Merriënboer, 1994; Sweller & Chandler, 1994; Sweller, Chandler, Tierney, & Cooper, 1990). In five different tests, learners viewed several slides in which printed text was placed close to the illustration. The degree of learning was compared to groups of students who viewed the same slides with the text placed at the bottom of the slide. In all five tests, the students who viewed the slides with contiguous text and graphics performed better on problem-solving tests, showing a median gain of 68% (Clark & Mayer, 2008).

The Segmenting Principle

Another principle in e-learning is the segmenting principle, in which complex lessons are separated into smaller parts that are presented one at a time. For example, teaching a procedure such as inserting an intravenous catheter could be separated into distinct sections that are easier to remember: gathering supplies, preparing the intravenous tubing system, selecting the insertion site, cleansing the skin, inserting the catheter, connecting the catheter to the intravenous tubing, anchoring the catheter, and dressing the insertion site. In using the segmenting principle, each small step would be presented with supporting visuals.

The use of the segmenting principle facilitates learning by allowing the student to process each segment before continuing to the next. This is essential when presenting complex or serial information as it prevents cognitive overload and permits the learner to absorb the material at his or her own pace. According to Clark and Mayer (2008), several studies found that learners who were given the material in segments performed better on tests of transfer of knowledge than those who received the information in a continuous presentation (Mayer & Chandler, 2001; Mayer, Dow, & Mayer, 2003). In a set of three studies reviewed by Clark and Mayer (2008), consistent positive effects for the use of segmenting were found, yielding a median effect size of 1 (p. 190). They conclude that preliminary evidence supporting segmenting is favorable but would benefit from additional research.

The Pretraining Principle

Use of the pretraining principle is another strategy for reducing the learner's cognitive load, which can be used alone or in combination with the segmenting principle. When using the pretraining principle, Clark and Mayer (2008) suggest that the teacher identify concepts or definitions that are essential to learning the procedure or the serial information. Key concepts are defined and the relationships between concepts are clarified prior to teaching the content (p. 193). The rationale underlying this principle is that providing pretraining will help the learner to manage the processing of complex material.

Research on the effectiveness of pretraining is promising. Clark and Mayer (2008) cite two separate tests by Pollock, Chandler, and Sweller (2002) and three studies by

Mayer, Mathias, and Wetzell (2002) that compared groups of students who were shown lessons with and without the use of pretraining. The pretraining groups significantly outperformed the no-pretraining groups in terms of transfer learning, with an effect size of 1 and .9, respectively. Thus, the use of pretraining principle shows promise as an effective means of reducing cognitive load when teaching new and complex material.

The Coherence Principle

Clark and Mayer (2008) emphasize that the coherence principle is perhaps the most essential aspect for providing effective teaching materials (p. 133). According to the coherence principle, when developing teaching materials, only materials that support the instructional goal should be included. Although this seems like a clear-cut recommendation, Clark and Mayer note that it is often violated (p. 133). Adding background music, audio clips, and graphics (either still or animated) for the sole purpose of making a presentation more interesting is not recommended. They suggest reviewing materials for any nonessential words, graphics, or sounds and removing them from the final presentation. Thus, the coherence principle focuses on keeping all information relevant and essential to the learning goal by reducing clutter in the form of extraneous text, visuals, and audio that does not directly provide needed information.

The rationale for the coherence principle is based on cognitive theory, which posits that working memory is limited and that extraneous background sounds and visuals can overload the cognitive system and distract the learner from the essential message of the presentation. This is especially crucial when the material is complex, unfamiliar, or covered at a fast pace (Clark & Mayer, 2008, p. 136). The coherence principle may seem to be in direct contradiction to the arousal principle, which proposes that learners who are more emotionally stimulated by the material will be more motivated and interested in learning the material. The arousal principle and coherence principle actually are compatable. Stimulating audio and visual effects can be used to enhance arousal if they are directly relevant to the learning goals and do not overload or distract the learner from the essential material. However, the tendency when using the arousal theory can be to enhance presentations by adding stimulating graphics or sounds just for the sake of arousal, rather than meeting the learning goals, thereby defeating the purpose.

Several studies support the benefits of eliminating extraneous words and sounds in learning material (Mayer, Sims, & Tajika, 1995; Moreno & Mayer, 2000). When students who studied presentations containing background music and sound effects were compared to those who viewed presentations with no extraneous sounds, a dramatic difference was observed (Moreno & Mayer, 2000, p. 139). Students studying the presentation with no extraneous audio scored between 61 and 149% better than those who viewed presentations with extraneous sounds, achieving an effect size of 1.66 (p. 139).

The coherence principle also advises against adding extraneous graphics such as color photos and video clips merely to make the presentation more interesting. The belief that extraneous visuals will facilitate learning is another faulty interpretation of the arousal principle. According to cognitive theory, the learner is trying to understand and make sense of the material presented. Adding extraneous visuals can actually detract from the process of understanding by: (1) overburdening the learner's visual processing capacity; (2) distracting the learner from relevant learning material; and (3) disrupting the learner's ability to generate appropriate connections between pieces of information (Clark & Mayer, 2008, p. 142).

Researchers have explored the use of graphics in presentations and textbooks to enhance learning. Mayer, Heiser, and Lonn (2001) compared students who viewed lessons containing video clips that were related to the topic but not essential to the learning objectives, with students who viewed the same lesson without the video clips. They found that those who did not receive video clips performed better in tests of problem solving. Sanchez and Wiley (2006) found similar support for not adding irrelevant graphics to scientific textbooks. By tracking the eye movements of learners as they viewed learning materials with irrelevant graphics, they found that lower ability students tended to spend more time looking at irrelevant graphics than the higher ability students; and lower ability students showed less significant levels of learning. In short, adding attention-grabbing but irrelevant sounds or images detracts from the learner's ability to process the relevant information. Including nonessential sounds and images can detract from the learning goals and should generally be avoided.

Although these principles were originally studied in the e-learning environment, many of the principles may be easily adapted to face-to-face presentations as well. Thus, applying the coherence, segmenting, and pretraining principles to the design of in-class presentations will result in greater presentation clarity and will likely enhance the student's ability to process the new information.

THEORY AND RESEARCH RELATED TO TEACHING STRATEGIES

In this section, several teaching strategies that can be integrated with lecture and discussion are presented along with the concepts of transformative and integrative learning that facilitate learning. Specific teaching strategies such as problem-based learning, Socratic questioning, concept mapping, and reflective journaling are introduced. Each of these theoretical perspectives and strategies share a common emphasis on making learning a deep, meaningful experience that taps the learner's higher-order thinking processes.

Transformative Teaching Strategies

Transformative learning involves "experiencing a deep, structural shift in the basic premises of thought, feelings, and actions . . . that dramatically and irreversibly alters our way of being in the world" (O'Sullivan, Morrell, & O'Connor, 2002, p. xvii). Many educators and researchers have used the theory of transformative perspective, originally developed by Mezirow (1978) to enhance learning. Mezirow believed that two dimensions were missing in existing educational theories. These included understanding how adults construct and validate meaning, and how they make sense of their experiences (1991, p. xii). Mezirow viewed reflection as a central process in transformative learning that enables the learner to address the missing dimensions (1991, p. 116). McGonigal (2005) concurred, noting that although some college courses lend themselves to assimilative learning, in which new information is fit into the student's preexisting knowledge structures, most college courses will require at least some level of transformative learning (p. 1). For that reason, says McGonigal, "presenting new information is not enough to guarantee optimal learning. Students must recognize the limitations of their current knowledge and perspectives" (2005, p. 1).

In nursing education, assimilative learning may be more dominant for students taking liberal arts and science courses, which lay a foundation for nursing practice. The need for transformative learning often becomes more essential as the student is faced with the need to think differently and apply what they have learned to human situations. For many nursing students, the nursing curriculum represents the first time they are expected to critically think and apply knowledge to ever-changing, real-life situations. Furthermore, as students gain clinical experience they may witness nursing practices that are contrary to those learned in the classroom. Using transformative learning approaches can help students gain knowledge that "teaches them to critique dominant and ritualized practices to better choose which ones to take up or replace" (McAllister, Tower, & Walker, 2007, p. 311). Transformative learning can teach students to challenge their nursing care habits and routines.

According to McGonigal (2005), transformational learning involves several predisposing conditions. First is an activating event, which exposes the student to the awareness of their limitations. This can be an activity, situation, or scenario in which the student engages in self-reflection. Second, the student needs to identify their current assumptions. Any metacognitive approach in which students talk through or write about their thinking can be used to help them identify their assumptions. One approach recommended by McGonigal is the use of a critical questioning technique in which students are asked to explain their reasoning. From there the teacher plays devil's advocate and offers different explanations. The third condition in the transformational learning approach involves encouraging critical self-reflection. In contrast to the process of identifying current assumptions, critical reflection involves thinking about and integrating what happened in the classroom or clinical and is thus more likely to occur outside of the classroom. Nursing clinical courses have often required students to write clinical journals that may be structured to encourage critical reflection. However, journaling does not need to be limited to clinical courses. McGonigal (2005) suggests that classroom journals can be used to prompt students to reflect on questions, insights, and confusing points. The journals can be read periodically by the instructor or can be exchanged with other students for comments.

A fourth predisposing condition in transformative learning is encouraging critical discourse. Asking students to explain and defend a perspective that differs from their own is one strategy to encourage critical discourse. Encouraging continued discussion outside of class using small groups or online discussions may be effective. However, it is important to note that discussion and debate in which the student's current perspective is reinforced, is not likely to be transformative.

The final part of the transformational learning process involves providing opportunities to apply and test the new perspective in a safe situation. Students can be asked to interpret readings, current events, or experiences using the new perspective they have acquired. Alternatively, students may respond to a problem, case study, or assignment using multiple perspectives. Role-playing, simulations, and debates that are deliberately focused on a new perspective are also useful (All & Havens, 1997).

The teaching strategies mentioned in the previous discussion on the predisposing components of transformative learning can be adapted to facilitate deeper, transformative learning, provided the learner is asked to think differently (Box 2-5). The ANE can foster transformative learning by integrating one or more of these strategies within a learning unit. The guiding principle is to provide learning experiences that allow the student to think differently about a situation, or event.

Teaching Strategies for Critical Thinking

The importance of facilitating student's critical thinking skills in nursing is widely acknowledged. Students often struggle with the challenges inherent in making critical assessments of their patients, analyzing assessment findings, and making decisions about interventions and patient care management. These clinical decision-making skills are typically a contrast to the linear types of analysis involved in previous learn-

---

BOX 2-5   Teaching Strategies for Transformative Learning

1. Critical self-reflection

2. Identify assumptions

3. Metacognitive activities

4. Critical questioning

5. Journaling

6. Discussion/debate taking a perspective different from own

7. Interpreting readings, current events and experiences

8. Responding to a problem using multiple perspectives

9. Incorporating a new perspective into role playing or simulation

Data from McGonigal, K. (2005) Teaching for transformation: From learning theory to teaching strategies. *Speaking of Teaching Newsletter, The Center for Teaching and Learning, Stanford University,* 14(2), 1–4. Retrieved from http://www.stanford.edu/dept/CTL/Newsletter/transformation.pdf.

---

ing settings. Facione (2007) defines critical thinking as the use of core thinking skills of analysis, interpretation, evaluation, inference, explanation, and self-regulation. Analysis involves looking at the components of an object, situation, or event and exploring relationships between the parts, and perhaps the similarities and differences between the parts. When interpretation skills are used, the person is able to understand the meaning and significance of an event or situation. Evaluation involves determining the value, usefulness, or the integrity of an object, situation, or event. Inference involves taking the information and forming conclusions or hypothesis. Skill in explanation incorpates the ability of the learner to describe the reasoning processes used.

In addition to the core skills of analysis, interpretation, evaluation, inference, and explanation, critical thinkers use their critical thinking skills for their own self-regulation (Facione, 2007). Persons who use critical thinking skills for self-regulation are able to monitor their thinking, and use the sub-skills of self-examination and self-correction of one's reasoning (Facione, 2007, p. 7). Scholars of critical thinking describe it as "providing conceptual tools for understanding how the mind functions, in it's pursuit of meaning and truth" (Paul & Elder, 2007, p. 36).

Problem-Based Learning

Problem-based learning (PBL) has emerged in healthcare education as a way to bring adult learning concepts into play and enhance higher-level thinking. PBL is defined as a teaching approach that uses realistic clinical scenarios as the focal point for students to gain problem-solving skills (Hmelo-Silver, 2004). Originally developed in 1969 at the School of Medicine in McMaster University in Canada, PBL has since been integrated into many curriculums in many countries (Johnson & Finucane, 2000). Over the years, more and more medical and nursing schools have changed from traditional lecture-based classes and memorization strategies to PBL.

Conducting a PBL session involves seven steps (Table 2-14). First, clinical information about a hypothetical patient is briefly presented. The presentation can be in the form of a brief written paragraph about the patient or a short recording of an interaction between a patient and health care provider. The second step involves asking the students to identify key information from the scenario. Information that can provide a clue to the patient's problem and appropriate management of the problem is extracted from the situation. In the third step, students brainstorm about possible underlying reasons for the client's condition, then generate and rank hypotheses based on the limited information they have about the client. The fourth step involves determining what additional information is needed to substantiate or refute each hypothesis. During this step, the teacher may or may not provide further information as requested by the students. The students then analyze the new information, revise their list of hypotheses, and again determine what additional information is needed. In the fifth step, the students determine the preferred hypothesis and, as a group, identify what they know and do not know about the science underlying the condition. This is the point at which the student identifies gaps in his or her knowledge, determines personal learning objectives, and engages in self-directed study related the learning objectives. In step six, after the students have explored the topics and engaged in self-study, they reconvene and report to their group to share their knowledge. The final step is to integrate the new knowledge to the client's situation and to consider the broader impact of the situation on ethical, legal, economic, and public health arenas (Johnson & Finucane, 2000).

The research reviewed by Johnson & Finucane (2000) supports the benefits of PBL in enhancing self-directed learning skills, creating a positive, student-centered learning environment, promoting interactions between students and faculty, and promoting deeper rather than superficial learning. The use of PBL helps the student develop what Hmelo-Silver (2004) refers to as flexible knowledge that can be applied to new situations. In addition, there is evidence that students develop self-directed learning and problem-solving skills through PBL.

TABLE 2-14 Seven Steps in Problem-Based Learning	
Steps in Problem-Based Learning	**Description of Steps**
1. Review clinical scenario	• Provide a brief, written, or verbal description of a patient scenario or a brief video of a patient nurse interaction
2. Have students identify factual information	• Instructor facilitates the students to identify the factual information of the case • Information is listed and displayed for the entire class
3. Have students brainstorm and generate hypotheses about the problem	• Instructor facilitates the students to think about possible causes • Possible causes may be listed and displayed for the entire class
4. Students determine additional information needed, analyze the new information, and revise hypothesis	• Using the lists of what is known and the possible causes, the students ask questions to obtain more data • The instructor may reveal or withhold specific information to facilitate exploration of specific problems
5. Students determine the preferred hypothesis and identify what is known and not known	• Use thinking skills to narrow the possibilities and determine additional information needed to confirm or disconfirm the hypothesis
6. Students engage in self-study	• Areas needing further study are divided among the students for self-study. Findings are then shared with the entire class • Self study information may lead to the acceptance of an hypothesis or the generate new hypotheses that need to be explored
7. Integrate new knowledge	• Once the hypothesis is accepted, the students determine the nursing care needed and how to manage the implications of the problem

Data from Johnson, S., & Finucane, P. (2000). The emergence of problem-based learning in medical education. *Journal of Evaluation in Clinical Practice, 6*, 281–291.

Socratic Questioning

According to Paul and Elder (2007), both critical thinking and the art of Socratic questioning share the ultimate goal of finding meaning and truth. Socratic questioning represents a systematic and in-depth process of questioning that uses the components of critical thinking to understand one's reasoning and the implications of that reasoning. The ability to analyze or break apart the components of thinking is essential to understanding. Paul and Elder (2007) outline categories of questioning that can provide in-depth analysis of a situation or event (Table 2-15). Some examples of questions using Socratic taxonomy are also provided; however, to be most effective, the instructor will need to tailor questions asked to meet the specific needs of the discussion topic. Teachers who use Socratic questioning will facilitate deeper understanding and will model the process of critical thinking to their students.

IDEALS Framework

Although critical thinking skills come naturally to some students, for others, the skills can be taught and learned. Facione identifies six steps in thinking critically and problem solving using the IDEALS acronym (Facione, 2007, p. 23). These steps take the learner through the core thinking skills of analysis, interpretation, self-regulation, inference, explanation, and evaluation discussed earlier. The first step identified in the IDEALS acronym is to determine the real Issue. The next is to Define the context by asking, "What are the facts of the situation?" Third is to Enumerate the choices by asking, "What are some reasonable options?" In the fourth step, the problem is Analyzed by asking the learner to determine the best course of action, weighing the pros and cons. The "L" in the acronym stands for "List reasons" or give rationale. The final step stands for Self-correct. This involves looking at the problem or situation and determining if the process has been completed satisfactorily. The ANE can teach students to apply this easy to remember seven-step process to a variety of situations that can facilitate learning.

Concept Mapping

The mental processes involved in concept mapping requires students to organize, analyze, and link data to construct new knowledge about a situation (All, Huycke, & Fisher, 2003). A concept map is a visual diagram of concepts usually linked by proposition statements. Concept maps may be categorized as spider, hierarchal, linear, or system structures. In the spider structure, subconcepts radiate outward from a central concept. In hierarchical maps, the most important concept is placed at the top and the subconcepts are beneath. Linear maps are nonhierarchical depictions linking one concept to the next. System maps depict multiple interrelationships between subconcepts. No matter the configuration used, the results represent the learner's conceptualization of the topic.

Concept maps can be used to facilitate learning and may be used by the teacher to organize and present content, and show the interrelationships between previous

TABLE 2-15 A Taxonomy of Socratic Questions		
Taxonomy	**Rationale**	**Examples of Questions**
Questions about goals and purpose	• Provides foundational understanding and helps clarify motivation	• What is the purpose of this situation, event, or condition? • What is the intended goal of this activity?
Questions that focus on questions in thinking	• "All thought is responsive to a question." (p. 36) • "To fully understand a thought requires understanding the question that gave rise to it." (p. 36)	• "What are the main questions that guide personal behavior in this situation?" (p. 36) • What is the best or most insightful way to phrase the question, or issue?
Questions about the information, data, or experiences	• All thoughts are founded on an information base • Understanding the information, data, and experiences, helps clarify the underlying thinking	• On what experience is the thinking based? • "Is there relevant information or data that has not been analyzed?" (p. 36). • Is the information reliable? • "Is the thinking based on facts or soft data?" (p. 37)
Questions about inferences and conclusions	• "No thought is fully understood until one understands the inferences that shaped it." (p. 37)	• "How was the conclusion reached?" (p. 37) • What are some other possible conclusions?
Questions about concepts and ideas	• All thought involves the use of concepts • "To understand a thought requires understanding the concepts inherent in that thought." (p. 37)	• What is the main concept or idea in this line of thinking? • Does the current way of thinking about the problem need to be reconceptualized?
Identifying assumptions	• All thoughts include inherent assumptions, or things taken for granted • Assumptions indicate the origins of the thought • Assumptions need to be identified and explored to understand the problem or issue	• What assumptions or beliefs underlie this situation? • Why is a particular assumption or belief made?

(continues)

TABLE 2-15 A Taxonomy of Socratic Questions (continued)

Taxonomy	Rationale	Examples of Questions
Questions about implications and consequences	• All thought is headed in a direction or has implications • All thought goes somewhere, or has consequences	• If such and such happens, what is the likely result? • If such and such happens, how could it affect ____?
Questions that explore viewpoints	• All thought takes place from a particular perspective or frame of reference	• What is the perspective in this situation? • What other perspectives are relevant? • What are the biases or prejudices within this viewpoint?

Data from Paul, R., & Elder, L. (2007). Critical thinking: The art of Socratic questioning. *Journal of Developmental Education, 31*(1), 36–37.

lessons and the current content. Concept maps are also useful strategies for students to use for note taking, for clinical preparation, or as a required course assignment. When used in the clinical setting, a concept map can allow the student and faculty to describe and analyze the patient situation and interrelationships from a holistic perspective. Studies from as early as the 1980s have found positive outcomes from the use of concepts maps to facilitate learning, promote discussion, improve writing and outlining skills, and increase retention (All & Havens, 1997).

Reflective Journaling

Many nursing programs incorporate journaling or clinical logs as a learning activity. When clinical journaling is constructed as a truly reflective endeavor using components of critical thinking (such as analysis, evaluation, and synthesis), insights may be identified and learning is likely to become internalized and meaningful. Blake's (2005) review of the literature on the goals and benefits of journaling clustered around nine themes that reflect the broad impact that journaling has on learning. The goals and benefits of journaling included: (1) discovering meaning, (2) caring for self, (3) making connections, (4) instilling values, (5) gaining perspectives, (6) reflecting on professional roles, (7) developing critical thinking skills, (8) developing affective skills, and (9) improving writing skills (p. 2). Although the themes were derived from predominantly qualitative research, "journaling continues to be valued by educators and students alike because of the ability to enhance the development of critical thinking and communication" (Blake, 2005, p. 10).

A study by Thorpe (2004) used two models of reflection as a framework for a series of reflective writings by nursing management students. The three stages of reflection model (Table 2-16) described by Scanlon and Chernomas (1997) and the three levels of reflection model (Table 2-17) described by Wong *et al.* (1997) and Kember *et al.* (1999) were used as frameworks to encourage high quality reflection in the journal entries. According to Thorpe (2004), the models provided a structure that was helpful for students writing the journals and allowed the students to gage their progress in developing reflective thinking. A study by Murphy (2005) also supports the concepts inherent in the models and found that those who were taught reflective journaling scored 29% higher than students who were not provided instruction in journaling.

Integrative Learning

Reflective journaling also provides an avenue for integrative learning experiences. Integrative learning is a relatively new concept that expands the concept of critical thinking to a new level. Huber *et al.* (2007) describe integrative learning as "the ability to make, recognize, and evaluate connections among disparate concepts, fields, or contexts" (p. 46). According to Huber's report, integrative learning includes connecting skills and knowledge from multiple sources and experiences. Integrative learning may occur in interdisciplinary courses, or by applying theory to practice in service learning experiences or practicums. Integrative learning explores diverse points of

TABLE 2-16 Three Stages of Reflection Model

Stages	Characteristics
1. Awareness	Characterized by curiosity, excitement and recognition of a need to know or need to be able to explain a situation
2. Critical analysis	Actively uses critical thinking skills to explore a situation or event
3. New perspective	The outcome of previous stages demonstrated by a change in affective or cognitive behavior

Data from Scanlon, J. M., & Chernomas, W. M. (1997). Developing the reflective teacher. *Journal of Advanced Nursing, 25,* 1138–1143.

TABLE 2-17   Three Levels of Reflection Model

Level of Reflection	Descriptive Characteristics
1. Non-Reflectors	Lower level reflection, may include: • "habitual action"—referring to using knowledge that has become automatic through repeated use • "thoughtful action"—involves making use of existing knowledge (book learning) without appraisal of that knowledge • "introspection"—involves the affective domain, exploring feelings and thoughts about one's self without exploring the soundness of one's prior knowledge
2. Reflectors	• Reflect on content, process or both content and process • Content reflection focuses on what the person thinks, feels, or does • Process reflection looks at how the person performs content reflection and how well it is carried out
3. Critical Reflectors	• Highest level of reflection focusing on premise reflection • Premise reflection requires the learner to examine assumptions in order to redefine the problem and take action

Data from Kember, D., Jones, A., Loke, A., McKay, J., Sinclair, K., Tse, H., Webb, C., Wong, F., Wong, M., & Yeung, E. (1999). Determining the level of reflective thinking from students' written journals using a coding scheme based on the work of Mezirow. *International Journal of Lifelong Education, 18*(1),18–30; and Wong, K., Loke, A., Wong, M., Tse, H., Kan, E., & Kember, D. (1997). An action research study into the development of nurses as reflective practitioners. *Journal of Nursing Education, 36*(10), 476–481.

view, seeks to understand the context underlying issues and positions, and helps students link affective and cognitive learning (Huber *et al.*, 2007).

THEORY AND RESEARCH RELATED TO THE LEARNING ENVIRONMENT

The learning environments in undergraduate nursing programs have expanded over the years. Classroom instruction is no longer limited to face-to-face instruction. More courses are being offered using blended or fully online formats in attempt to accommodate technology savvy learners, reach a broader geographic area, and circumvent scheduling difficulties inherent in face-to-face classes. Changes in clinical and skills laboratory instruction have also occurred. There is increased competition for clinical sites and students need to learn to care for patients with higher levels of acuity than in the past. These changes, coupled with the expectation that nursing students will have a certain level of clinical skill prior to stepping onto a nursing unit, have lead to changes in the clinical teaching environment. Today, there is a growing emphasis on providing realistic clinical laboratory practice and testing, and on the use of diverse clinical sites in the community and hospital specialty units. In this section, theory and research related to the four major learning settings, face-to-face classrooms, e-learning, skill laboratory, and clinical practicum, are reviewed.

The Face-to-Face Classroom

Teaching in a face-to face classroom setting involves interacting with students in real time, in the same physical locality. As with all educational settings, teaching in the face-to face classroom can be influenced by principles and characterized by strengths and drawbacks. In this section, awareness of selected principles of learning and attributes of the classroom environment that impact face-to-face teaching are discussed.

Principles for Effective Face-to Face Teaching

Fink (2003) outlined six principles of significant learning that have implications for the face-to-face learning environment. First, the student needs foundational knowledge, a conceptual understanding of the most important knowledge in the course. For the teacher, this means identifying the main ideas and the relationships between those main ideas. Second, is the principle of application, making the information useful in the classroom setting and beyond. Third, is the principle of integration or connecting what has been learned to previous knowledge and to future learning. The forth principle, called the human dimension, recognizes that effective learning is social. Learning requires interaction with the content, the teacher, and or other learners. Fink (2003) identified caring as the fifth principle. Caring in the learning context refers to the learner's motivation, which serves to energize the learner and provide an impetus for learning. For the instructor, the ability to make the learning environment welcoming and interactive; plus being clear about the usefulness of the content will help infuse the principle of caring into the learning situation. Learning how to learn is the final principle for significant learning. This involves becoming a life-long learner and becoming comfortable navigating through the educational system. For an example of the application of Fink's principles in nursing education, please refer to Magnussen (2008).

Limitations of the Physical Classroom

Most educators agree that student participation and engagement in the learning process enhances learning. Yet there are environmental factors such as class size, classroom seating, and characteristics of the interpersonal environment that can detract from the student's ability and willingness to engage in the learning process. According to Faust & Courtenay (2002), the physical and interpersonal environment of the classroom is a significant factor that can either enhance or detract from participation and the ability of the learner to focus on learning.

Class size is an environmental factor that the instructor may not be able to control. However, class size can affect participation and classroom dynamics. Therefore, the instructor needs to recognize the underlying issues and utilize strategies that will enhance classroom dynamics. Students in large classes tend to participate less often for a variety of reasons. An obvious reason is that in large classes students may feel inhibited and may be less likely to engage in discussion or actively participate. One way to deal with this is to provide opportunities early on for students to get to know each other. Faust and Courtenay (2002) found that when faculty provided such opportunities, students reported feeling more comfortable participating. Thus, one strategy may be to engage the students in dyads or small groups early on, so the students can get know each other and feel comfortable discussing within their groups.

Another environmental issue, according to Faust and Courtenay (2002), is that large class size makes it more difficult to see and hear students who are speaking. In addition, the ability to have eye contact with the instructor and classmates is more limited in larger classes and in classes where students are seated in rows. Seating arranged in a horseshoe configuration is ideal for classes that rely heavily on discussion because it affords students clear visibility of each other and closer proximity to the instructor. If the classroom seating cannot be reconfigured, strategies to encourage participation include having the instructor move about the room during lecture and discussions, repeating students' comments for the entire class to hear, or dividing the class into small groups to work on specific assignments. Another option is using the think-pair-share activity in which the student is asked to write a response in one or two minutes to the instructor's statement or question. Each student then pairs with a student nearby, and shares their thinking with their partner (Angelo & Cross, 1993). The instructor can then ask a few pairs to share their conclusions with the entire class. Using think-pair-share gives students who may be reluctant to share in a large group the opportunity to get to know and interact one-on-one, with another classmate.

In large classrooms, where engagement with students can be problematic, the ANE's ability to create a positive context for learning depends on multiple factors. Long and Coldren (2006) suggest several strategies that can be used to create a positive learning context, such as (1) model and explain the thinking processes used to make decisions; (2) create a team atmosphere—when addressing the class refer to "we" instead of "you"; (3) use relevant anecdotes and stories; (4) speak in a conversational style and allow students to respond; (5) use mistakes as opportunities to learn;

(6) show enthusiasm for the topic; and (7) use communication strategies that engage the learner such as eye contact and warm tone of voice.

Student Response Systems

In large lecture classes, it is difficult for students to become engaged in learning through discussion, feedback, and active involvement (Trees & Jackson, 2007, p. 22). Electronic student response systems, or clickers, are a newer technology designed to increase student participation and provide student and instructor feedback. Clickers are handheld electronic devices that allow individual students to respond to questions posed by the instructor. The student responses are received and recorded electronically, then tabulated and projected back to the students and teacher as aggregate data. The ANE can use the student response system to stimulate discussion or to provide opportunities for higher-order thinking by replying to problem-solving and decision-making scenarios or solving drug calculations. Clickers also can provide students formative feedback on their thinking and understanding of material. Thus, by asking students to respond to questions using clicker technology, active participation and active learning are enhanced, even in large lectures.

Several studies have explored the effectiveness of student response systems in facilitating learning. Trees and Jackson (2007) conducted a study of over 1500 students enrolled in seven courses that used clicker technology. The researchers found that students with the most positive perception of the clicker technology tended to value feedback, tended to have a less favorable impression of large lecture classes, and had a strong desire for engagement in the class (p. 32). Interestingly, the student's level of learning and involvement was related to the number of clicker questions typically asked during a class session. Students reported the lowest level of learning and involvement in classes that incorporated an average of 1–3 clicker responses and higher levels of learning and involvement when an average of 4–9 responses were solicited (p. 34).

Another interesting finding related to the use of clickers and point allocation for responses. Those enrolled in courses in which student responses were part of the course grade reported greater motivation to attend class. Burnstein and Lederman (2001) found attendance levels around 90% when the student responses accounted for at least 15% of the course grade, and Woods and Chiu (2003) found a positive relationship between attendance and student responses when the responses were worth as little as 5% of the course grade (p. 36). In addition, the use of clickers encouraged students to be more prepared for class, especially when responses were part of the course grade.

The Skill Laboratory Environment

Prior to placement of students in a clinical practicum setting, students generally practice skills in a simulated setting. Mannequins, models, other students, and standardized patients are often used as a focus for practice. Three areas of growing interest in teaching skills are reviewed in this section including the use of programmable high-fidelity human patient simulators, standardized patients, and computer-based virtual clinical scenarios.

Clinical Simulation

Clinical simulation has been used in nursing education to prepare students before clinical experiences for decades. From the crudest form of simulation such as giving an injection to an orange, to high-fidelity human patient simulators, the use of simulation is here to stay. Many nursing programs today integrate several types of simulation, using body part models and static full body mannequins for learning isolated skills such as tracheostomy care, catheterization, wound care, injections, and intravenous infusions.

The growing need to assure students have a beginning level of knowledge and competency in managing specific situations, along with the difficulty in providing each student with those experiences, has resulted in many nursing programs providing full-scale scenario-based simulations prior to the clinical practicum. Thus, after students have practiced the skills in isolation, a realistic, scenario-based simulation is provided to allow the student to perform multiple psychomotor skills, integrated along with clinical decision-making skills.

Full-scale simulations may involve the recreation of a realistic scenario using human actors or standardized patients, virtual computer aided instruction (CAI), and/or high-fidelity human patient simulators. Waldner & Olson (2007) note that most research on the effectiveness of simulation, when compared to traditional lecture and clinical instruction, remains inconclusive (p. 4). For example, Madorin & Iwasiw (1999) found an initial increase in student self-confidence in those who used a computer–assisted instruction (CAI) simulation to learn a skill; however, there was no difference between the control group and treatment group after they had performed the skill in the clinical setting. In contrast, another study found that combining CD-ROM based simulations with other learning methods (such as lecture and clinical) was more effective than using each method alone (Bauer & Huynh, 2001). Additionally, some researchers have reported improved performance with the use of human patient simulators (Alinier, Hunt, & Gordon, 2004; Yoo & Yoo, 2003), but others have reported no difference or a decrease in knowledge (Griggs, 2002; Ravert, 2004).

Despite the lack of consensus on the objective effectiveness of simulations, there is a consensus on the perceived satisfaction and perceived value of simulation experience. A study by Bremner, Aduddell, & Amason (2008) explored the effect of human patient simulator experience on 149 nursing students prior to their first clinical experience. They found that 97% of the students agreed the simulation component should be included in the nursing curriculum as a required component. Seventy-one percent reported gaining confidence with physical assessment skills and 42% were less anxious about their first clinical experience (p. 7). Additionally, several research reviews have reported numerous studies of students and faculty that support the perceived benefits and value of high-fidelity patient simulators (Feingold, Calaluce, & Kallen, 2004; Waldner & Olson, 2007). A benefit of using high-fidelity human patient simulations is that they afford students the opportunity to integrate and practice skills in a controlled and nonthreatening environment prior to clinical placement. As a result, students and faculty have generally found that these simulations provide a valuable and realistic learning experience.

Standardized Patients

An alternative approach for simulating clinical experiences is the use of standardized patients (SP). SPs are "individuals who have been carefully trained to present an illness or scenario in a standardized, unvarying manner" (Becker, Rose, Berg, Park, & Shatzer, 2006, p. 103). SPs have been used to portray patients with a variety of conditions, allowing the opportunity to teach and evaluate student skills in therapeutic communication, interviewing, assessment, and patient teaching (Becker *et al.*, 2006).

According to Becker *et al.* (2006) the accuracy and realism of the SP has been tested by several researchers who found SPs more than 90% accurate in portraying the condition they were contracted to represent. In a mental health rotation, Becker *et al.* used SP scenarios to evaluate student's communication skills, and knowledge and evaluation of depression. The researchers found no difference in test scores on communication knowledge between the control group and the experimental group. However, the experimental group who interviewed the SP reported that the experience helped them think critically. In addition, having the students interview the same patient provided a benchmark for faculty assessment of student learning and for the student's personal self-assessment (p. 108). The realism, uniformity, and controllability afforded by SP scenarios provides an effective bridge from classroom book knowledge of skills, to the application of knowledge and skills in the clinical setting.

There are several advantages of using SPs in the skills laboratory. It allows students to practice skills in a more realistic yet less threatening environment than the clinical setting, and allows the student and faculty to obtain immediate feedback on the student's performance from the patient's perspective (Becker *et al.*, 2006, p. 104). For faculty, the SP can be developed to meet specific course objectives and provide a clinical type of experience that is uniform for all students. Unlike the clinical setting, the instructor can control the complexity of the SP situation, keeping it consistent for all students, which enhances the reliability of evaluation of skill performance. Furthermore, when using SPs, the instructor does not have to rely on the unpredictable availability of patients in a clinical setting. As with the use of high fidelity human patient simulators, SPs provide a relatively constant scenario for students to respond to without risk of harm to a real patient.

Virtual Clinical Simulation

Virtual clinical simulations use realistic clinical scenarios on interactive CDs to provide exposure to a variety of clinical situations. Jeffries (2000) developed and tested the hyperlearning model for designing effective, interactive CDs for teaching nursing skills. The model incorporated four dimensions that are integrated into the lessons: general principles, processes, critical thinking, and professional application. Application of general principles involves the use of learning activities and resources that allow students to vary the cognitive load and provide an array of connections from which they can build their knowledge. A baseline of reading assignments, presentations, and Web sites is provided for all students and is supplemented by additional sources and activities for students to use if they are having difficulty with the material. The process dimension allows the learner to self-assess their learning and determine individual learning needs. The learner is free to select and explore the general principles and process aspects of the lesson. However, completion of the critical thinking and professional application dimensions is required. The learning activities included in the critical thinking and professional application dimensions were "designed to develop metacognitive skills: planning, predicting, evaluating, and revising methods of self-regulation" (p. 74). Since Jeffries' study in 2000, the model has been used by others to develop interactive CDs for learning clinical knowledge and skills (Sternberger, 2002; Sternberger & Meyer 2001).

The Clinical Learning Environment

As a practice profession, nursing relies on providing real-time, hands-on experiences for students. This involves performing skills in the clinical arena in which complex tasks and procedures are carried out under a sense of time pressure, on patients who are ill and distraught. To get the students to a point at which they perform under these conditions with relative ease is quite an accomplishment. Optimal clinical environments are essential for application and development of knowledge and skills in acute care, long-term care, and community settings.

Influence of the Clinical Instructor

The nature of the clinical environment is strongly influenced by the clinical instructor and the attitudes, behaviors, and relationships established with clinical staff. To explore the attributes of good clinical instructors, Hanson and Stenvig (2008) conducted a grounded theory study. They identified three attribute categories of good clinical instructors: knowledge, interpersonal, and teaching strategies. The instructor's knowledge consisted not only of practice knowledge, but also knowledge of the facility and students. Knowing the students' backgrounds and needs were seen as valuing and respecting students. Interpersonal attributes included displaying a positive, professional attitude and an encouraging demeanor, as well as being an organized, approachable, and accessible resource person (p. 41). Good clinical instructors also demonstrated teaching strategy attributes that challenged the students, and they were able to manage paperwork and postconference planning effectively. Cook (2005) found that if students perceived the instructor's clinical teaching behaviors as inviting by communicating respect, caring, trust, and optimism, the students had lower state anxiety (p. 160). Likewise, higher state anxiety significantly correlated with disinviting instructor behaviors such as demeaning or defeating comments, uncaring, condescending, sexist, or racist behaviors.

Cook (2005) suggests that faculty interested in being proactive in terms of creating a positive clinical environment can survey their students early in the clinical rotation. The 44-item Clinical Teaching Survey (CTS) used in the study can provide formative feedback that can be used by the ANE to create an inviting clinical atmosphere. The survey was originally develop by Ripley (1986) using an established tool called the Invitational Teaching Survey to address clinical teaching specifically. The CTS has under gone a process of content validity review and tested high in internal consistency (Cook, 2005; Ripley, 1986).

The Distance Learning Environment

The proliferation of distance learning, e-learning, or online learning courses has resulted in a unique type of learning environment. With the absence of face-to-face contact with the instructor and other students, the technology used to create the courses has become the vehicle for creating a positive, effective classroom environment. This shift in delivery methods coupled with the need to create a positive, interactive, connected, learning environment has sparked a reexamination and clarification of the core goals, purposes, theories, and principles in education. Although the concepts discussed in this section were originally intended for application to a distance learning, technology-based learning environment, many if not all of the ideas have relevance to face-to-face teaching environments, as well.

Clark and Mayer (2008) identify three types of e-learning based on the overall educational goal. If the goal is to inform or update the learner, the receptive, show and tell type of format works well. For teaching procedures and tasks, the directive, "tell and do" approach is most appropriate. When the educational goal is to enable the learner to transfer the knowledge and skills to real life situations, the problem-solving guided-discovery type of e-learning is appropriate.

Clark and Mayer (2008) also outline three categories of e-learning with associated roles of the learner and teacher (p. 34). First is the response strengthening view of learning, which is concerned with the strengthening of associations (i.e., behaviorism perspective). The learner takes a passive role and the instructor takes the role of controlling the learning by dispensing rewards and punishments. The second category of learning emphasizes knowledge acquisition and memory (i.e., cognitivism perspective). Here, the learner is also passive and the instructor is an active dispenser of information. The final category of learning is viewed as knowledge construction (i.e., constructivism perspective) and is concerned with the mental representation that the learner creates. From this perspective, the roles of student and teacher are reversed. The student is active in the process and the teacher functions as a cognitive guide. Although Clark and Mayer (2008) point out that there is merit in each perspective, the main goal of effective instruction today emphasizes knowledge construction. For the ANE this means facilitating and guiding active learning and thinking processes used by the student.

Competencies for Distance Teaching

Competencies for distance teaching have been established and validated by the International Board of Standards for Training, Performance, and Instruction (Darabi, Sikorski, & Harvey, 2006). An initial list of 20 competencies were identified from the literature and rated in terms of importance, frequency of performance, and perception of time spent on task, by distance learning professionals and subject matter experts. Interestingly, the competencies related to communication and interaction with the students were ranked highest, whereas all of competencies related to technology including using technology effectively, using various methods of distance education, and accommodating problems with technology, were rated in the bottom fifth of all competencies.

These findings validate the importance of instructor communication and interaction in creating effective distance learning environments. Swan (2004) provides further support in a review of research related to interaction. Swan summarized the research and identified four types of interaction: (1) interaction between the student and content, (2) between the student and instructor, (3) between other students, and (4) between the student and the course interface. In terms of interaction with content, online discussion that focuses on divergent thinking, complex cognitive understanding, and reflection, was found more effective than face-to-face discussion. Two possible reasons for this include a sense of anonymity in online discussions and the asynchronous structure of online discussions. The sense of anonymity and being able to discuss with written versus spoken words may decrease student's inhibitions and place timid students on par with more assertive students. The asynchronous structure of discussions allows students time to think and research various perspectives and formulate more articulate and well thought out responses. Swan recommends engaging in activities early on that allow the students to get to know each other and develop a sense of trust. Developing grading rubrics for the desired cognitive behaviors and modeling the desired behaviors will help facilitate learning.

Both the quantity and quality of interactions between student and teacher and evidence of teaching presence are important in online learning environments. Teaching presence can be established through optimal design and organization of the learning environment, by facilitating discussion, providing direct instruction, and by providing opportunities for ongoing assessment of learning and feedback (Swan, 2004). The instructor can provide timely feedback using automated testing and feedback when appropriate, engaging public discussion forums, private e-mail, or phone calls to individual students.

Interaction with classmates in the online learning environment also facilitates learning. According to Swan (2004), research supports that learning is enhanced in classes in which there is a sense of community. However, there is generally greater variability in how students rate their sense of community in online courses as compared to face-to-face courses, indicating a need to focus efforts on community building activities. Swan recommends that teachers model "immediacy behaviors" in their interactions with students. Verbal immediacy behaviors such as responding to students in online discussions by name, sharing personal stories, and using a conversational tone in course correspondence will enhance the learner's sense of connection with the teacher.

The final area of interaction that Swan (2004) identifies as important is the student's interaction with the course interface. Some of the aspects of the course interface are within the instructor's direct control such as allowing the learner to control the pace of presentations and formatting presentations using principles of e-learning to minimize cognitive load. Other aspects of the course interface such as the orientation to the course interface, provision of 24/7 online support, and using a consistent template for course structure may be dictated by the academic institution. Swan recommends that all courses in a program should use a consistent interface so that students do not spend time learning to navigate new systems. Adhering to the principles of multimedia design and e-learning proposed by Mayer (2001) will also help ensure that effective presentations and learning materials are provided.

To identify and tie all of the aspects relevant to effective online teaching together, Ryan, Hodson-Carlton, & Ali (2005) developed a Model for Faculty Teaching Online (p. 363). The model identifies antecedent conditions, context, strategies, and consequences of online learning. Antecedent conditions refer to aspects that need to be developed and in place for effective implementation. Support structures, resources, technology partnerships, access to hardware, software, and technical skills training are needed for effective implementation of online teaching. Once these are in place, policies to guide the implementation of these factors into the distance learning environment are needed. The antecedent conditions interact with the context of the learning environment. Contextual considerations include the nature of the online curriculum, the unique aspects of the online environment (such as portability and convenience), and around the clock access to learning.

The antecedents and context of learning help inform the next category in the model, called strategies. When considering strategies, the role of the faculty and the way courses are designed and managed may need to be reconceptualized. In lieu of the regular face-to-face contact typically found in a non-online course, the Model for Faculty Teaching Online recommends integrating diverse opportunities for frequent communication. Instead of in-person presentations and class sessions, attention to the design of course media and presentations so that they are engaging, informative, motivating, and user friendly is emphasized. Unlike face-to-face classes, online courses need to be prepared ahead of time and modules need to be made available to students who like to work ahead of schedule. Periodic adjustments to new technology and software will also be required.

The aspects of antecedents, context, and strategies then influence the final aspect of the model—consequences. The model recognizes both positive and negative consequences of online learning such as changes in faculty roles, adjustments to teaching online, changes in the nature of relationships with students, and the collaborative nature of the learning environment. A validation study conducted by Ryan *et al.* (2005) supports the model as a useful guide for faculty who are redesigning courses into an online format. The model can be useful for anticipating issues, needs, resources, and processes that should be addressed prior to and during implementation.

Online Discussion

The importance of discussion in online learning has led many to explore the various aspects of discussion. Han & Hill (2006) have delineated the types of online discussion and Dixson, Kuhlhorst, & Reiff (2006) have identified the optimal roles of the instructor and student in online discussion. Others have developed models for facilitating online discussion (Murphy, Mahoney, Chen, Mendoza-Diaz, & Yang, 2005). The types of discussion used, the roles of the faculty and students in the discussion process, and the adoption of models for facilitating discussion, are largely influenced by the instructor's values and beliefs, which are in turn reflected in the various educational perspectives previously discussed. For example, instructors operating from a social constructivist perspective may involve students in discussions, not only as contributors, but also as facilitators, as this allows the student to mold the direction of the discussion and construct knowledge.

Murphy *et al.* (2005) developed a model for facilitating student discussion that is consistent with the constructivist perspective. The model is similar to using a train-the-trainer approach. The instructor serves as the primary trainer for the teaching assistants (TA) and student facilitators. The TA in turn serves as a coach and facilitator for the student discussion leaders. According to the model, the instructor teaches the TA and discussion leaders the strategies for discussion such as identifying areas of agreement and disagreements, and ways to encourage and reinforce participation, and ways to reach consensus (p. 354). The instructor also teaches the TA how to coach and facilitate the student discussion leaders in their new roles. In essence, Murphy and colleagues see the instructor's role as involving various combinations of mentoring, coaching, and facilitating actions, which provide opportunities for active learning and help form cognitive scaffolding that permits the students to assume more responsibility for their learning.

Testing of the model revealed that student facilitators were able to clarify areas of agreement and disagreement. They were able to help the participants reach a consensus, make connections between others, comments and the readings, and help students understand points of view different from their own. Other activities of the facilitators included encouraging participation and elaboration of ideas, acknowledging comments, and querying students by their names. The study by Murphy *et al.* (2005)

supports the findings of earlier studies, which found that student-led discussions demonstrated greater levels of student participation and student satisfaction than instructor-led discussions (p. 355).

Applying the Personalization Principle

Creating positive online learning environments can be facilitated by using a positive tone when providing instructional dialog. The personalization principle refers to the use of a conversational style when designing text-based presentations. Three subcomponents are included in the personalization principle. These involve (1) writing on-screen instructions and audio narration in first and second person, using you and I when appropriate; (2) using an active voice (i.e., present tense); and (3) using what Clark and Mayer (2008) refer to as polite speech. When giving online instructions, an example of using polite speech would be to say, "You may click the enter key now" versus "Click the enter key," which is more abrupt and less personal.

Research reviewed by Clark and Mayer (2008) supports the use of the personalization principle. In five out of five experimental studies that compared transfer of learning, those who received the personalized onscreen text performed better than those who received the formal type of onscreen text. For example, the following impersonal sentences, "During systole, the ventricles contract. The right ventricle pumps blood to the lungs and the left ventricle pumps blood to the rest of the body" can be personalized by substituting the word "your" for "the" as follows: "During systole *your* ventricles contract. *Your* right ventricle pumps blood to *your* lungs and *your* left ventricle pumps blood to the rest of *your* body" (Clark & Mayer, 2008, p. 165). The effectiveness of personalization was studied in a series of three experiments by Mayer, Fennell, Farmer, & Campbell (2004). According to Clark and Mayer, the researchers created a personalized script for teaching students about lung function by changing the word "the" to "your" in eleven places. They found improvement in transfer of learning that produced an effect size of .79.

Another component of the personalization principle involves the use of on-screen agents, also called coaches or characters, who guide the learning process during an e-class. The agent may be a cartoon-like character; a virtual reality avatar fashioned after a real person, or simply a voice or printed text that provides guidance. According to Clark and Mayer (2008), preliminary research on the effects of using agents in two separate studies found that the agent group generated 24–48% more solutions in testing than the no-agent group.

Another benefit of applying the personalization principle is that it helps provide the teacher with a sense of presence in the online classroom. Clark and Mayer (2008) point out that instructional text that uses a formal, impersonal, third-person style tends to make the author seem invisible. Conversely, a conversational style and the use of first-person narrative makes each student feel as though the teacher is communicating directly with them. Other ways to improve the personalization aspects in e-learning involve implementing strategies to make the teacher real and provide a visible presence in the online classroom. Some examples may include providing a photo and instructor biography, asking the learner questions during onscreen presentations, and sharing personal experiences related to the lesson. Clark and Mayer reported on several studies that support the value of making the author visible. In a study of high school students, Paxton (2002) found that using techniques that made the author visible promoted deeper engagement in the learners, and they were able to write longer essays that showed greater sensitivity than those whose class materials did not make the author visible. Similarly, Inglese, Mayer, & Rigotti (2007) found that college students wrote more and provided richer answers when they received course materials in which the authors were made visible.

In online as well as face-to-face courses, researchers agree that learners who interact with faculty and each other receive multiple benefits. "However, interaction is not a guarantee that students are cognitively engaged in an educationally meaningful manner" (Garrison & Cleveland-Innes, 2005, p. 135). Furthermore, interaction alone is not sufficient for deep learning to occur. Deep, higher-order learning requires the integration of social, cognitive, and teaching presence (p. 134). A study comparing four course designs with varying degrees of overall interaction (social presence), reflective assignments (cognitive presence), and instructor involvement (teaching presence), found that the quality of interaction and teaching presence were essential for deep learning to occur (p. 141).

Principles for Designing e-Learning Activities

Incorporating practice exercises in e-learning supports social presence and the psychological and cognitive processes involved in learning. Practice activities can engage the learner, draw attention to key information covered, integrate the new knowledge with previous knowledge, and help to implant the new knowledge into long-term memory (Clark & Mayer, 2008). When designing practice activities for e-learning, Clark and Mayer recommend utilizing five practice principles. First, mirror the job. This means identifying the ways the learner is expected to use the information and providing practice activities that mirror those applications. For example, in clinical nursing courses, it is expected that course content be developed that emphasizes planning, providing care, and problem solving. Therefore, presenting activities that allow the learner to make decisions about nursing care and problem solve, such as case studies and simulations would "mirror the job."

The second practice principle is to provide explanatory feedback. This gives the learner more than just the knowledge of whether they choose the right or wrong answer (i.e., corrective feedback). Explanatory feedback provides a rationale that will help the student correct misconceptions and build the right mental model (Clark & Mayer, 2008, p. 239). A third related practice principle is to "adapt the amount and placement of practice to job performance requirements" (p. 242). Researchers have established that practice completed early in the learning sessions is more likely to lead to improved performance. To decide how much practice is required to reap the desired outcomes most efficiently, the ANE needs to determine the nature of the task and determine how critical it is that the student performs proficiently. According to Clark and Mayer (2008), there is consistent evidence that "the greatest amount of learning accrues on the initial practice event" . . . and that "Large amounts of practice will build automaticity [in skill performance], but offer diminishing performance improvements" (p. 248). In addition, practice that was distributed throughout a learning event rather than concentrated in one time or place was found most effective (p. 248).

The fourth practice principle involves applying the instructional design principles for multimedia presentations. This involves incorporating several principles discussed earlier—specifically, the principles of modality, redundancy, contiguity, and coherence (see Table 2-13). Using these principles will help ensure that the online environment is conducive to learning.

R2D2 Model

R2D2 is an acronym that stands for Read/listen, Reflect/write, Display, and Do (Bonk & Zhang, 2006). Using the R2D2 model enables online educators to create an optimal online environment in terms of in the types of tasks, activities, and instructional materials integrated into online modules.

The R2D2 model recognizes the importance of addressing visual, auditory, and kinesthetic learning styles and the active processes of knowledge creation inherent in reflection, writing, displaying, and doing. The first part of the model denotes reading and listening activities that focuses on acquisition of knowledge (p. 255). Learners may experience lectures, read textbooks, watch streaming videos, and listen to podcasts as part of this phase. During the second part of the model learners engage in reflective or observational activities such as asynchronous discussion, course related blogs, reflection papers, or summary writings. Instructors may also integrate reflective and observational activities within the sessions by using self-tests, reflective questioning, or observation and reflection on videos or clinical experiences. The third part of the model is concerned with displaying information and is especially useful for visual learners. Bonk and Zhang note that the instructor can create (or can have the student create) visual representations of the content. Creating concept maps and writing summaries are appropriate strategies for the display part of the model and they have an additional benefit of requiring the student to reflect on what they have learned. When conducting synchronous discussions, the instructor may use interactive whiteboards to summarize and emphasize important concepts. The final aspect of the R2D2 model involves doing or applying what has been learned. The doing phase of the model is compatible with the needs and preferences of kinesthetic learners who benefit from engaging in authentic, real-world activities. Having learners collect and analyze data, conduct interviews, perform procedures or skills are strategies that emphasize the doing phase of the model.

Bonk and Zhang (2006) suggest using the R2D2 model (Read, Reflect, Display, Do) as an organizational guide to create a learning environment that addresses the needs of students with diverse learning styles. Each part of the model may be used separately, at different times throughout a course, or all four aspects may be used as part of a problem solving process. Using the model to guide the organization and structure of online modules will help address the needs of online learners of all major learning styles and will provide a wide range of learning activities. More information on creative teaching strategies for the R2D2 model can be found in the text entitled, *Empowering Online Learning: 100+ Ideas for Online Reading, Reflecting, Displaying, and Doing* by Bonk and Zhang (2008).

Using Distance Learning Technologies

The 2008 Horizon Report describes the results of a collaborative research project published by The New Media Consortium and Educause Learning Initiative (2008). The report identifies emerging technologies and the impact of these on education. Each year since 2004, a handful of technologies are selected based on their potential influence on education. The 2008 Horizon Report profiled six promising technologies including grassroots video, collaboration webs, mobile broadband, data mashups, collective intelligence, and social operating systems. This section reports on the educational uses of those technologies, as well as, webcasting, podcasting, reusable learning objects, and new applications of the Internet.

Grassroots Video

Educators are familiar with the concept of videos and DVDs. However, recent technological advances have improved the ease of recording, editing, and disseminating videos. Tools for recording and editing video clips are inexpensive or free, thus removing the high costs of production, which were barriers in the past. The ease with which nontechnically-trained individuals can create, edit, and disseminate videos makes the use of grass roots videos a growing phenomenon in education. Students are able to use the video capture function on mobile phones and digital cameras to create video clips, which can be integrated into class assignments. This opens up a new arena for constructing digital-based assignments and projects. Faculty can incorporate video-based assignments and the development of video logs to document service and field work activities. Students can also create digital portfolios to document their learning.

Not only can faculty create digital-based assignments for students, they can use existing video clips to supplement course content. Because of the ease of creating, editing, and posting videos, educators and subject matter experts can easily create and post brief video clips and tutorials in repositories such as YouTube and i Tunes U. The details of encoding and searching for videos are handled by the hosting site, thus reducing the demand for high tech knowledge or skills. According to the Horizon Report (The New Media Consortium and Educause Learning Initiative, 2008), custom branding, which allows educational institutions to make their presence known on such sites, is projected to further increase the production and distribution of grassroots videos by educational institutions. The Video Toolbox site listed in the resources section provides an annotated list of over 150 tools to assist educators in all phases of the video creation, production, and distribution process.

Collaboration Webs

Web-based applications allowing virtual, real-time meetings for conferencing and project work have been available for a while, however the costs of implementing have been prohibitive for many (The New Media Consortium and Educause Learning Initiative, 2008). Developments in the area of collaboration tools have resulted in programs that allow individuals to work collaboratively on projects, presentations, papers, and written assignments. Another area of development is in the creation of virtual workspaces in which people can gather information, share resources, and discuss the project. These virtual workspaces can be used for students enrolled in a single college course, or for students to engage with experts outside the institution, or even for students from different campuses to "meet," share information, and collaborate on projects. The combination of these developments in collaborative programs and workspaces have fostered the creation of collaborative webs that can enable interactive learning to occur in the virtual environment.

Mobile Broadband

For several years, collaborators for the Horizon Report have been tracking the development and uses of mobile devices in education (The New Media Consortium and

Educause Learning Initiative, 2008). Over the years, cellular phones have progressed from being merely portable phones to devices that can capture images, transmit multimedia, and store information, to networking devices enabling expanded communication and connection options via Internet and e-mail. The uses of these devices in education are numerous. Authors of the Horizon Report site several examples of educational uses of mobile broadband in a variety of disciplines. For example, in engineering, "broadband cell phones can be used to remotely monitor structures, equipment, and processes used in real time" (p. 18). In service learning projects, students can use mobile broadband to collaborate with community agency personnel. For fieldwork in the socials sciences, students can take notes, photos, and videos of their project, upload them to a course blog, and receive feedback from the instructor . . . all without access to a traditional computer. Mobile broadband phones can also download educational media used in a course such as audio files or podcasts, and PDF files.

Mashups

A mashup has been defined as "a combination of data from multiple sources into a single tool" (The New Media Consortium and Educause Learning Initiative, 2008, p. 20). Others have defined it as, "a combination of separate, stand-alone technologies into a novel application" (Educause Learning Initiative, 2006, p. 1), or a Web-based application that integrates two or more sources of information into a single learning activity (Lamb, 2007, p. 14). One example of a mashup available from the Harvard-MIT Division of Health Sciences and Technology is a healthmap designed to depict global infectious disease outbreaks. The healthmap "brings together disparate data sources to achieve a unified and comprehensive view of the current global state of infectious diseases and their effect on human and animal health" (Freifeld & Brownstein, 2007, para 1). The healthmap site combines news data sources with World Health Organization, and Euro Surveillance sources to create color-coded maps indicating severity of outbreaks.

According to Berlind, executive director of ZDNET, a comprehensive technology Web site, mashups represent the "fastest growing ecosystem on the Internet" (Berlind, 2009). The 2008 Horizon Report identifies mashups as one of the top six emerging technologies with significant implications for education. According to the report, mashups will become even more common as new authoring tools are developed that will easily allow nonprogrammers to create new mashups. Many Web-based tools for creating mashups are now available that are free and simple to use. "The power of mashups for education lies in the way they help us reach new conclusions or discern new relationships by uniting large amounts of data in a manageable way" (The New Media Consortium and Educause Learning Initiative, 2008, p. 21). Mapping mashups that combine the geographical context with a specific subject matter can be useful in a variety of subjects including nursing. Although most mashups currently "focus on the integration of maps with a variety of data, it is not difficult to picture broad educational and scholarly applications for mashups" (The New Media Consortium and Educause Learning Initiative, 2008, p. 20). The potential applications for nursing education are endless. Whenever it is useful to depict global or regional trends in disease, trauma, healthcare access, demographics, and more, mapping mashups may help students internalize the significance of the data by "helping them see patterns and movements that explain ideas and their significance" (Educause Learning Initiative, 2006, p. 2). Additional examples of mashups that the ANE may find helpful, along with resources for creating mashups for course content are presented by Skiba (2007) and the 2008 Horizon Report.

Collective Intelligence

The term collective intelligence refers to "the knowledge embedded within societies or large groups of individuals" (The New Media Consortium and Educause Learning Initiative, 2008, p. 23). Collective intelligence stems from the collaboration and competition of many people. This knowledge or information can be explicit as in online encyclopedias (e.g., Wikipedia and Celliphedia) created and update by thousands of individuals, or collective intelligence can be implicit. Implicit knowledge allows the discovery of new knowledge through ongoing analysis of patterns and correlations over time. Implicit intelligence is used whenever a search term is entered onto a Web browser. The search engine determines which pages are most relevant to the query. Google for example, uses a PageRank system that looks at the number of pages linked to a Web site and explores the patterns within those links to determine which sites are likely to be most relevant (The New Media Consortium and Educause Learning Initiative, 2008, p. 23). Another example of implicit intelligence is when you search an online store catalog for a particular item. The system links your search with others who searched for that item and based on the patterns detected provides suggestions for other items you might like to purchase.

The implications for the use of explicit and implicit collective intelligence sources and processes in education are growing. These knowledge sources provide students the opportunity to explore topics, engage in independent study, and use critical thinking to analyze, evaluate, and even construct new knowledge. It is projected that the combination of mashups with new knowledge generated by collective intelligence will become more common, providing greater understanding of our world (The New Media Consortium and Educause Learning Initiative, 2008, p. 4).

Social Operating Systems

The final technology featured in the 2008 Horizon Report is the development of social operating systems. Defined as the next generation of social networking, social operating systems represent a conceptual shift from sharing files and applications to a focus on relationships and connections. Social network sites such as classmate.com, MySpace, and Facebook focus on sharing interests and/or activities and exploring the interests and activities of others. The social operating systems "will change the way we search for, work with, and understand information by placing people at the center of the network" (p. 26).

Several potential applications to the field of education are provided to help clarify what social operating systems are and how they may be useful in the future. In a graduate online course, a student could click next to the name of their classmate to discover information about other areas the student has studied. This can help students feel connected by being able to share common interests and could deepen online discussions by enabling the teacher and students to easily draw on the experiences of the group. When groups of students work collaboratively on a paper or presentation, social operating systems could also be beneficial. For example, by touching the cursor to the document, a display of who has worked on the document previously would appear. Based upon the social and interest profiles of the users, suggestions on who to contact for further information would be made. Another example cited by the Horizon Report is the Xobni application, which extends the functions of Microsoft Outlook. The application tracks and analyzes e-mail interactions. By selecting an e-mail message, the application automatically summarizes key points about your e-mail history including listing attachments that have been sent and received. This type of social operating system can be extremely useful when communicating with students enrolled in online courses. In essence, social operating systems applied to the online classroom will create a place other than home, work, or the face-to-face classroom in which individuals with similar interests can meet. This information will come to the individual rather than the individual searching for it online.

Webcasting

Webcasting is technology that enables the learner to play a streaming audio or a combination of streaming audiovisual, which is broadcast on the Internet and viewed from a personal computer (Baecker, Moore, & Zijdemans, 2003, p. 896). Streaming refers to the transmission process, which in this case involves playing the media through your computer Web browser, rather than downloading the file and playing it from your desktop. Webcasting enables the delivery of real-time audio-video presentations using the Internet. Thus, webcasting can provide synchronous learning in which a local audience and speaker come together via streaming video, face-to face. The speaker and the local audience can interact as they would in a traditional classroom and can be joined simultaneously by a remote audience who view the webcast from their personal computer. Webcasts also can be archived on the Internet for later viewing, which provides an asynchronous format enabling the learners to access, pause, and repeat the presentation at their own pace.

Enhancing the instructor's presence through interactivity is essential for both synchronous and asynchronous webcast formats. Using a component of a webcasting system called e-presence, Baecker and colleagues (2003) outline the types of interactivity that can enhance the experience of presence in webcasts. Interactivity between the lecturer and the remote audience includes polling the audience and receiving responses electronically, and responding to text-based queries from the audience. The use of chat areas can provide a mechanism whereby remote viewers can dialog with one another without distracting the speaker or other classmates. Interactivity between the speaker and the local audience includes traditional verbal and nonverbal communication plus responding to polling questions posed by the speaker. The use of wireless mobile devices will enable local audience members to participate in chat room sessions and engage in private messaging to others in the class and at a distance. There are also mechanisms for interactivity among the asynchronous audience members who view the archived presentation using post-presentation chat and discussion boards. Baecker and colleagues (2003) note that webcasting is transforming the way lectures are experienced. The use of features available in webcast systems such as ePresence, may assist in creating a stronger knowledge base and enhance learning (p. 896).

To facilitate implementation of webcasting, the faculty at West Virginia University School of Nursing have provided a thorough account of their experience transitioning from using interactive TV (ITV) and WebCT formats (DiMaria-Ghalili, Ostrow, & Rodney, 2005). They piloted four graduate nursing classes as webcasts and gathered feedback from the students after each class. They described the feedback from the students ($n = 27$) as largely positive, with many citing that they enjoyed the interactivity of polling students and the convenience of not having to travel great distances to attend class. The faculty noted that webcasting provided a learning environment very similar to face-to-face classes in that faculty and students could interact in real time, ask and answer questions, and engage in group work using the bulletin board functions of WebCT.

Podcasting

For students enrolled in distance education, the geographic distance factor may be a major factor contributing to a sense of isolation (Lee & Chan, 2007). The geographical distance between students and faculty often precludes social interactions that oc-cur on campus. The lack of a set meeting time as occurs in asynchronous online courses may add to the perception of isolation and lack of interaction and connected-ness. Podcasting is an inexpensive tool used to broadcast audio files that can bridge the sense of isolation. Podcasting allows audio content from really simple syndication (RSS) feeds to be automatically downloaded to a learner's home computer, iPod, or MP3 player. Because podcasts are based on RSS, once the content is downloaded, the user can filter and search the content, listening only to the messages of interest.

Although the use of audio recordings may have limited appeal to visual and kines-thetic learners, Lee and Chan (2007) point out that using podcasts may have some ad-vantages. Podcasts that convey noncomplex information in brief segments (under 5 minutes) are more beneficial than longer podcasts, which cover more dense or com-plex subject matter. Because there is no need for the learner to fixate visually on a screen to obtain the information, listening to podcasts frees the learner's eyes and hands and allows the learner to be fully mobile. This can be advantageous for kines-thetic learners, as well as generation Y learners, who are accustomed to multitasking.

WebQuests

The Internet is useful tool for conducting inquiry activities referred to as WebQuests. The concept of a WebQuest, originally developed by Bernie Dodge in 1995, involves the exploration of a topic that is divided into clearly defined steps or processes (Sky-lar, Higgins, & Boone, 2007, p. 20). According to Dodge (2001) a well-designed WebQuest will focus on critical thinking strategies of analysis, comparing and con-trasting, synthesis, and evaluation of the information. WebQuests are structured us-ing six components, an introduction, description of the task, an outline of the processes involved, a list of Web site resources, an evaluation, and a conclusion.

The goal of a WebQuest assignment emphasizes the effective use of the informa-tion rather than the process of searching for the information. Conducting a WebQuest calls for a structured environment with specific steps identified for per-forming a WebQuest, a list of appropriate Web sites for the learner to explore, and instructions for how the Internet research should be compiled. Dodge (2001) defines the types of WebQuests as short-term, which focuses on knowledge acquisition and integration; and long-term, which involves the higher-order processes of analyzing and transforming data into a new form.

WebQuests are learner-centered activities that can be designed to accomplish a variety of learning tasks. Dodge (2002) developed a taxonomy of WebQuest tasks to describe the goal, purpose, and focus of specific types of WebQuest assignments (Box 2-6). At the most basic level is "retelling," which involves conveying information

---

BOX 2-6   A Taxonomy of WebQuest Tasks

1. Retelling—No transformation of information involved. Used to develop background knowledge of a topic

2. Compilation—gathering information, some transformation of data occurs

3. Mystery—requires synthesis of information from a variety of sources

4. Journalistic—incorporates different perspectives

5. Design tasks—"creating a product or plan of action that accomplishes a pre-determined goal and works within specified constraints" (para. 22)

6. Creative product—similar to design tasks but more open-ended and unpredictable

7. Consensus building—involves considering and expressing differing views

8. Persuasion—development of a convincing case

9. Self-Knowledge—personal exploration to improve self-understanding

10. Analytical—determining relationships between components

11. Judgment—rating, ranking items and providing rationale for decision

12. Scientific—using the scientific method to explore a topic

Data from Dodge, B. (2002). WebQuest taskonomy: A taxonomy of tasks. Retrieved from http://webquest.sdsu.edu/taskonomy.html.

---

without transforming the information in any way. The remaining terms involve some degree of data transformation and therefore require higher-order cognitive tasks. According to Dodge, all students, even those with learning disabilities, can participate in WebQuests. However, students with learning disabilities would benefit from the inclusion of study guides, advance organizers, and graphic organizers (p. 23).

Reusable Learning Objects

Another strategy for the online learning environment involves the creation and use of "reusable learning objects" (RLO), defined as "digital, reproducible resources for performing or supporting learning activities" (Jesse, Taleff, Payne, Cox, & Steele, 2006, p. 1). Koper offers a further distinction, defining learning objects as "any digital, reproducible, and addressable resource used to perform learning activities or learning support activities, made available for others to use" (2003, p. 4). To conceptualize the idea more clearly, individual RLOs have been compared to LEGO blocks that can be stacked and connected to create a structure, and then reused to create another structure. Similarly, RLOs in the form of video clips, audio clips, animations, or text could be combined to form a unit of instruction for one class and combined with other RLOs and used in a different unit of instruction.

According to Ruiz, Mintzer, and Issenberg (2006), "to make e-learning more effective, instructional resources must be adaptable to varying contexts, learners, and educators" (p. 599). In our rapidly changing digital-age teaching environment, the use of reusable learning objects may fill this need. Ruiz and colleagues identify the minimal criteria for learning objects as:

1. able to stand alone or be useful to achieve a specific learning outcome without combining it with another object,
2. be reusable by diverse groups of learners,
3. require interaction with the learner,
4. able to be linked with other objects to form new learning objects, lessons, or modules,
5. be highly interoperable with other software and platforms, and
6. be accessible by tagging with metadata, which allows them to be located easily (p. 600).

Using learning objects that have the attributes identified by Ruiz *et al.* (2006) provides several benefits. For the ANE these benefits include reduced time and effort devoted to developing or searching for learning resources, the reusability of material in different courses, and the ability to track the students' use of materials. For the learner, reusable learning objects help to meet a variety of learning style preferences, and can increase the student's comfort with online learning by providing a consistent appearance and feel to the resources. Instructors who are interested in developing or using RLOs can find further information in the resource section.

Technologies such as the ones reviewed in this section can be used to enhance the distance learning environment by adding interactivity, encouraging knowledge construction, adding a sense of instructor presence in the virtual world, and enhancing the students' sense of connection. These and other technologies assist the instructor in providing distance learning sessions in a manner that reflects many of the 20 distance learning competencies identified by Darabi *et al.* (2006).

CONCLUSION

Facilitating learning involves demonstrating skills in multiple areas that impact learning such as assessing learners, using principles to guide content development, applying teaching strategies for transformative learning, and fostering critical think-ing. The ANE applies these skills in a range of settings including the face-to face classrooms, online formats, the skills laboratory, and in diverse clinical learning set-tings. The ANE also uses knowledge of the self as teacher, plus knowledge and skills related to the learner, the content, teaching strategies, and the learning environment to create optimal learning experiences for students.

SUMMARY

- To facilitate learning, the ANE applies knowledge and skills related to the teaching–learning process to create an optimal learning environment, design the content, and implement selected teaching strategies.
- Figure 2-1 depicts factors that facilitate learning including: (1) research and theory; (2) the learning environment, learning content and teaching strategies; and (3) student/teacher attributes and preferences.
- Educational theories reflect unique perspectives based on differing assumptions, values, and beliefs about teaching, learning, and the learning process.
- Behaviorism is a theoretical perspective that views learning as a change in behavior that is influenced by the environment.
- Cognitivism is a theoretical perspective that emphasizes the internal thinking processes involved in learning.
- Information processing theory focuses on how the individual stores and remembers information.
- Social Learning Theory is a synthesis of behaviorism and cognitivism that values the influence of the environment on learning and sees learning as a social process in which the individual can learn vicariously or deliberately by observing others.
- Gestaltism is a theoretical perspective that emphasizes the person's ability to see the whole, rather than focus on the parts.
- Constructivism represents a theoretical perspective that views learning as constructed by the learner by building on previous learning.
- Adult Learning Theory, or andragogy, describes a set of assumptions and principles that can be used to tailor learning to the unique motivations and experiences of adult learners.
- The humanist perspective emphasizes motivation to learn a particular topic as central to the learning process and values the learner's sense of self-esteem.
- Parse's Human Becoming Teaching–Learning Process views learning as "a cocreated journey."

- Connectivism describes an emerging theory that emphasizes how learners acquire knowledge in the digital age.
- Principles of learning represent the core values, beliefs, and practices that underlie many of the major educational theories (see Table 2-1).
- Each principle of learning describes aspects that can be utilized to shape positive learning experiences and facilitate learning.
- Seven principles of good practice in undergraduate education include: (1) encourage student-faculty contact, (2) encourage cooperation among students, (3) encourage active learning, (4) give prompt feedback, (5) emphasize time on task, (6) communicate high expectations, and (7) respect diverse talents and ways of learning.
- Assessment of learners involves determination of learning styles and preferences; learning strengths and weaknesses; knowledge and experience; the influence of social, cultural, and cohort attributes; and environmental characteristics.
- Learning style refers to inner characteristics and preferences that influence the way learners think and learn. Learning style preferences may change over time.
- Each person has one or more preferred ways of receiving and processing information.
- Myers-Briggs personality types include 16 combinations of four dichotomous personality attributes including: (1) introvert–extravert, (2) sensing–intuitive, (3) thinking–feeling, and (4) perceiving–judging.
- Keirsey synthesized the Myers-Briggs personality types into four temperaments types referred to as the artisan, guardian, idealist, and rationalist.
- The VAK Learning Styles Model proposes that visual learners learn best by seeing and reading, auditory learners by hearing, and kinesthetic learners by touching and doing.
- Multiple intelligences are preferred ways of receiving and processing information described as linguistic, spatial, kinesthetic, musical, logical/mathematical, personal, and naturalistic.
- Individuals have capabilities in all modes of multiple intelligence; however, one mode will usually be dominant, and three to four others will be strong.
- Kolb's Model of Experiential Learning describes four processes of engagement and interaction with the learning: (1) concrete experience, (2) reflective observation, (3) abstract conceptualization, and (4) active experimentation.
- Four Learning Styles derived from Kolb's Model of Experiential Learning include convergent, divergent, assimilator, and accommodator.

- Convergent learners rely on abstract conceptualization and active experimentation.
- Divergent learners do well with brainstorming and interactive learning activities.
- Assimilators use abstract conceptualization and reflective observation.
- Accommodators rely on concrete experience and active experimentation as dominant learning modes.
- Emotional intelligence (EI) involves the ability to perceive, use, understand, and manage one's emotions. EI and IQ work in conjunction to enable the individual to function effectively in society.
- Generational theories are based on the premise that persons born and raised during certain time periods share common history, values, and culture. These shared experiences affect the person's learning style.
- The Dunn & Dunn Learning Style model integrates ideas from VAK and brain dominance theories, and recognizes environmental, social, and psychological preferences in learning.
- The Dunn and Dunn Learning Style Inventory can be used to determine learning style preferences and the strength of those preferences.
- The Felder-Silverman Learning Style Model is an integrative model that synthesizes concepts from VAK, brain dominance, and Myers-Briggs theories.
- Felder-Silverman Learning Style Model describes learners as having preferences in four dichotomous areas: (1) active/reflective, (2) sensing/intuitive, (3) visual/verbal, and (4) sequential/global.
- Critical thinkers explain their thinking and reasoning in a clear, coherent manner and use their critical thinking skills for their own self-regulation.
- Self-regulation of learning involves the student's ability to monitor their thinking and use the subskills of self-examination and self-correction of one's reasoning.
- Teaching styles, like learning styles, stem from one's perspective, personal strengths, and preferences.
- Grasha's Teaching Styles include the expert, formal authority, personal model, facilitator, and delegator. Each teaching style is characterized by specific teacher attributes and associated with specific teaching methods.
- Mosston's Spectrum of Teaching Styles depicts a continuum of student/teacher involvement in the teaching and learning of psychomotor skill-based content.
- Self-reflection emphasizes that learning is a personal, internal process of meaning making that can be used to validate and clarify what has been learned.

- Role modeling involves a continuum of learning from observation to participation.
- Processes involved in learning through role modeling include attention, retention, motor reproduction of the behavior, and determining the degree of motivation needed to replicate the behavior.
- Content domains reflect cognitive, affective, and psychomotor learning. Each domain has one or more taxonomies that can be used to develop learning objectives.
- Designing e-learning presentations can be guided by using the modality, redundancy, contiguity, segmenting, pretraining, multimedia, and coherence principles (see Table 2-13).
- Transformative learning becomes more essential as the student is faced with the need to think differently and apply what has been learned to real life situations.
- Predisposing conditions for transformative learning include (1) an activating event that exposes the student to their limitations, (2) identification of current assumptions, (3) the process of critical self-reflection, and (4) critical discourse.
- Problem-based learning (PBL) is a teaching method that enhances higher-level thinking.
- Socratic questioning is a process of questioning and guiding students to higher level thinking and discovery.
- The IDEALS framework takes the student through the critical thinking processes of analysis, interpretation, self-regulation, inference, explanation, and evaluation.
- Concept mapping is a learning activity that involves creating a visual to organize, analyze, and show the relationships between concepts.
- Reflective journaling provides an avenue for integrative learning experiences.
- Stages of reflective learning include awareness, critical analysis, and a new perspective.
- Levels of reflective thinking include: (1) nonreflectors, (2) reflectors, and (3) critical reflectors.
- Integrative learning includes connecting skills and knowledge from multiple sources and experiences.
- Six principles of significant learning that have implications for the face-to-face learning environment include: (1) providing foundational knowledge; (2) application of information; (3) integration or connecting what has been learned to previous knowledge and to future learning; (4) recognizing that effective

learning is social; (5) caring about learner motivation and the learning environment; and (6) learning how to learn.

- Student response systems, or clickers, are a technology designed to increase student participation and provide student and instructor feedback.
- Clinical simulation has evolved to encompass full-scale simulations involving the creation of realistic scenarios using standardized patients, high-fidelity human patient simulators, or virtual clinical scenarios.
- Learning in the clinical environment is influenced by the clinical instructor and the attitudes, behaviors, and relationships established with clinical staff.
- Competencies for distance learning instructors emphasize the instructor's communication, interaction, and use technology, to create effective learning environments.
- The quantity and quality of interactions between student and teacher and evidence of "teaching presence" are important in online learning environments.
- R2D2 (Read, Reflect, Display, Do) is as an organizational guide for creating an online learning environment that addresses diverse learning styles.
- Emerging educational technologies identified by the Horizon Report include: (1) grassroots videos, (2) collaborative webs, (3) mobile broadband, (4) mashups, (5) collective intelligence, and (6) social operating systems.
- Webcasting is a technology that enables the learner to play a streaming video from the internet on a personal computer.
- Podcasting allows audio files from RSS feeds to be downloaded to the learner's home computer, iPod, or MP3 player.
- WebQuests are instructor-designed, learner-centered activities in which the learner uses Web sites to explore a topic.
- Reusable learning objects are digital, addressable, and reusable learning materials that can be used alone or combined with other learning objects to form new learning objects.

RECOMMENDED RESOURCES

General Teaching–Learning Resources

- McMaster University, home of the problem-based learning (PBL) initiative, sponsors the Center for Leadership in Learning Web site at http://cll.mcmaster.ca. The site features extensive resources and information about PBL.

- The 16-minute video "Restoring Meaning to Teaching" is available for free viewing at the SEDL Web site at http://www.sedl.org/pubs/catalog/items/teaching08.html.
- The Foundation for Critical Thinking Web site at http://www.criticalthinking.org/ houses a wealth of information and resources on critical thinking. The "Where to Begin" menu provides in-depth coverage for specific academic areas, including nursing and higher education. Under the "Online Learning" menu the Foundation features online lessons and has a YouTube channel with excerpts from their video collections.
- The Carnegie Foundation for the Advancement of Teaching web site at http://www.carnegiefoundation.org/ features an e-library of downloadable articles and reports dating back to the Flexner Report published in 1910.
- Information on integrative learning is available in at the Carnegie Foundation Web site at http://www.carnegiefoundation.org/files/elibrary/integrativelearning/index.htm.
- Access to "Change: A Magazine of Higher Learning" is available at http://www.changemag.org/. The magazine features downloadable articles on a wide array of educational topics.
- The Center for Teaching and Learning at Stanford University publishes an excellent online newsletter on teaching available at http://ctl.stanford.edu/Newsletter/.
- The publication, "Seven Principles of Good Practice in Education" may be downloaded from the Washington Center for Improving the Quality of Undergraduate Education http://learningcommons.evergreen.edu/pdf/fall1987.pdf.

Learning Style Resources

- The Center for Applications of Psychological Types at http://www.capt.org provides a searchable bibliography containing over 11,000 references on research, test interpretation, and applications of the Myers-Briggs Type Inventory.
- The Myers & Briggs Foundation at http://www.myersbriggs.org/ provides background information on the Myers-Briggs Type Inventory tool, as well as information on testing, interpretation of the tool, and general resources.
- Information about the Keirsey Temperament Sorter (KTS-II) and the four temperament types is available at http://www.keirsey.com/. The site contains a link for taking the KTS-II and obtaining a free mini-report of your results.

- A Learning Style Inventory for visual, auditory, and kinesthetic learners is available at http://www.puc.edu/__data/assets/pdf_file/0003/13395/Learning-Styles-Inventory.pdf. The site also contains suggestions for learning and studying for each specific style and ways to expand and develop one's learning style.
- A free downloadable e-book titled *Educating the Net Generation* is available from the Educause Web site at http://www.educause.edu/educatingthenetgen.

Technology Resources

- Massachusetts Institute of Technology (MIT) sponsors the MIT World Web site at http://mitworld.mit.edu/. The site provides free videos of significant public events held at MIT such as conference speakers and expert panels, which may be of interest to persons outside the MIT campus. Browse the MIT World's video index of more than 500 videos.
- The Harvey Project funded by the National Science Foundation has produced reusable learning objects depicting concepts related to human physiology. These may be used freely by educators. Available at http://opencourse.org/Collaboratories/harveyproject.
- HEAL is the Health Education Assets Library, a national repository for digital education resources. Educational materials are peer reviewed and free access is available at http://www.healcentral.org/.
- The Knowledge Exchange Exhibition and Presentation (KEEP) Toolkit is a set of free Web-based tools that help teachers and students from all levels of institutions develop well-designed knowledge materials for the web. The KEEP Toolkit is available from the Carnegie Foundation Web site at http://www.cfkeep.org/static/index.html.
- The annual Horizon Report describes emerging technologies likely to have a large impact on teaching learning. An extensive annotated list of examples, Web sites, and links to resources for further learning is provided. To find out more about these technologies and download the 2008 Horizon Report and reports from previous years, go to http://www.nmc.org/pdf/2008-Horizon-Report.pdf.
- The e-book "Theory and Practice in Online Learning" published in 2008 by Anderson and Elloumi, is available for free download at http://www.aupress.ca/books/Terry_Anderson.php.
- A brief video about mashups featuring David Berlind, editor of ZDNET is available at http://news.zdnet.com/2422-13569_22-152729.html.

- An excellent article entitled "7 Things you want to know about mapping mashups" is available from the Educause Learning Inititave at http://net. educause.edu/ir/library/pdf/ELI7016.pdf.
- The Web site "Connectivism Networked and Social Learning" contains many papers and presentations about connectivism available at http://www. connectivism.ca/ under the wiki menu.
- e-learn space everything e-learning, is just what the name implies—resources and information galore. The site was developed by connectivism theorist, George Siemens and can be accessed at http://www.elearnspace.org/.
- Learn more about WebQuests at http://webquest.org/. The site contains tutorials with step-by-step instructions on how to develop a WebQuest, a searchable database of WebQuests, informative reports, and resources.
- For information on reusable learning objects, how to locate, use, and/or develop them, see the article by Ruiz, Mintzer, & Issenberg (2006) entitled, "Learning Objects in Medical Education," listed in the reference section or see the *Journal of Interactive Media in Education* (April 2003), for a special issue on Reusing Online Resources: A Sustainable Approach to e-Learning available online at http://www-jime.open.ac.uk/2003/1/.

REFERENCES

1. Akerjordet, K., & Severinsson, E. (2007). Emotional intelligence: A review of the literature with specific focus on empirical and epistemological perspectives. *Journal of Clinical Nursing*, *16*, 1410–1416.
2. Alinier, G., Hunt, W., & Gordon, R. (2004). Determining the value of simulation in nursing education: Study design and initial results. *Nurse Education in Practice, 4*, 200–207.
3. All, A. C., & Havens, R. L. (1997). Cognitive/concept mapping: A teaching strategy for nursing. *Journal of Advanced Nursing, 25*, 1210–1219.
4. All, A. C., Huycke, L. I., & Fisher, M. J. (2003). Instructional tools for nursing education: Concept maps. *Nursing Education Perspectives, 34*, 311–317.
5. Anderson, L., Krathwohl, D., Airasian, P., Cruikshank, K., Mayer, R., Pintrich, P., *et al.* (2001). *A taxonomy for learning teaching and assessing: A revision of Bloom's taxonomy of objectives.* New York: Addison Wesley Longman.
6. Angelo, T., & Cross, P. (1993). *Classroom assessment techniques: A handbook for college teachers* (2nd ed.). San Francisco: Jossey Bass.
7. Arhin, A., & Cormier, E. (2007). Using deconstruction to educate generation y nursing students. *Journal of Nursing Education, 46*(12), 562–567.
8. Arhin, A., & Johnson-Mallard, V. (2003). Encouraging alternative forms of self-expression in the generation y student: A strategy for effective leaning in the classroom. *The ABNF Journal, 14*(6), 121–122.

9. Armstrong, N. (2008). Role modeling in the clinical workplace. *British Journal of Midwifery, 16*(9), 596–603.

10. Armstrong, T. (1994). Multiple intelligences: Seven ways to approach curriculum. *Educational Leadership, 52*(3), 26–28.

11. Ausubel, D. P. (1968). *Educational psychology: A cognitive view.* New York: Holt.

12. Babcock, D., & Miller, M. (1994). *Client education: Theory and practice.* St. Louis: Mosby.

13. Baecker, R., Moore, G., & Zijdemans, A. (2003). *Proceeding of HCL international 2003, vol 1,* Mahwah, NJ: Lawrence Erlbaum Associates.

14. Bandura, A. (1977). *Social learning theory.* New York: General Learning Press.

15. Bandura, A. (2001). Social cognitive theory: An agentic perspective. *Annual Review of Psychology, 52,* 1–26.

16. Bauer, N., & Huynh, M. (2001). Teaching blood-pressure measurement: CD-ROM versus conventional classroom instruction. *Journal of Nursing Education, 40*(3), 138–141.

17. Becker, K., Rose, L., Berg, J., Park, H., & Shatzer, J. (2006). The teaching effectiveness of standardized patients. *Journal of Nursing Education, 45*(4), 103–111.

18. Benziger, K. (2000). The basics. Everything you need to know before considering KBA. Retrieved November 15, 2008 from http://www.benziger.org/articles/pdf/the_basics.pdf.

19. Berlind, D. (2009). *What is a mashup?* Video. Retrieved on April 10, 2009 from http://news.zdnet.com/2422-13569_22-152729.html.

20. Billings, D. (2004). Teaching learners from varied generations. *The Journal of Continuing Education in Nursing, 35*(3), 104–105.

21. Billings, D., Skiba, D., & Connors, H. (2005). Best practices in web-based courses: Generational differences across undergraduate and graduate nursing students. *Journal of Professional Nursing, 21*(2), 126–133.

22. Blake, T. K. (2005). Journaling: An active learning technique. *International Journal of Nursing Scholarship, 2*(1), 1–13.

23. Bloom, B. (Ed.). (1956). *The classification of educational goals, handbook I: Cognitive domain.* New York: David McKay.

24. Bonk, C. (2007). *USA today leads to tomorrow: Teachers as online concierges and can Facebook pioneer save face?* Retrieved on February 20, 2009, from http://travelinedman.blogspot.com/.

25. Bonk, C., & Zhang, K. (2006). Introducing the R2D2 model: Online learning for the diverse learners of this world. *Distance Education, 27*(2), 249–264.

26. Bonk, C., & Zhang, K. (2008). *Empowering online learning: 100+ activities for reading, reflecting, displaying, and doing.* San Francisco: Jossey-Bass.

27. Bremner, M., Aduddell, K., & Amason, J. (2008). Evidence-based practices related to the human patient simulator and first year baccalaureate nursing students' anxiety. *Online Journal of Nursing Informatics, 12*(1), 10 p.

28. Brown, J. S. (2005, January 18). Learning in the digital age (21st century): Catalyzing creativity by artful making & by honoring the vernacular of today's students. Retrieved April 4th, 2009 from http://pict.sdsu.edu/JSB_digital_learning.pdf.

29. Bruner, J. (1964). The course of cognitive growth. *American Psychologist, 19,* 1–15.

30. Burnstein, R. A., & Lederman, L. M. (2001). Using wireless keypads in lecture classes. *The Physics Teacher, 39,* 6–11.

31. Caudron, S. (1997). Can generation Xers be trained? *Training and Development, 3,* 20–24.

32. Chandler, P., & Sweller, J. (1991). Cognitive load theory and the format of instruction. *Cognition and Instruction, 8*(4), 293–332.

33. Cherniss, C., Extein, M., Goleman, D., & Weissberg, R. (2006). Emotional intelligence: What does the research really indicate? *Educational Psychologist, 41*(4), 239–245.

34. Chickering, A., & Gamson, Z. (1987). Seven principles for good practice in undergraduate education. *The Wingspread Journal, 9*(2), 1–4.

35. Clark, R., & Mayer, R. (2008). *E-learning and the science of instruction: Proven guidelines for consumers and designers of multimedia learning* (2nd ed). San Francisco: Pfeiffer.

36. Clausing, S., Kurtz, D. L., Pendeville, J., & Walt, J. (2003). Generational diversity—The nexters. *AORN Journal, 78*, 373–379.

37. Cook, L. J. (2005). Inviting teaching behaviors of clinical faculty and nursing students' anxiety. *Journal of Nursing Education, 44*(4), 156–161.

38. Corkill, A. J. (1992). Advance organizers: Facilitators of recall. *Educational Psychology Review, 4*, 33–67.

39. Darabi, A., Sikorski, E., & Harvey, R. (2006). Validated competencies for distance teaching. *Distance Education, 27*(1), 105–122.

40. Dave, R. (1970). Psychomotor levels. In R. J. Armstrong (Ed.). *Developing and writing behavioral objectives*. Tucson, AZ: Educational Innovators Press.

41. Dewey, J. (1910/1997). *How we think*. Mineola, NY: Dover.

42. DiMaria-Ghalili, R., Ostrow, L., & Rodney, K. (2005). Webcasting: A new instructional technology in distance graduate nursing education. *Journal of Nursing Education, 44*(1), 11–18.

43. Dixson, M., Kuhlhorst, M., & Reiff, A. (2006). Creating effective online discussions: Optimal instructor and student roles. *Journal of Asynchronous Learning Networks, 10*(4), 15–28.

44. Dodge, B. (2001). Five rules for writing a great webquest. *Learning & Leading with Technology, 28*(8), 6–9 & 58.

45. Dodge, B. (2002). WebQuest taskonomy: A taxonomy of tasks. Retrieved November 10, 2008 from http://webquest.sdsu.edu/taskonomy.html.

46. Dunbar-Wells, R. (2003). Using appropriate language modes and explicit teaching aids. *Australian Voice 2003,9*, 63–68.

47. Dunn, R. (1992). Strategies for teaching word recognition to disabled readers. *Reading, Writing Quarterly: Overcoming Learning Difficulties, 8*, 157–177.

48. Dunn, R., & Dunn, K. (1993). *Teaching secondary students through their individual learning styles: Practical approaches for grades 7–12*. Boston: Allyn & Bacon.

49. Dunn, R., Dunn, K., & Price, G. E. (1989). *Learning style inventory*. Lawrence, KS: Price Systems.

50. Dunn, R., Griggs, S. A., Olson, J., Gorman, B., Beasley, M., & Gorman, B. S. (1995). A meta-analytic validation of the Dunn and Dunn learning styles model. *Journal of Educational Research, 88*(6), 353–361.

51. Dunn, R., & Griggs, S. A. (Eds.). (1998). *Learning styles and the nursing profession*. New York: NLN Press.

52. Educause Learning Initiative. (2006). Seven things you should know about mapping mashups. Retrieved November 28, 2008 from http://net.educause.edu/ir/library/pdf/ELI7016.pdf.

53. Facione, P. (2007). Critical thinking: What it is and why it counts. *Insight Assessment*, 1–23.

54. Faust, D., & Courtenay, B. (2002). Interaction in the intergenerational freshman class: What matters. *Educational Gerontology, 28*, 401.

55. Feingold, C. E., Calaluce, M., & Kallen, M. A. (2004). Computerized patient model and simulated clinical experiences: Evaluation with baccalaureate nursing students. *Journal of Nursing Education, 43*, 156–163.

56. Felder, R., & Silverman, L. (1988). Learning and teaching styles. *Journal of Engineering Education, 78*(7), 674–681.

57. Fink, L. D. (2003). *Creating significant learning experiences: An integrated approach to designing college courses.* San Francisco: Jossey-Bass.

58. Freifeld, C., & Brownstein, J. (2007). Healthmap global disease alert map. Retrieved Feburary 20, 2009 from http://www.healthmap.org/en.

59. Freshwater, D., & Stickley, J. (2004). The heart of the art: Emotional intelligence in nursing education. *Nursing Inquiry, 11*(2), 91–98.

60. Gagné, R. M. (1985). *The conditions of learning and theory of instruction.* (4th ed.). New York: Holt, Rinehart, and Winston.

61. Gagné, R. M., Wager, W. W., Golas, K.C., Keller, J. M. (2005). *Principles of instructional design* (5th ed.). Belmont, CA: Thomas/Wadsworth Publishing.

62. Galbraith, D., & Fouch, S. (2007, September). Principles of adult learning: Application to safety training. *Professional Safety, 52*(9), 35–40.

63. Gardner, H. (1983). *Frames of mind: The theory of multiple intelligences.* New York: Basic Books.

64. Gardner, H. (1999). *Intelligence reframed: Multiple intelligences for the 21st century.* New York: Basic Books.

65. Gardner, H. (2004). *Frames of mind: The theory of multiple intelligences* (10th Anniversary ed.). New York: Basic Books.

66. Gardner, H., & Moran, S. (2006). The science of multiple intelligences theory: A response to Lynn Waterhouse. *Educational Psychologist, 41*(4), 227–232.

67. Garrison, D. R., & Cleveland-Innes, M. (2005). Facilitating cognitive presence in online learning: Interaction is not enough. *American Journal of Distance Education, 19*(3), 133–148.

68. Gestalt Center of Gainesville, Inc. (2009). What is gestalt? An online tutorial. Retrieved February 19, 2009 from http://www.afn.org/~gestalt/.

69. Giles, J., Ryan, D. A. J., Belliveau, G., De Freitas, E., & Casey, R. (2006). Teaching style and learning in a quantitative classroom. *Active Learning in Higher Education, 7*, 213–225.

70. Goleman, D. (1998). *Working with emotional intelligence.* New York: Bantam Books.

71. Goleman, D. (2001). Issues in paradigm building. In C. Cherniss, & D. Goleman, (Eds.), *The emotional intelligent workplace: How to select for, measure, and improve emotional intelligence in individuals, groups, and organizations* (pp. 13–26). San Francisco: Jossey Bass.

72. Goleman, D. (2005). *Emotional intelligence.* (10th Anniversary ed.). New York: Bantam Books.

73. Graf, S., Viola, S., Leo, T., & Kinshuk, (2007). In-depth analysis of the Felder-Silverman learning style dimensions. *Journal of Research on Technology in Education, 40*(1), 79–93.

74. Graham, C., Cagiltay, K., Lim, B., Craner, J., & Duffy, T. (2001). Seven principles of effective teaching: A practical lens for evaluating online courses. *The Technology Source*, March/April. Retrieved December 1, 2008 at http://sln.suny.edu/sln/public/original.nsf/0/b495223246cabd6b85256a090058ab98.

75. Grasha, A. F. (1996). *Teaching with style.* Pittsburgh: Alliance Publishers.

76. Grasha, A. F. (2003, July/August). The dynamics of one-on-one teaching. *The Social Studies*, *94*(4), 179–187.

77. Griggs, R. (2002). *The effects of the use of a human patient simulator on the acquisition of nursing knowledge in undergraduate nursing students at a university in Illinois.* Doctoral Dissertation: Southern Illinois University at Carbondale.

78. Han, S., & Hill, J. R. (2006). Building understanding in asynchronous discussions: Examining types of online discourse. *Journal of Asynchronous Networks, 10*(4), 29–50.

79. Hand, H. (2005). Promoting effective teaching and learning in the clinical setting. *Nursing Standard, 20*(39), 55–63.

80. Hanson, K., & Stenvig, T. (2008). The good clinical nursing educator and the baccalaureate nursing clinical experience: Attributes and praxis. *Journal of Nursing Education, 47*(1), 38–42.

81. Harris, P. (2005, May). Boomer vs. echo boomer: The work war? *Training and Development, 22*(10), 44–46, 48–49.

82. Harrow, A. J. (1972). *A taxonomy of the psychomotor domain.* New York: David McKay Co.

83. Hmelo-Silver, C. (2004). Problem-based learning: What and how do students learn? *Educational Psychology Review, 16*(3), 235–266.

84. Hooper, B., & Hurry, P. (2000, December). Learning the MI way: The effects on students' learning of using the theory of multiple intelligences. *Pastoral Care*, 26–32.

85. Howe, N., & Strauss, W. (2000). *Millennials rising: The next great generation.* New York: Vintage Books.

86. Huber, M. T., Brown, C., Hutchings, P., Gale, R., Miller, R., & Breen, M. (Eds.). (2007, January). *Integrative learning: Opportunities to connect.* Public Report of the Integrative Learning Project sponsored by the Association of American Colleges and Universities and The Carnegie Foundation for the Advancement of Teaching, Stanford, CA. Retrieved January, 17, 2009 from http://www.carnegiefoundation.org/files/elibrary/integrativelearning/index.htm.

87. Huitt, W., & Hummel, J. (1997). An introduction to operant (instrumental) conditioning. *Educational Psychology Interactive.* Valdosta, GA: Valdosta State University. Retrieved November 1, 2008 from http://chiron.valdosta.edu/whuitt/col/behsys/operant.html.

88. Inglese, T., Mayer, R. E., & Rigotti, F. (2007). Using audiovisual TV interviews to create visible authors that reduce the learning gap between native and non-native language speakers. *Learning and Instruction, 17*(1), 67–77.

89. Jeffries, P. (2000). Development and test of a model for designing interactive CD-ROMS for teaching nursing skills. *Computers in Nursing, 18(3)*, 118–124.

90. Jesse, D. E., Taleff, J., Payne, P., Cox, R., & Steele, L. L. (2006). Reusable learning units: An innovative teaching strategy for online education. *International Journal of Nursing Education Scholarship, 3*(1), 1–12.

91. Johnson, S., & Finucane, P. (2000). The emergence of problem-based learning in medical education. *Journal of Evaluation in Clinical Practice, 6*, 281–291.

92. Kalyuga, S., Chandler, P., & Sweller, J. (1999). Managing split-attention and redundancy in multimedia instruction. *Applied Cognitive Psychology, 13*(4), 351–371.

93. Kalyuga, S., Chandler, P., & Sweller, J. (2000). Incorporating learner experience into the design of multimedia instruction. *Journal of Educational Psychology, 92*(1), 126–136.

94. Kalyuga, S., Chandler, P., & Sweller, J. (2004). When redundant on-screen text in multimedia technical instruction can interfere with learning. *Human Factors, 46*(3), 567–581.

95. Keirsey.com. (2008). About the Keirsey temperament sorter. Retrieved November 18, 2008 from http://Keirsey.com.

96. Keirsey, D. (1998). *Please understand me II. Temperament, character, intelligence.* Del Mar, CA: Prometheus Nemesis Book Company.

97. Kember, D., Jones, A., Loke, A., McKay, J., Sinclair, K., Tse, H., *et al.* (1999). Determining the level of reflective thinking from students' written journals using a coding scheme based on the work of Mezirow. *International Journal of Lifelong Education, 18*(1), 18–30.

98. Kim, C. (2008). Using email to enable e^3 (effective, efficient, and engaging) learning. *Distance Education, 29*(2), 187–198.

99. Knowles, M. (1984). *The adult learner: A neglected species* (3rd ed.). Houston: Gulf Publishing.

100. Knowles, M., Holton, E., & Swanson, R. (2005). *The adult learner: The definitive classic in adult education and human resource development.* Burlington, MA: Elsevier.

101. Kolb, D.A. (1984). *Experiential learning: Experience as the source of learning and development.* Englewood Cliffs, NJ: Prentice-Hall.

102. Koper, R. (2003). Combining re-usable learning resources to pedagogical purposeful units of learning (Ch. 5). In A. Littlejohn & S. S. Buckingham. (Eds.), Reusing online resources: A sustainable approach to e-learning. *Journal of Interactive Media in Education* special issue (1). Retrieved February 16, 2009 from http://www.jime.open.ac.uk/2003/1.

103. Krathwohl, D. R., Bloom, B., & Masia., B. B. (1964). *Taxonomy of educational objectives. The classification of educational goals Handbook II: Affective domain.* New York: David McKay.

104. Kuiper, R. A. (2005). Self-regulated learning during a clinical preceptorship: The reflections of senior baccalaureate nursing students, *Nursing Education Perspectives, 26*(6), 351–356.

105. Kuiper, R., & Pesut, D. (2004). Promoting cognitive and metacognitive reflective reasoning skills in nursing practice: Self-regulated learning theory. *Journal of Advanced Nursing, 45*(4), 381–391.

106. Kuit, J. A., Reay, G., & Freeman, R. (2001). Experiences of reflective teaching. *Active Learning in Higher Education, 2,* 128–142.

107. Lamb, B. (2007). Dr. mashup: Or why educators should learn to stop worrying and love the remix. *Educause Review, 42*(4), 12–15.

108. Lee, M. J., & Chan, A. (2007). Reducing the effects of isolation and promoting inclusivity for distance learners through podcasting. *Turkish Online Journal of Distance Education, 8*(1), Art.7. Retrieved March 12, 2007, from http://tojde.anadolu.edu.tr/tojde25/articles/Article_7.htm.

109. Letcher, D. C., & Yancey, N. R. (2004). Witnessing change with aspiring nurses: A human becoming teaching-learning process in nursing education. *Nursing Science Quarterly, 17,* 36–41.

110. Livsey, R., & Palmer, P. (1999). *The courage to teach: A guide for reflection and renewal.* San Francisco: Jossey-Bass.

111. Long, H., & Coldren, J. (2006). Interpersonal influences in large lecture-based classes: A socioinstructional perspective. *College Teaching, 54*(2), 237–243.

112. Loughran, J. J. (1996). *Developing reflective practitioners: Learning about teaching and learning through modeling.* London: Falmer.

113. Lovelace, M. K. (2005). Meta-analysis of experimental research based on the Dunn and Dunn model. *The Journal of Educational Research, 98*(3), 176–183.

114. Luiten, J., Ames, W., & Ackerson, G. (1980). A meta-analysis of the effects of advance organizers on learning and retention. *American Educational Research Journal, 17*(2), 211–218.

115. Madorin, S., & Iwasiw, C. (1999). The effects of computer-assisted instruction and self-efficacy on baccalaureate nursing students. *Journal of Nursing Education, 38*(6), 282–285.

116. Magnussen, L. (2008). Applying the principles of significant learning in the e-learning environment. *Journal of Nursing Education, 47*(2), 82–86.

117. Martin, J. (2004). Self-regulated learning, social cognitive theory, and agency. *Educational Psychologist, 39*(2), 135–145.

118. Maslow, A. H. (1968). *Toward a psychology of being* (2nd ed.). New York: Van Nostrand.

119. Mayer, R. E. (1989). Systematic thinking fostered by illustrations in scientific text. *Journal of Educational Psychology, 81*, 240–246.

120. Mayer, R. E. (2001). *Multimedia learning.* New York: Cambridge University Press.

121. Mayer, R. E., Dow, G. T., & Mayer, S. (2003). Multimedia learning in an interactive self-explaining environment: What works in the design of agent-based microworlds? *Journal of Educational Psychology, 95*(4), 806–813.

122. Mayer, R. E., Fennell, S., Farmer, L., & Campbell, J. (2004). A personalization effect in multimedia learning: Students learn better when words are in conversational style rather than formal style. *Journal of Educational Psychology, 96*(2), 389–395.

123. Mayer, R. E., Heiser, J., & Lonn, S. (2001). Cognitive constraints on multimedia learning: When presenting more material results in less understanding. *Journal of Educational Psychology, 93*(1), 187–198.

124. Mayer, J., & Salovey, P. (1997). What is emotional intelligence? In P. Salovey & D. Sluyter, (Eds.), *Emotional development and emotional intelligence: Educational implications* (pp. 3–31). New York: Basic Books.

125. Mayer, J., Salovey, P., & Caruso, D. (2004). Emotional intelligence: Theory, findings, and implications. *Psychological Inquiry, 15*(3), 197–215.

126. Mayer, R. E., Steinhoff, K., Bower, G., & Mars, R. (1995). A generative theory of textbook design: Using annotated illustration to foster meaningful learning of science text. *Educational Technology Research and Development, 43*, 31–43.

127. Mayer, R. E., & Chandler, P. (2001). When learning is just a click away: Does simple user interaction foster deeper understanding of multimedia messages? *Journal of Educational Psychology, 93*, 390–397.

128. Mayer, R. E., Mathias, A., & Wetzell, K. (2002). Fostering understanding of multimedia messages through pre-training: Evidence for a two-stage theory of mental model construction. *Journal of Experimental Psychology, 8*(3), 147–154.

129. Mayer, R. E., Sims, V., & Tajika, H. (1995). A comparison of how textbooks teach mathematical problem solving in Japan and the United States. *American Educational Research Journal, 32*(2), 443–460.

130. McAllister, M., Tower, M., & Walker, R. (2007). Gentle interruptions: Transformative approaches to clinical teaching. *Journal of Nursing Education, 46*(7), 304–312.

131. Mccann, E., & Turner, J. (2004). Increasing student learning through volitional control. *Teachers College Record, 106*(9), 1695–1714.

132. McGonigal, K. (2005) Teaching for transformation: From learning theory to teaching strategies. *Speaking of Teaching Newsletter, The Center for Teaching and Learning, Stanford University, 14*(2), 1–4.

133. McInerney, D. (2005). Educational psychology—theory, research, and teaching: A 25-year retrospective. *Educational Psychology, 25*(6), 585–599.

134. Mezirow, J. (1978). Perspective transformation. *Adult Education, 28*(2), 100–110.

135. Mezirow, J. (1991). *Transformative dimensions of adult learning.* San Francisco: Jossey-Bass.

136. Miller, G. (1956). The magical number seven, plus or minus two: Some limits on our capacity for processing information. *Psychological Review, 63,* 81–97.

137. Moreno, R., & Mayer, R. E. (1999). Cognitive principles of multimedia learning: The role of modality and contiguity. *Journal of Educational Psychology, 91,* 358–368.

138. Moreno, R., & Mayer, R. E. (2000). A coherence effect in multimedia learning: The case for minimizing irrelevant sounds in the design of multimedia instructional messages. *Journal of Educational Psychology, 92*(1), 117–125.

139. Morse, J. S., Oberer, J., Dobbins, J., & Mitchell, D. (1998). Understanding learning styles: Implications for in-service educators. In R. Dunn & S. A. Griggs, (Eds.), *Learning styles and the nursing profession.* New York: NLN Press.

140. Mosston, M. (1966). *Teaching physical education.* Columbus, OH: Charles Merrill.

141. Mosston, M., & Ashworth, S. (1990). *The spectrum of teaching styles: From command to discovery.* White Plains, NY: Longman.

142. Mosston, M., & Ashworth, S. (2002). *Teaching physical education.* Columbus, OH: Charles Merrill.

143. Mullen, P. (2007). Use of self-regulated learning strategies by students in the second and third trimesters of an accelerated second-degree baccalaureate nursing program. *Journal of Nursing Education, 46*(9), 406–412.

144. Murphy, J. (2005). How to learning, not what to learn: Three strategies that foster life-long learning in clinical settings. In M. Oermann & K. Heinrich, (Eds.), *Annual review of nursing education* Vol 3 (pp. 37–55). New York: Springer.

145. Murphy, K., Mahoney, S., Chen, C., Mendoza-Diaz, N., & Yang, X. (2005). A constructivist model of mentoring, coaching, and facilitating online discussions. *Distance Education, 26*(3), 341–366.

146. Myers & Briggs Foundation. (n.d.). MBTI basics. Retrieved September 30, 2008 from http://www.myersbriggs.org/.

147. National League for Nursing, Task Group on Nurse Educator Competencies. (2005). Core competencies of nurse educators with task statements. Retrieved September 10, 2008 from http://www.nln.org/facultydevelopment/pdf/corecompetencies.pdf.

148. Nussbaum-Beach, S. (2008). No limits. *Technology & Learning, 28*(7), 14–16, 18.

149. Oblinger, D. G., & Oblinger, J. L. (Eds.), (2005). *Educating the net generation.* Boulder, CO: Educause. Retrieved November 17, 2009 from http://www.educause.edu/ir/library/pdf/pub7101.pdf.

150. O'Shea, E. (2003). Self-directed learning in nurse education: A review of the literature. *Journal of Advanced Nursing, 43*(1), 62–70.

151. O'Sullivan, E. V., Morrell, A., & O'Connor, M. A. (Eds.), (2002). *Expanding the boundaries of transformative learning: Essays on theory and praxis.* New York: Palgrave Press.

152. Paas, F., & Van Merriënboer, J. (1994). Instructional control of cognitive load in the training of complex cognitive tasks. *Educational Psychology Review, 6*(4), 351–371.

153. Palloff, R., & Pratt, K. (2003). *The virtual student: A profile and guide to working with online learners.* San Francisco: Jossey-Bass.
154. Parse, R. (2004). A human becoming teaching learning-model. *Nursing Science Quarterly, 17,* 33–35.
155. Paul, R., & Elder, L. (2007). Critical thinking: The art of Socratic questioning. *Journal of Developmental Education, 31*(1), 36–37.
156. Paxton, R. (2002). The influence of author visibility on high school students solving a historical problem. *Cognition and Instruction, 20*(2), 197–248.
157. Piaget, J. (1972). Intellectual evolution from adolescence to adulthood. *Human Development, 15,* 1–12.
158. Piaget, J. (2003). Part I: Cognitive development in children: Piaget: Development and learning. *Journal of Research in Science Teaching, 40* (Suppl 1), S8–S18.
159. Pollock, E., Chandler, P., & Sweller, J. (2002). Assimilating complex information. *Learning and Instruction, 12*(1), 61–86.
160. Ravert, P. (2004). *The use of human patient simulator with undergraduate nursing students: A prototype evaluation of critical thinking and self-efficacy.* Doctoral dissertation. Salt Lake City, UT: University of Utah.
161. Ripley, D. (1986). Invitational teaching behaviors in the associate degree clinical setting. *Journal of Nursing Education, 25,* 240–246.
162. Rogers, C. (1961). *On becoming a person: A therapist's view of psychotherapy.* London: Constable.
163. Rogers, C. (1980). *A way of being.* Boston: Houghton Mifflin.
164. Rogers, C. (1983). *Freedom to learn for the 80's.* New York: Charles Merrill.
165. Rogers, C., & Freiberg, H. J. (1994). *Freedom to learn* (3rd ed.). New York: Charles Merrill.
166. Ruiz, J. G., Mintzer, M. J., & Issenberg, S. B. (2006). Learning objects in medical education. *Medical Teacher, 28*(7), 599–605.
167. Ryan, M., Hodson-Carlton, K., & Ali, N. (2005). A model for faculty teaching online: Confirmation of a dimensional matrix. *Journal of Nursing Education, 44*(8), 357–365.
168. Salovey, P., & Mayer, J. (1990). Emotional intelligence. *Imagination, Cognition, and Personality, 9,* 185–211.
169. Sanchez, C. A., & Wiley, J. (2006). An examination of the seductive details effect in terms of working memory capacity. *Memory & Cognition, 34*(2), 344–355.
170. Scanlon, J. M., & Chernomas, W. M. (1997). Developing the reflective teacher. *Journal of Advanced Nursing, 25*(6), 1138–1143.
171. Schunk, D. H. (2008). *Learning theories: An educational perspective* (5th ed.). Englewood Cliffs, NJ: Prentice-Hall.
172. Sharp, J. G., Byrne, J., & Bowker, R. (2007). The trouble with VAK. *Educational Futures, 1,* 76–93. Retrieved November 18, 2008 from http://www.besajournal.org.uk/journals/200706/sharp.pdf.
173. Siemens, G. (2005). Connectivism: A learning theory for the digital age. *International Journal of Instructional Technology and Distance Learning, 2*(1), 20 p.
174. Siemens, P. (2008). Learning and knowing in networks: Changing roles for educators and designers. Retrieved February 14, 2008 from http://it.coe.uga.edu/itforum/Paper105/Siemens.pdf.

175. Simpson, E. J. (1972). *The classification of educational objectives in the psychomotor domain* (1st ed.). Washington, DC: Gryphon House.

176. Skiba, D. J. (2007). Nursing education 2.0: Are mashups useful for nursing education? *Nursing Education Perspectives, 28,* 286–288.

177. Skiba, D., & Barton, A. (2006). Adapting your teaching to accommodate the net generation of learners. *Online Journal of Issues in Nursing, 11*(2), 6p.

178. Skylar, A., Higgins, K., & Boone, R. (2007). Strategies for adapting webquests for students with learning disabilities. *Intervention in School and Clinic, 43*(1), 20–28.

179. Slavin, R. E. (2006). *Educational psychology: Theory and practice.* New York: Pearson.

180. Sternberger, C. (2002). Using a hyperlearning model for web course development. *Nursing Education Perspectives, 23,* 72–75.

181. Sternberger, C., & Meyer, L. (2001). Hypermedia-assisted instructions: Authoring with learning guidelines. *Computers in Nursing, 19,* 69–74.

182. Stone, C. L. (1983). A meta-analysis of advance organizer studies. *Journal of Experimental Education, 51,* 194–199.

183. Swan, K. (2004). *Relationships between interactions and learning in online environments.* Needham, MA: The Sloan Consortium.

184. Sweller, J., & Chandler, P. (1994). Why some material is difficult to learn. *Cognition and Instruction, 12*(3), 185–233.

185. Sweller, J., Chandler, P., Tierney, P., & Cooper, M. (1990). Cognitive load as a factor in the structuring of technical material. *Journal of Experimental Psychology, 119*(2), 176–192.

186. The New Media Consortium and Educause Learning Initiative. (2008). *The horizon report 2008 edition.* Austin, TX: The New Media Consortium. Retrieved November 10, 2008 from http://www.nmc.org/pdf/2008-Horizon-Report.pdf.

187. Thorpe, K. (2004). Reflective learning journals: From concept to practice. *Reflective Practice, 5*(3), 327–343.

188. Trees, A. P., & Jackson, M. H. (2007). The learning environment in clicker classrooms: Student processes of learning and involvement in large university-level courses using student response systems. *Learning, Media, and Technology, 32*(1), 21–40.

189. Van Wynen, E. A. (1998). How do you think? Two sides to every story. In R. Dunn, & S. A. Griggs (Eds.), *Learning styles and the nursing profession* (pp. 41–52). New York: NLN Press.

190. Waldner, M., & Olson, J. (2007). Taking the patient to the classroom: Applying theoretical frameworks to simulation in nursing education. *International Journal of Nursing Education Scholarship, 4*(1), 1–14.

191. Walker, J., Martin, T., White, J., Elliott, R., Norwood, A., Mangum, C., *et al.* (2006). Generational (age) differences in nursing students' preferences for teaching methods. *Journal of Nursing Education, 45*(9), 371–374.

192. Waterhouse, L. (2006). Inadequate evidence for multiple intelligences, Mozart effect, and emotional intelligence theories. *Educational Psychologist, 41*(4), 247–255.

193. Western Nevada College. (2001, July). Learning styles and personality types. Retrieved November 15, 2008 at http://www.wnc.edu.

194. Wong, K., Loke, A., Wong, M., Tse, H., Kan, E., & Kember, D. (1997). An action research study into the development of nurses as reflective practitioners. *Journal of Nursing Education, 34*(10), 476–481.

195. Woods, H. A., & Chiu, C. (2003, September/October). Wireless response technology in college classrooms. *Technology Source.* Retrieved February 20, 2009 from http://www.technology source.org/article/wireless_response_technology_in_college_classrooms/.

196. Yoo, M., & Yoo, I. (2003). The effectiveness of standardized patients as a teaching method for nursing fundamentals. *Journal of Nursing Education, 42*(10), 444–448.

CHAPTER 3

Facilitate Learner Development and Socialization—Competency 2

OBJECTIVES

1. Identify learning needs and successful teaching and advising approaches for multicultural, disadvantaged, at risk, and second degree students.
2. Explore examples of positive learning environments.
3. Compare taxonomies for cognitive, affective, and psychomotor learning.
4. Examine adult learning and social learning theories.
5. Explore the impact of peer and self-evaluation, role modeling, mentoring and communication styles on learner development and socialization.

KEY TERMS

Andragogy
Bandura's social learning theory
Benner's novice to expert theory
Developmental advising
Giger-Davidhizar's transcultural theory
Kohlberg's theory of moral development

Mentoring
Prescriptive advising
Rest's Theory of Morality
Role modeling
Service learning

DEFINITION AND DESCRIPTION OF COMPETENCY

The second competency, facilitate learner development and socialization, represents an extension of competency 1 which was discussed in Chapter 2. Both competencies emphasize the facilitation role of the teacher; however, competency 1 is focused on teaching clinical and didactic content and dealing with factors that influence initial learning. Competency 2 is concerned with helping the student function effectively in the nursing role and dealing with factors that can adversely effect the transition into the profession.

To demonstrate competency 2, the academic nurse education (ANE) needs to be able to identify students with unique learning needs and implement approaches that will build on the learner's strengths and effectively deal with any limitations (National

League for Nursing [NLN] Task Group on Nurse Educator Competencies, 2005). The ANE also needs to draw on interpersonal skills to provide academic counseling, effective role modeling of professional behaviors, and create learning environments that support the student's self-reflection and professional socialization (NLN, Task Group on Nurse Educator Competencies, 2005).

THEORY AND RESEARCH RELATED TO COMPETENCY

Several theories previously discussed in Chapter 2, andragogy and social learning, are particularly relevant to learner development and socialization and will be reviewed from the context of facilitating learner development and socialization. Andragogy is relevant because of its emphasis on the learner and the valuing of the experiences and background of the learner, whereas social learning theory is applicable because of its emphasis on acquisition of professional behaviors through observation. Benner's Novice to Expert Theory and Giger-Davidhizar's Model of Transcultural Assessment are explored to provide the ANE with greater understanding of the student and the processes used to enhance development and socialization into the nursing role. The moral development theories of Kohlberg, Gilligan, and Rest are also discussed to provide understanding and guidance for interacting with learners who are at various stages of development.

Andragogy

The term andragogy, referring to the methods or techniques used to teach adults, was popularized in 1990 by Malcolm Knowles in his book *The Adult Learner: A Neglected Species*. The principles underlying andragogy represented a shift from instructor-driven learning processes to ones that involve the learner in a mutual process of assessing, determining learning objectives, planning, implementing, and evaluating learning. In andragogy, importance is placed on understanding student behavior and on the teacher-student relationship. See Chapter 2 for discussion of the assumptions and principles of andragogy.

Operating from an andragogical perspective, the ANE is able to assist the learner to function as a self-directed learner and experience transformative learning. According to Mezirow's transformative learning theory (1991, 2000), as a practitioner of andragogy, the ANE should strive to decrease the learner's dependency on the teacher, thereby preparing the learner for clinical practice. The educator can facilitate what Mezirow calls a perspective transformation by helping the learner analyze and solve problems and consider alterative perspectives. In teaching from an andragogical per-

---

BOX 3-1   Strategies for Facilitating Transformative Learning

Ask learners to:

• Examine their beliefs (i.e., the history, context, and consequences of their beliefs).

• Reflect on their problem solving processes.

• Bracket their assumptions and preconceived ideas.

• Openly consider other's perspectives.

• Reassess and critique their own premises.

Data from Mezirow, J. (1991). *Transformative dimensions of adult learning* (p. 215). San Francisco: Jossey-Bass.

---

spective, the ANE may use processes of role modeling, questioning, and self-reflection. These teaching strategies assist in achieving the desired outcome of transformative learning and can ". . . help learners construe experiences in a way that allows them to understand more clearly the reasons for their problems and the action options open to them . . ." (Mezirow, 1991, p. 203). Suggestions for fostering transformative adult learning are summarized in Box 3-1. These guidelines can be easily adapted as a framework for students' written reflection assignments or used to guide face-to-face or online discussions.

Bandura's Social Learning Theory

The core components of social learning theory identified by Bandura (1977) include the person, the environment, and behavior in reciprocal relationships (pp. 9–10). Bandura (1977) views the attributes of the environment and the individual as "reciprocal determinants" of each other (p. vii). This depiction of social learning theory as reciprocal influences of person, environment, and behavior is simple, yet it accounts for the complexity of modeled behaviors. The person's unique processing and interpretation of an observed behavior explains in part why, if two people observe the same event, one will learn and repeat the behavior while the other will not.

Social Learning Theory shares the behaviorist's emphasis on the importance of the external environment in influencing behavior. It also recognizes the complexity of behavior and the impact of personal attributes such as cognitive abilities and self-regulation. Bandura notes that the use of cognitive abilities is essential for acquiring knowledge. "Through verbal and imagined symbols people process and preserve experiences in representational forms that serve as guides for future behavior. . . . Without symbolizing powers, humans would be incapable of reflective thought" (Bandura 1977, p. 13). The process of social learning is also influenced by personal factors that provide self-regulatory processes. "People are not simply reactors to external influences. They select, organize, and transform the stimuli that impinge upon them" (Bandura, 1977, p. vii). This perspective views the person as neither completely controlled by external environmental factors nor as a totally self-regulated being who is free of environmental influence.

It is important to recognize that social learning is probably always occurring to some degree, as long as the person is observing behaviors of others. In applying social learning concepts to teaching nursing, the ANE recognizes that social learning can be deliberately taught, through conscious role modeling and conscious reflection on the modeled or observed behavior. Awareness of the ongoing nature of social learning enables the ANE to be proactive in helping students interpret the benefits and detractors of modeling specific behaviors. The degree to which the environment and personal attributes influence the student's modeling of an observed behavior will vary depending upon (1) the interactions of multiple environmental and personal factors, (2) the individual's interpretation of the behavior, and (3) the rewards and detriments associated with the behavior. Therefore, the ANE can play an active role in helping the student learn from observation by using deliberate discussion and reflection on the positive and negative consequences of the behavior.

Benner's Novice to Expert Theory

Benner's classic work *From Novice to Expert: Excellence and Power in Clinical Nursing Practice* is based on a descriptive study that delineated characteristics of five levels of nursing competency (Benner, 1984). The five levels of competency, originally described in Dreyfus' theory of skill acquisition, include the novice, advanced beginner, competent, proficient, and expert (Benner, 1984, p. 13). These five levels represent progression in three aspects of skill performance: (1) the novice moves from reliance on principles to the use of past experiences, (2) the novice moves from the perception of equally relevant parts to the perception of the complete whole and discernment of relevance of the parts, and (3) the novice moves from a detached observer to an involved performer (p. 13).

To study how the Dreyfus model applied to nursing, Benner conducted interviews with 21 preceptee/preceptor pairs from three different hospitals and conducted participant observation and interviews with an additional 51 experienced nurses and 15 students and new graduate nurses. The participants were asked about critical patient care incidents, and accounts of the same incidents between preceptor and preceptee were compared.

Benner's findings delineate the attributes of nursing students and nurses in each of the fives stages of skill acquisition (1984). In the first stage, the novice is described as operating from rule-based textbook guidelines. The novice is not comfortable with clinical practice and is not able to consider contextual variations within the setting. The novice has book knowledge of how to manage patient care but has limited direct experience (p. 21). Student nurses, new graduates, and even seasoned nurses who are practicing in an area that is unfamiliar to them may be classified as novice practitioners.

The second stage of skill performance is the advanced beginner. This stage includes students who have had some real experiences that enable them to identify selected aspects of the clinical situation. The advanced beginner can formulate guidelines that acknowledge the aspects of the situation. However, the guidelines tend to "ignore the differential importance" and treat all aspects as equally important (Benner, 1984, p. 23). When faced with performance of a task, the advanced beginner will need to focus on the task and typically is not able to focus on other aspects of the situation.

The competent level of skill performance in nursing is typically seen in nurses who have worked in the same clinical area for several years (Benner, 1984). The nurse functioning at the competent level is able to determine which aspects of care are most important, prioritize care, and establish a plan of action. This stage is characterized by "conscious deliberate planning" (p. 27) and the achievement of a measure of organization and efficiency not seen in the advanced beginner stage.

As the nurse progresses to the proficient level of practice, a shift in perspective occurs. The proficient nurse has moved from viewing aspects of the patient situation to seeing the situation as a whole and appreciating the long-term implications (Benner, 1984, p. 27). Nurses at the proficient level of practice also base their care on knowledge derived from past experiences. Past nursing care experiences enable the proficient nurse to create a picture of what constitutes a normal, expected, patient care situation. The expected situation can then be compared to what is actually observed. Benner describes this stage as using maxims or subtle nuances to guide nursing care (p. 29).

The final stage of skill proficiency is the expert clinician who has many years of nursing experience in a specific specialty. The expert has progressed from using rules, guidelines, and maxims in providing patient care to using intuition (Benner, 1984, p. 32). The expert nurse "now has an intuitive grasp of each situation and zeros in on the accurate region of the problem without wasteful consideration of a large range of unfruitful alternative diagnoses and solutions" (p. 32). Benner describes several unique characteristics of the expert nurse. First, an expert nurse's actions are based on an intuitive grasp of the situation. Therefore, the nurse often has difficulty describing how he or she knows that his or her interpretation of the situation is accurate, or on what information a particular decision is based. Second, the clinical performance of expert nurses may not be easily captured by traditional performance evaluation criteria that value stepwise, analytical processes (p. 34).

Each of the five stages of skill proficiency describes the nurse's progressive development of characteristics and perception. These alter the way the nurse interacts with patients, and identifies and manages patient care issues. During each stage, Benner suggests specific teaching approaches that will enhance the nurse's learning and development. The ANE can use knowledge of the stages to frame expectations for student learning. In entry level nursing programs where the students have no previous nursing experience, the ANE will see progression of the student from the novice to advanced beginner stage and will find the teaching approaches listed in Table 3-1 helpful. However, for students who have previous nursing experience, such as those in a baccalaureate completion or graduate program, the student's stage will depend on the match between previous experience and the subject matter. Returning nursing students who had attained the competent, proficient, or even expert stage in their area of specialization, will not function at the same level in a new practice area. Therefore, the teaching approaches will need to be individualized for returning nursing students. Facilitating the student's progression through the stages of novice to expert enhances learner development and socialization into nursing practice.

Moral Development Theories

Many authors have identified dealing with unethical student behavior as a growing concern (Begley, 2006; Johnson & Martin, 2005; Kolanko *et al.*, 2006). Theories of moral development can be useful for understanding the student's behavior and for planning ways to assist the student's moral development. Baxter & Boblin (2007) discuss unethical classroom and clinical behaviors in terms of the moral development theories of Kohlberg, Gilligan, and Rest, and offer strategies to facilitate students' moral development.

Kohlberg's Theory of Moral Development

According to Kohlberg's (1981) theory, individuals progress through three levels of moral development: (1) preconventional, (2) conventional, and (3) post conventional. Individuals progress sequentially through successive levels, and once a level is

TABLE 3-1   **Characteristics of Novice to Expert Nurses and Teaching Approaches**

Stage	Characteristics	Teaching Approaches
Novice	Nursing student with little nursing experience. Rule governed behavior, task focused, unable to appreciate the contextual nuances of a situation (pp. 20–21).	To increase comfort and assist the student in moving beyond this stage, provide multiple diverse opportunities for skill performance and patient contacts.
Advanced beginner	Typical of a nursing student toward the end of nursing program or a graduate nurse. Able to consider aspects of the situation but tends to treat all aspects as equally important (pp. 22–23).	Discuss clues and guidelines that can be used to help the advanced beginner differentiate aspects that are important (p. 23).
Competent	Typically a nurse with 2–3 years experience in a specific area. Characterized by planned patient care, and ability to prioritize needs and cope with the unexpected (pp. 26–27).	Decision-making games and simulations will enhance the competent nurse's ability to initiate plans of care for multiple complex patient care situations (p. 27).
Proficient	Perceives situations as wholes rather than focusing on aspects. "Has learned from experience what typical events to expect in a given situation and how plans need to be modified in response to these events" (p. 28). Uses maxims or nuances of a situation to guide decisions and responses.	Use inductive approaches focusing on clinical experiences. Use challenging and realistic case studies that provide insufficient information for decision making or provide irrelevant information (p. 31).
Expert	Demonstrates an intuitive grasp of the situation with a "deep understanding" (p. 32) and is able to focus quickly on the priority problem. Provides nursing care in a fluid, flexible manner.	Explore "critical incidents from their practice that illustrate expertise or breakdown in performance" (p. 35).

Data from Benner, P. (1984). *From novice to expert. Excellence and power in clinical nursing practice.* Menlo Park, CA: Addison-Wesley.

reached there is no regression to an earlier level (Table 3-2). Students in the preconventional level tend to see the fairness and rightness of a situation only in terms of their own needs. Because learners in this level are greatly influenced by authority figures, they may prioritize their actions based on which authority figure is mostly likely to evoke punishment (Baxter & Boblin, 2007). At the conventional level the student is concerned with other's feelings and may rationalize unethical behavior if the behavior preserves other's feelings. Baxter and Boblin give the example of a student falsely documenting patient care because the student does not want to disturb a patient who is sleeping and does not want to create a conflict with instructors and staff. The ANE can determine the student's level of moral development by simply asking the student to explain the reasons why a given situation would be right or wrong.

According to Kohlberg (1981) most adults reach the conventional level of moral reasoning but few reach the third level (postconventional), which is characterized by the ability to take principled action. This may involve making decisions and taking actions that may be in conflict with the norms of a group. Principled action means ultimately being guided by broad ethical principles.

TABLE 3-2   Stages of Moral Development

Categories of Moral Development	Stages and Characteristics
Preconventional thinking: Behavior is based on rules and labels of good/bad, right/wrong.	Stage 1: Moral behavior is based on fear of punishment and deference to authority. Stage 2: Moral behavior is rule based and meets immediate needs (p. 54).
Conventional thinking: The individual values maintaining family or other groups' expectations.	Stage 3: Moral behavior is guided by concern for other's feelings and being loyal. Behavior is often judged by the intention behind it. Stage 4: Moral behavior is guided by needs of society, fulfilling expectations of society.
Postconventional thinking: Develops moral values and principles that go beyond the individual's identification with a group	Stage 5: Characterized by upholding rights of society as agreed on by the whole society, even in the face of conflict with other groups. Stage 6: Guided by broader, universal ethics base on principles of justice, reciprocity, and equality of human rights and respect for human dignity (p. 55).

Data from Kohlberg, L, & Hersh, R. H. (1977). Moral development: A review of the theory. *Theory into Practice, 16*(2), 54–55.

The ANE can use Kohlberg's stages of moral development not only as a basis for understanding moral development of students but as a framework for analyzing ethical issue in the clinical and classroom settings. Presenting situations in which the student can challenge his or her way of thinking can facilitate progression to a higher level of moral reasoning (Allen, 2003). Teaching students the stages outlined by Kohlberg, then asking them to reflect and analyze their perspective on an issue using Kohlberg's framework, can facilitate the students' self-understanding and acquisition of advanced levels of moral reasoning.

Gilligan's Theory of Moral Development

Gilligan, a student of Kohlberg, developed a different perspective that emphasized how moral development of women is achieved. Based on a study of three different morally challenging situations, Gilligan (1982) concluded that unlike men, women evaluate their morality based on their ability to care. Accordingly, moral development depends on the connection between the person's sense of responsibility and personal relationships. Gilligan's theory suggests that female nursing students may engage in unethical actions because they do not fully understand the relationships and the interdependence of people. Strategies the ANE can use to assist the learner involve having the students reflect on their role, interactions, and relationships with others in the healthcare system. Role playing and simulation are also useful strategies for modeling caring and concern and helping students see their interconnectedness.

Rest's Theory of Morality

A third theory of moral development described by Rest (1986, 1994) integrates the concept of justice, which is central to Kolhberg's theory, and the concept of care that is emphasized by Gilligan. According to Rest (1986), "the function of morality is to provide basic guidelines for determining how conflicts in human interests are to be settled and for optimizing mutual benefit of people living together in groups" (p. 1). The ability to deal with conflicts underlying moral issues is an important component of socialization to the role of nursing. Faculty who understand the processes involved in moral decision making and behavior can teach students the processes, thus preparing them for challenges in the work setting.

In Rest's Theory of Morality, he proposes four interactive psychological components including: (1) moral sensitivity, or one's interpretation of the situation; (2) moral judgment, or deciding which action is morally right or wrong; (3) moral motivation, involving prioritizing values; and (4) moral character, referring to the strength of a person's will (Rest, 1986 & 1994). A central notion is that knowledge of a situation is essential to interpretation of the situation. Therefore, the nurse's moral reasoning can be enhanced by increased knowledge through formal education (Baxter & Boblin, 2007).

In analyzing research on moral development, Rest notes that development of moral judgment is fostered by awareness of the broader social context and the individual's relationship within society. A meta-analysis of 56 studies found that education increased scores on the defining issues test used to measure the development of moral reasoning (Rest, 1994). Those who develop moral judgment tend to seek learning opportunities, enjoy intellectual challenges, engage in reflective activity, and see themselves as within a broad, interconnected, social perspective (Rest, 1986, p. 57). A general pattern of social/cognitive development occurs in those who develop moral judgment. Rest describes the pattern as one of career satisfaction, continued intellectual stimulation, interest in social issues, and community involvement (p. 57). Providing learning opportunities that broaden the individual's awareness of interrelationships with society along with reflective learning activities are beneficial. This can help learners establish a pattern of social/cognitive development that enhances the learner's professional development and socialization into nursing.

Building on the model moral action identified by Rest (1982; 1984; 1986; and 1994), Duckett and Ryden (1994) provide a five-component model that can be used by the ANE to facilitate the development of ethical nursing practice (Table 3-3). Each of the four components, according to Duckett and Ryden, is related to the concept of caring that is integral to nursing practice. The first component, moral sensitivity, is shown through "perspective taking, empathy, and genuineness" (p. 60). Moral reasoning involves considering the relationships and the context of the situation. Taking multiple relationship and contextual factors into account implies caring. Moral commitment also infers the underlying principle of caring. The nurse demonstrating moral commitment must have a strong enough desire to take action that is perceived as morally right even in the face of professional repercussions. The fourth component, moral character, refers to personal attributes that can be developed and used as the foundation for moral reasoning. Caring can be one of these, along with attributes such as strength, courage, and perseverance (p. 61). The fifth component that Duckett and Ryden added to Rest's model is implementing a moral decision. The process of implementation involves interpersonal communication skills that demonstrate caring, including "warmth, empathy, compassion, and connectedness" (p. 61). Duckett and Ryden (1994) conclude that "Ethics education in nursing is possible for students whose prior development has been such that they are capable of normal moral emotions such as empathy, care, concern, and love. Moral theory can be learned; sensitivity and reasoning skills can be enhanced; and effective ways of implementing moral

TABLE 3-3 Five Component Model for Moral Action and Teaching Strategies		
Moral Component	**Definition**	**Teaching Strategy**
Moral sensitivity	The ability to empathize and see a situation from another person's perspective	• Teach foundational communications skills of empathy and genuineness. • Apply the skills in role playing and clinical situations.
Moral reasoning	The ability to consider relationships and contextual factors and apply moral principles when making decisions	• Extend role playing to incorporate decision making processes and application of principles. • Class discussion on reasoning processes used.
Moral commitment	The willingness to follow through with what the individual judges to be morally right even though the actions may not be supported by others.	• Class discussion using "what if" scenarios in which the individual will encounter opposition or conflict concerning the moral action taken.
Moral character	Personal attributes including ego strength, perseverance, conviction, and courage	• Discussion with others who demonstrate these attributes • Role modeling by persons with these attributes
Interpersonal implementation skills	The interpersonal process in which the moral decision is communicated and carried out	• Builds on therapeutic communication skills, assertive communication, and conflict resolution skills. • Apply the skills in role playing and clinical situations.

Data from Duckett, L. J., & Ryden, M. B. (1994). Education for ethical nursing practice. In J. Rest & D. Narvaez (Eds.), *Moral development in the profession* (pp. 51–69). Hillside, NJ: Erlbaum.

Teaching Ethics

Approaches to teaching ethics to healthcare professionals typically involve one of three formats: (1) ethics courses can be taught outside of nursing by philosophy or theology departments; (2) ethics courses can be taught within the nursing department; or (3) ethics content can be integrated into one or more nursing courses. Duckett and Ryden (1994) documented the implementation and evaluation of a fourth approach called multicourse sequential learning (MCSL). In the MCSL approach, the content is referred to as a vertical course with units embedded in existing courses throughout the curriculum (p. 55). However, MCSL differs from integration of content into existing courses in several ways. In the MCSL approach, "The content is carefully sequenced from course to course in the various levels of the program so as to provide a good fit with student development and to build on previous learning" (p. 55). Another difference is that the responsibility for the MCSL content and evaluation rests with a specific faculty or group of faculty who teach the content throughout the individual courses.

According to Duckett & Ryden (1994), a faculty member teaching in a specific course in which the MCSL units are embedded serves as a reinforcer, facilitator, and advisor for the MCSL (pp. 56–57). The course faculty reinforce the content by referring to the content as they teach subsequent topics in the course. The course faculty facilitate the students in applying knowledge and skills from the MCSL to clinical experiences. Course faculty also serve as advisors to the MCSL faculty by keeping them apprised of the course progression, student experiences, and noting when adjustments in the curriculum may be needed.

Over a 4-year period, the effect of an ethics MCSL was evaluated by comparing student's initial and exit knowledge using a test of moral reasoning developed by Rest (1979). All student groups showed an increase in exit scores, with three of the four

---

BOX 3-2   Affective Dispositions of Critical Thinking

1. Independent thinking

2. Fair-mindedness

3. Insight into egocentric, sociocentric beliefs

4. Intellectual courage

5. Intellectual humility

6. Perseverance

7. Confidence in reasoning

8. Inquisitiveness

9. Self-reflection on thoughts and feelings

Data from Allen, J. (2003). Fostering ethical competence in nursing education. *Clinical Research and Regulatory Affairs, 20*(4), 373–377; Paul, R. (1993). Ethics without indoctrination. Retrieved April 4, 2009 from http://www.criticalthinking.org/articles/ethics-wo-indoctrination.cfm.

student groups showing a significant difference in moral reasoning (Duckett & Ryden, 1994, p. 62). Scores on the moral reasoning test were found to account for 34% of the variance in CET scores, thus supporting a relationship between moral reasoning and clinical performance (p. 65).

According to Allen (2003), "Unresolved ethical issues or unsatisfactory resolution of ethical issues, results in moral distress for the practicing nurse" (p. 374). Allen notes that the processes involved in ethical decision making share similarities to the nursing process and critical thinking. Therefore, teaching affective dispositions of critical thinking (Box 3-2) identified from the works of Richard Paul (1993) also can provide the student with tools for ethical reasoning. Paul emphasizes that although teaching these dispositions is difficult and is hampered by lecture-based teaching strategies that do not offer opportunities for discussion and reflection, the development of these dispositions is essential for effective practice in today's complex environment.

THEORY AND RESEARCH RELATED TO LEARNER ATTRIBUTES

Characteristics that the learner brings to the learning situation also impact the learner's development and socialization to the profession. Factors such as communication and help-seeking skills, and cultural/academic background including whether the student is a high or low achiever or has achieved degree completion are explored in this section.

Communication Skills

Communication is the vehicle through which nursing care is delivered and managed. Therefore, effective communication skills are essential for safe nursing practice and socialization to the role of professional nursing. The Joint Commission on Accreditation of Healthcare Organizations (JCAHO) identified one of its major goals as improving communication between healthcare providers (JCAHO, 2006). At one end of the spectrum are miscommunications that contribute to critical events such as patient death or injury, and at the other end are miscommunications that do not adversely affect patient safety. However, communication difficulties at any point along the spectrum may undermine the student or new graduate's effective socialization into practice.

The Commission recommends teaching students the SBAR communication framework to enhance effective communication in practice. SBAR is an acronym that stands for Situation-Background-Assessment-Recommendation (Box 3-3). Teaching students to use the SBAR communication framework provides a systematic

---

BOX 3-3   The SBAR Framework for Clinical Communication

S = Describe the Situation

B = Provide Essential Background

A = Present Current Assessment Findings

R = State Recommendations

Data from The Joint Commission on Accreditation of Healthcare Organizations. (2006). *Meeting the joint commission's 2007 national patient safety goals.* Joint Commission Resources, p. 26.

---

and comprehensive process for communicating within professional practice situations. SBAR enhances clear and effective clinical communication which in turn can directly impact the student's socialization into nursing practice. Check the resource section for information on an SBAR tool kit developed by Arizona Hospital and Healthcare Association.

Cultural Characteristics

Each student has unique learning needs that are shaped by multiple factors including the individual's age, gender, race, religious beliefs, socioeconomic status, regional influences, and personal history. These factors and many more come together to shape the learner's cultural background, "to form one's self identity—how one understands health and illness, how one relates to authority figures, and how one comes to know" (Ruth-Sahd, 2003, p. 130). The ANE who is sensitive to the impact of cultural background on learning will be able to disseminate knowledge and create learning environments that reduce barriers to learning, thereby enhancing the learner's socialization to the profession. In this section, several theory-based teaching approaches are presented that can be useful for teaching culturally diverse groups of students.

Giger-Davidhizar's Model of Transcultural Assessment

The Giger-Davidhizar's Model of Transcultural Assessment has been widely used in nursing education for teaching students about cultural factors to assess in their clients. The model also can be easily adapted by faculty to assess cultural diversity of their students (Davidhizar & Shearer, 2005). According to the model, cultural assessment involves exploring six aspects: (1) communication; (2) time orientation; (3) space, or distance preferences during interactions; (4) values and beliefs of influential social organizations; (5) the amount of personal control the individual feels over the environment; and (6) biological variations. When using this model to assess students, the first five aspects have direct application for the ANE and the approaches used in teaching.

According to Davidhizar & Shearer, communication can be a source of significant problems between instructor and student, especially when English is not the shared primary language. Difficulties may involve not understanding pronunciation of words and not fully understanding the meanings of words. All international students are required to complete the Test of English and Foreign Language (TOEFL), which is used as a screening and placement tool to determine language ability. The instructor can use the TOEFL score to gage language proficiency. The ANE also may conduct mini assignments early in the course to reveal difficulties the student may have in communication. Creating assignments that require the student to understand written or verbal instructions and produce a product verbally or in writing can be used to screen for communication problems.

The ANE and student nurse may also experience communication problems when English is the primary language of both parties. The words and phrases used when teaching and explaining concepts may not always be easily grasped by nursing students, especially early in their nursing program. Lack of familiarity with terminology coupled with a heighten stress response can contribute to misunderstandings. The ANE can implement a variety of strategies such as the pretraining principle and advance organizers discussed in Chapter 2, to enhance clarity and understanding of information. To determine the effectiveness of specific strategies, the ANE can use a variety of assessments such as (1) the RSQC2 activity in which the student is asked to recall, summarize, question, comment, and connect information presented in class, or (2) identify the muddiest point in a reading or presentation, or (3) have students submit a list of questions they have. These and other assessment strategies are available from Angelo & Cross (1993) and Silberman (1996), listed in the resource section.

Cultural groups can also differ in terms of time orientation, emphasizing either social or clock time. In the United States, adherence to clock time is valued and is the expectation for classroom and clinical attendance and job performance. Expectations concerning punctuality in terms of class attendance and assignments should be explained in writing in the syllabus and explained verbally during the first class meeting. Periodically, the expectations for attendance and submission of assignments may need to be repeated.

In cultural assessment, the concept of space refers to the physical distance and intimacy techniques used when communicating (Davidhizar & Shearer, 2005, p. 359). Cultural groups differ in the amount of personal space needed. Individuals with greater needs for personal space may show signs of anxiety in large crowded class-rooms or may back away if others approach too closely. Violation of a student's personal space can be distracting for the student and if severe enough, can be a source of anxiety leading to poor performance.

Each culture shares an emphasis on certain social organizations (such as school, church, family, employers) and on individuals who fulfill social roles in those organizations. Exposure to individuals within specific social organizations helps to shape the individual's values, beliefs, and expectations. For example, various cultures hold differing beliefs and expectations for men and women, old and young, wealthy and poor, and people with specific religious and political affiliations. Davidhizar and Shearer recommend using a simple student profile form to gather data about social organizations that are meaningful for the student. The ANE can use this background information to enhance understanding of the students as individuals, and provide meaningful examples and situations that relate to the learner's experiences.

The amount of environmental control that the student perceives can also have an impact on learning. How much control and whether the control is perceived as internal or external can influence the student's motivation, independent problem solving, and initiative (Davidhizar & Shearer, 2005, p. 360). Ginsberg (2005) also supports the importance of the learning environment for motivation noting that "classrooms are likely to be more effective in developing the capacity of students . . . if teachers understand how culture can shape learning and how teachers can develop classrooms that tap into the intrinsic motivation of culturally diverse learners" (p. 218). Students who perceive little control over their learning environmental may have less motivation to try to improve a situation because they perceive it as outside of their control or view the situation as fate.

Ginsberg's Framework for Culturally Responsive Teaching

According to Ginsberg (2005) a variety of cultural factors are important in the motivation of a student's learning. Furthermore, Ginsberg states that "Every instructional plan ought to be motivationally conceived from beginning to end" (p. 221). Factors such as "language, ethnic and racial history, experience with political and economic oppression, sense of opportunity, values, and perceptions converge in the (student's) response to teaching and learning" (p. 220).

To address the cultural influences on student motivation, Ginsberg (2005) developed a motivational framework for culturally responsive teaching. She identified four conditions that work together to support learning including: inclusion, competence, attitude, and meaning. Inclusion refers to creating a learning environment where both the teacher and student feel connected to one another and interact with a sense of respect. Competence refers to engaging in practices that help students be effective. This may involve providing clear criteria for achieving success and multiple ways to meet the criteria. Attitude involves creating a positive atmosphere where learning is relevant to students. This means a place where they can share experiences, opinions, and make choices about their learning experiences. The meaning component of the model involves challenging students to create meaning through active participation. Ginsberg sees all four components as stimulating the development of intrinsic motivation in students regardless of cultural affiliation.

Suggestions for teaching culturally diverse students are described in Table 3-4. These suggestions mirror the nursing process. Actions should be informed and founded on an assessment of students so that appropriate options can be implemented. The implementation of the actual teaching approaches should be reinforced verbally and in writing when teaching ESL students. Feedback from students is important in determining if the instruction is understood. However, in some cultures a more distant, authoritarian relationship with the teacher is the tradition. In these cases, students may need frequent encouragement to interact, share, and express opinions. The last three suggestions represent formal or informal options to provide support and interaction for students. According to Ginsberg "the response a person has to a learning activity reflects his or her cultural background, talents that have been nurtured, and peer group relations . . ." (2005, p. 223). The frameworks and suggestions provided in this section reflect these three aspects and can provide useful guidelines for teaching culturally diverse students.

High Achieving Students

Students with a GPA below a B level have been recognized as at risk for failing courses and also at risk for failing the licensure examination. However, students with a high GPA are also at risk. Rollant, who has authored several texts that focus on test taking, proposes that those with high GPA may fail NCLEX because they do not possess critical thinking skills needed to figure out the answer (Rollant, 2007). Because of their past success in school, high GPA students may not see the need for learning new critical thinking skills that will enable them to solve problems when they do not know all the answers.

For others, low test scores may be the result of high anxiety during testing. For these students Rollant (2007) offers the "Five Cs for Test Success," which the ANE can use to help students prepare for testing (Table 3-5).

TABLE 3-4 Recommendations for Teaching Culturally Diverse Students

Strategies	Rationale
1. Assess the student's traditional learning practices, expectations, and responses to teaching efforts.	• Obtaining baseline information will enable the ANE to be proactive in planning ways to meet the educational needs of students.
2. Use a variety of teaching strategies, not just the spoken word (p. 361).	• ESL students may not comprehend lecture and verbal discussion sessions as quickly as naturalized students. • Use print materials and media that can be played back to enhance comprehension. Encourage recording classroom lectures.
3. Solicit feedback and encourage in-person consultation.	• Some cultural groups may keep faculty/student interaction more distant and reserved. • Offer students frequent encouragement to ask questions in class and outside of class.
4. Offer a "Nursing Success" course.	• Course can address a variety of topics such as test taking, study habits, note taking, and time management (p. 361).
5. Encourage ESL students to join study groups and network with others classmates.	• Interaction with other classmates will reduce isolation. • Discussion with classmates may clarify expectations for assignments and tests.
6. Provide faculty and or student mentors.	• Students may be more comfortable asking questions in a one-on-one relationship with a faculty member who is not currently serving as their teacher. • Students may benefit from peer mentors who have worked through similar experiences.

Some data from Davidhizar, R., & Shearer, R. (2005). When your nursing student is culturally diverse. *The Health Care Manager, 24*(4), 361–362.

The ANE can use the 5 Cs to help students identify learning and testing strategies that will facilitate successful testing by asking them questions about (1) content, (2) confidence, (3) control, (4) common sense, and (5) comparison. The ANE may ask students to reflect on their knowledge of the content and their degree of confidence in what they know. The students' confidence may be reinforced by reminding them

TABLE 3-5   Using the Five Cs for Test Success

The 5 Cs	Questions to Ask the Student
Content	What test question topics or subject matter do you feel most comfortable answering?
Confidence	How confident are you that your response to a question is correct?
Control	During testing do you feel anxious? Bored? Tend to loose concentration? When do these tend to occur?
Common sense	Think about each test item response and determine if there one response that makes more sense than the others.
Comparison	For difficulty choosing between two responses ask how each response is different from the other.

Data from Rollant, P. (2007). "How can I fail the NCLEX-RN with a 3.5 GPA?" Approaches to help this unexpected high risk group. In M. Oermann & K. Heinrich (Eds.), *Annual review of nursing education volume 5, 2007: Challenges and new directions in nursing education* (pp. 259–273).

of what they have learned in terms of content and test taking skills. The third C deals with the learner's mental and emotional control during testing. Does the student feel anxious, upset, bored, or lose focus during testing? Identifying the presence of these feelings, as well as when these control issues occur during a test, can be helpful. Students who identify the timing of these control issues will be able to initiate relaxation and refocusing strategies appropriately. According to Rollant (2007), 90% of students experience boredom and loss of focus before reaching question number 35 (p. 267). Teaching students to do a simple physical activity when they reach their focus capacity, such as deep breathing or having them reposition themselves in their seat, will help them refocus.

The fourth C, common sense, is really directing the student to reflect, think, and use the information provided in the test question to identify the best response. Once the possible responses have been narrowed to two, the fifth C guides the student to compare responses. Often it is difficult for a student to choose the best response because she or he does not see the key difference between the responses or has not identified the key issue in the stem of the question that would help determine the correct response. During the process of reading the test question, specific strategies such as rewording the question, identifying the problem underlying the question, and then comparing options may be helpful. By looking at what is different about each response, the student's ability to select the best response may be enhanced (Rollant,

2007, p. 266). Teaching the student these test taking strategies boosts their confidence in their knowledge base and provides analytical skills that can be useful in adapting to clinical practice.

Developing content knowledge and confidence in that knowledge are ongoing processes that occur throughout the program. The remaining three Cs can be used early on in the nursing curriculum. Control, common sense, and compare strategies are test taking strategies that can be taught the first day and reinforced throughout the program.

Degree Completion Students

Facilitating learner development and socialization of RN to BSN students centers around expanding and enriching their professional roles and values. RN to BSN students already come to the learning environment with unique backgrounds and experiences in nursing. For these students, researchers Morris and Faulk (2007) found that transformative learning experiences that incorporate critical self-reflection and create cognitive dissonance or a conflict of values, were effective. The study was based on Mezirow's (1991) transformation theory, which views learning as occurring when the learner's perspective changes as a result of unexpected events. When unexpected events or dilemmas create cognitive dissonance, the ANE can encourage and guide the learner in the process of critical reflection to developing new understandings, insights, and ways of thinking. This is what Mezirow refers to as perspective transformation.

Other ways to promote perspective transformation may be as straightforward as integrating assignments for clinical and nonclinical experiences. Whenever the student is exposed to new situations, the ANE can encourage and guide them in conducting verbal or written self-reflection. Assignments such as attending and analyzing legislative sessions, participating in professional organizations, and discussing issues on professional listservs may provide experiences that serve as a stimulus for perspective transformation.

THEORY AND RESEARCH RELATED TO TEACHER ATTRIBUTES

Teacher attributes that are helpful in facilitating learner development and socialization to nursing include teaching styles, skills in academic advising and counseling, mentoring, and role modeling. In this section, each of these topics is discussed and suggestions for application to teaching practice are provided.

Teaching Styles

Grasha (2003) defined teaching style as the attitudes and behaviors that the teacher displays when interacting with learners. The five teaching styles developed by Grasha, which were initially discussed in Chapter 2, are also relevant for facilitating learner development and socialization. Grasha identified five distinct teaching styles using the One-on-One Teaching Style Inventory. The expert style focuses on the student's acquisition of knowledge and competence, and strives to maintain status as an expert in the subject matter. The teacher with senior status who is seen as an authority figure may function within the formal authority teaching style, which emphasizes established learning expectations and standards. The personal model style values teaching by personal example and showing the learner how to accomplish tasks. According to Grasha, the goal of the facilitator teaching style is to help the learner develop independence, initiative, and responsibility (2003, p. 186). The facilitator seeks to meet learning needs through interaction with students, by asking questions, and by exploring alternatives. The delegator is also concerned with the student developing initiative and responsibility. However, unlike the facilitator, the delegator assumes a less interactive approach, being available as a resource, and occasionally reviewing student's progress.

Realistically, students will have differing abilities and needs in terms of learner development and socialization. Therefore, awareness of a range of teaching styles will enable the ANE to provide teaching approaches which are congruent with student needs. As with learning styles, flexibility and adaptability in the use of teaching styles are keys to effective teaching practice.

Academic Advisement and Counseling Skills

Providing academic advising and counseling for students has great potential to impact the student's growth and development. In the advising relationship, the teacher guides and directs the student in selection of courses, and over time may develop a relationship in which they discuss nursing career options and role expectations of various nursing specialties. Sharing knowledge of role expectations with students can help prepare them for clinical practice and facilitate socialization nursing.

Bland (2004) draws several contrasts between two advising approaches, referred to as prescriptive and developmental, which facilitate socialization into nursing (Table 3-6). Prescriptive advising emphasizes course selection and meeting the requirements of the program of study. The relationship between the advisor and student focuses on solutions for academic problems and is unidirectional with advice flowing from the

TABLE 3-6	Comparison of Prescriptive and Developmental Advising	
	Prescriptive Advising	**Developmental Advising**
Goals	Focused on problem solving and meeting registration requirements	Focused on student's life and career goals
Nature of advising sessions	Unidirectional relationship Advisor controls the agenda	Mutual responsibility and empowerment

Data from Bland, S. (2004). Advising adults: Telling or coaching? *Adult Learning, 14*(2), 6–9.

faculty to the student. Developmental advising uses a holistic approach with the goal to empower the student to achieve personal, academic, and career success. The relationship between the student and advisor is one of shared responsibility, which requires ongoing communication, whereas prescriptive advising is more advisor directed and controlled (p. 7). The developmental advising approach facilitates the growth and development of the student and facilitates the learner's socialization to nursing (Bland, 2004).

A comprehensive advising program incorporates both developmental and prescriptive activities. Prescriptive advising includes scheduling classes, selecting courses, and designing of a program of study. Developmental advising includes tasks such as exploring career goals, life goals, values, abilities, interests, and limitations (Freeman, 2008, p.13).

Implementing a Developmental Advising Approach

Advising practices typically reflect the institution's orientation, mission, and philosophy. Implementation of an advising approach is also influenced by structural support and resources for advisors. Bland (2004) suggests that building a developmental advising system is a crucial element of the developmental advisor's role. Faculty advisors need to work within the governing structure of the institution to incorporate developmental advising in the institution's mission and philosophy statements, and in the institution's ongoing strategic plan.

Institutions that wish to adopt a developmental advising infrastructure from the ground up may find the processes used by other institutions helpful. One example of the formation of a developmental advising structure occurred at a community college in Florida. They used a five-stage conceptual model, referred to as LifeMap, to reorganize the support services and programs and to engage faculty, staff, and students in an environment that focused on career and educational planning (Shugart & Romano, 2006). Using the LifeMap model the faculty, staff, and college resources were integrated into a system that fostered interaction yet allowed the student to become more self-sufficient in managing their educational information.

On a smaller scale, if the institutional infrastructure already supports developmental advising, that approach may be implemented by simply educating faculty about its key components. Whatever the nature of the advising system, having a structure for decision making, problem solving, and communication is helpful. The American Association of Colleges and Universities studied the practices of 16 universities and identified seven principles of advising excellence:

1. Aim high.
2. Give students a compass.
3. Teach the art of inquiry and innovation.
4. Engage the big questions.
5. Connect knowledge with choices and action.
6. Foster civic, intercultural, and ethical learning.
7. Assess students' ability to apply learning to complex problems (LEAP, 2008).

These principles represent a shift from emphasis on "course categories and titles to the quality and level of work students are actually expected to accomplish" (LEAP, 2008, p. 7). The first principle, "aim high," refers to seeking excellence by using learning outcomes as a framework for the student's program of study and linking education to the student's work and life experiences. Giving the students a compass refers to using the learning outcomes to guide the student's program of study and providing mechanisms for assessing student progress in achieving those outcomes. Principle 3 values the importance of thinking and creative processes in learning. The remaining principles relate to the student's application of knowledge and skills to issues outside the classroom. Principle 4, "engage the big picture" emphasizes learning from a broader scope by exploring "far-reaching and enduring issues" (p. 5). The next principle, "connect knowledge with choices and action," focuses on preparing the student for life in the work world by learning about real-world problems. The importance of developing personal and social responsibility is reflected in Principle 6. For this principle, learning opportunities are provided that enable the learner to integrate cultural and ethical components into real world situations. The final principle ensures that learning opportunities are provided to assess the student's ability to engage in complex problem solving. The principles are designed to be applied "by any college, community college, or university. They are intended to influence practice across disciplines, as well as in general education programs" (LEAP, 2008, p. 7).

Role Modeling and Mentoring

Role modeling and mentoring by nurse educators are effective teaching practices to enhance learner development and socialization. Educators are involved in modeling professional behaviors to students either intentionally through deliberate mentoring actions; or unintentionally through passive observation. Role modeling is discussed further in Chapter 2 (see Bandura's Theory of Social Learning).

According to McKinley (2004), the mentoring process follows progressive stages referred to as the three R's; reflection, reframing, and resolving (Table 3-7). During the reflection stage, active listening, sharing personal background information, and taking time to get to know the mentee are foundational activities. Later, the reflection stage expands to include reviewing experiences that the mentor and mentee have shared and asking open-ended questions about the mentee's perception of the experience. The mentor may demonstrate skills or techniques, give constructive feedback, or share personal experiences with the mentee. The next stage in the mentoring process, called reframing, is more deeply interactive. In this stage the mentor encourages new ways of problem solving and goal setting that enable the mentee to move to the resolving stage with greater understanding and more options. Resolving is "empowering the individual to problem solve and identify progress toward positive outcomes" (p. 209).

By using the three R's as a guide, the ANE can develop and maintain a successful mentoring relationship. As the ANE embarks on a mentoring relationship, the emphasis should be on gaining understanding of the mentee. This process is facilitated

TABLE 3-7   The Three Rs of Mentoring

Mentoring Processes	Definition
Reflection	Introductory phase of relationship characterized by information sharing, establishing ground rules, setting goals, and sharing past experiences
Reframing	The working phase characterized by giving feedback and challenging the mentee
Resolving	Involves using new ways of thinking to problem solve and develop a plan for taking action

Data from McKinley, M. G. (2004). Mentoring matters: Creating, connecting, empowering. *AACN Clinical Issues, 15*, 205–214.

by asking the mentee appropriate reflective questions about his or her experiences. As the ANE learns how the mentee thinks and responds to situations, the mentee can be assisted in reframing situations. This enables the mentee to respond and resolve situations differently. The reframing process assists the mentee in understanding the experience and viewing the situation or problem from an alternative perspective. As the mentee acquires new insights and understandings of the situation, the ANE's role as mentor shifts to assisting the mentee to set new goals, problem solve, and implement strategies to achieve the new goals.

THEORY AND RESEARCH RELATED TO CONTENT

Educators and professional regulatory agencies have traditionally placed great emphasis on the content knowledge required for effective nursing practice. Accreditation organizations have established criteria that describe successful program outcomes, and licensure organizations have developed test blueprints delineating content emphasis for RN licensure. In addition, researchers have surveyed the major practice settings to determine competencies needed for specific practice areas. In this section guidelines from accreditation and licensure organizations and researchers will be explored. Each of these sources serves as a guide for nursing program content that will ultimately enhance learner development and socialization.

Essential Content for Nursing Education

The American Association of Colleges of Nursing has established the Essentials for Baccalaureate Education for Professional Nursing Practice which describes nine essentials for practice-focused outcomes (AACN, 2008). The National Council of State Boards of Nursing (2006) has developed a test plan that reflects knowledge deemed essential for safe nursing practice. Each set of guidelines shares commonalities and differences (Table 3-8). For example, both detail a strong emphasis on direct patient care, health promotion, and communication. Differences relate predominantly to the broader scope of education required of baccalaureate students compared with the basic expectations for all levels of RN preparation. In addition to the competencies and outcomes established by national nursing organizations, many individual state boards of nursing have established entry level competencies. These entry level competencies reflect another type of outcome that nursing programs must evaluate. Typically, state board of nursing competencies are integrated into the program's evaluation plan with documentation of achievement required upon completion of the program. Check the Web site of your state board of nursing for specific competency requirements.

TABLE 3-8   Guidelines for Nursing Program Content

AACN Essentials for Baccalaureate Education	NCSBN Test Content Categories for RN Licensure*
1. Liberal Education	1. Safe and Effective Care Environment, Management of Care, and Safety and Infection Control
2. Organizational and Systems Leadership for Quality Care and Patient Safety	2. Health Promotion and Maintenance
3. Scholarship for Evidence-based Practice	3. Psychosocial Integrity
4. Information Management and Application of Patient Care Technology	4. Physiological Integrity: – Basic Comfort Care – Pharmacological and Parenteral Therapies – Reduction of Risk Potential
5. Health Care Policy, Finance, and Regulatory Environments	5. Physiological Adaptation
6. Interprofessional Communication and Collaboration	* Nursing process, Caring, Communication, Documentation, and Teaching-Learning processes are integrated into each category.
7. Clinical Prevention and Population Health	
8. Professionalism and Professional Values	
9. Generalist Nursing Practice	

Data from American Association of Colleges of Nursing. (2008, October). *Essentials of baccalaureate education for professional nursing practice.* Available from http://www.aacn.nche.edu/education/pdf/BaccEssentials08.pdf, pp. 3–4; and National Council of State Boards of Nursing. (2006). *NCLEX-RN Test plan for the national council licensure examination for registered nurses.* Available from https://www.ncsbn.org/RN_Test_Plan_2007_Web.pdf.

Research on Nursing Competencies

As the healthcare environment and patient demographics change, the learning needs and competencies for nursing practice also have evolved. In a survey of hospital, nursing home, and home care agency administrators, Utley-Smith (2004) found that competencies of nursing staff clustered into six categories: (1) health promotion, (2) direct care, (3) interpersonal communication, (4) supervision, (5) computer technology, and (6) case load management. Interestingly, administrators at each setting rated health promotion, direct care, and interpersonal communication as most important. The other competencies varied in importance depending on the setting. Nursing home administrators valued supervision more than hospital and home care agencies, and hospital administrators valued computer and caseload management competencies more than nursing home and home care agency administrators. Facilitating students' development of knowledge and skills in each competency area will help ensure students develop the skill sets needed for socialization to the role expectations for specific practice settings.

Teaching Affective Content

The cognitive, psychomotor, and affective learning domains serve as a framework for course and program objectives and outcomes, as well as individual learning goals. Educators typically emphasize cognitive and psychomotor domains of learning that are easily measurable. However, learning in the affective domain is equally important because it impacts the student's philosophy, values, and manner of interaction with clients and families. Furthermore, affective learning has a great impact on the student's ability to socialize into nursing practice.

By incorporating learning objectives, assignments, and experiences that address progressively higher-order affective knowledge and skills, the ANE can facilitate the student's development and socialization into nursing. According to Van Valkenburg and Holden "the purpose of teaching and learning in the affective domain is to assist the learner in internalizing desirable professional and humanistic characteristics" (2004, p. 347). They point out that the affective domain is linked to the cognitive domain. Although "cognition stimulates active thinking," affective processes are "the psychological processes that reorganize learned structures as a result of the interaction" (p. 347). This interrelationship forms the basis for critical thinking and action learning. Affective learning manifests in behaviors, values, beliefs, and attitudes that are not easily quantified but serve as a foundation for clinical decision making, communication, and interpersonal relationships.

Learning in the affective domain is particularly relevant to the learner's development and socialization as it reflects the learner's values and beliefs. Krathwohl, Bloom, & Masia (1964) outlined a taxonomy for the affective domain that reflects progressive higher-order affective learning. The taxonomy progresses from the receiving level which includes passive involvement, to the characterization level which includes integration and internalization of new values and behaviors. The affective learning taxonomy and examples of objectives are presented in Table 3-9.

TABLE 3-9   Affective Learning Taxonomy and Examples of Objectives

Affective Taxonomy Level	Examples of Learning Objectives
Receiving: 1. Awareness 2. Willingness to receive 3. Acquiescence	1. Develops awareness of cultural differences 2. Appreciates cultural diversity 3. Follows recommendations for providing culturally sensitive care
Responding: 1. Willingness to respond 2. Satisfaction in response	1. Takes actions to acquaint self with social issues 2. Enjoys providing health education to the under privileged
Valuing: 1. Acceptance 2. Preference 3. Commitment	1. Continuously displays a desire to understand the experiences of the homeless 2. Deliberately examines a variety of viewpoints on a controversial topic with the intent of forming opinions about them (p. 181) 3. Demonstrates commitment to perform nursing care of vulnerable clients with respect and integrity
Organization: 1. Conceptualization of a value 2. Organization of a value system	1. Identifies personal attributes of professional behavior 2. Evaluates alternative policies for healthcare access
Characterization by a value or value complex: 1. Generalized set 2. Characterization	1. Responds to ethical dilemmas by applying principles 2. Demonstrates behaviors consistent with professional nursing practice

Some data from Krathwohl, D. R., Bloom, B., & Masia, B. B. (1964). *Taxonomy of educational objectives. The classification of educational goals handbook II: Affective domain.* New York: David McKay Co.

A major aspect of affective learning is reflected in the professional and ethical behavior of students. Professionalism is the milieu through which practitioners become socialized to their profession. Cruess and Cruess (2006) discuss the processes and principles involved in teaching professionalism to students. They emphasize two processes that are necessary for teaching this content effectively. First, provide foundational cognitive knowledge of professionalism, including definitions, understanding the characteristics of professional behavior, and the obligations inherent in being a professional (p. 205). The second process for teaching students' professionalism is to provide "opportunities for internalization of values and behaviors" (p. 205). Providing role modeling of professionalism and ample opportunities for the student to engage in self-reflection on their clinical experiences and observations is essential. Cruess and Cruess also emphasize that instruction and opportunities to internalize aspects of professionalism should be ongoing and included throughout the curriculum. This integration will provide "growth of both explicit and tacit knowledge of professionalism . . . in parallel with growth of knowledge in other areas" (p. 206).

Cruess and Cruess describe the use of several principles embedded in situational learning theory as useful in guiding students to establish a professional role. Situational learning theory holds that "learning should be embedded in authentic activities which help transform knowledge from the abstract and theoretical to the usable and useful" (2006, p. 205). This principle emphasizes the value of a cognitive knowledge base as well as opportunities for experiential learning. Self-reflection is a major aspect of experiential learning that warrants a separate principle. Therefore, Cruess and Cruess note that "Self-reflection . . . is essential to the acquisition of experiential learning" (p. 205).

THEORY AND RESEARCH RELATED TO TEACHING STRATEGIES

Socialization to the nursing profession is concerned with providing students with knowledge, skills, and values that will help them effectively deal with issues that arise in clinical practice. Teaching strategies that expose the learner to real-world situations, build upon foundational knowledge, utilize problem-solving skills, and emphasize affective or value-oriented learning will help prepare the learner to function in nursing practice. Several teaching strategies that emphasize these aspects are presented in the following section, including problem-based learning, self-reflection, peer review, and service learning. This is not an exhaustive list of options but will provide a starting point for ANEs who wish to provide greater emphasize on learner development and socialization.

Problem-Based Learning

One approach originally used in medical education to enhance cognitive learning is problem-based learning (PBL). PBL is an instructor-facilitated, learner-directed approach characterized by the use of patient problems as a focus for student problem solving, small group work, and self-directed study. Many studies have found that using PBL enhances cognitive learning and critical thinking skills (Beers, 2005; Brown, Matthew-Maich, & Royle, 2001; Hmelo-Silver, 2004; Johnson & Finucane, 2000; Lyons, 2008; Williams, 2001; Zubaidah, 2005). PBL has been found equally effective as lecture in terms of student learning (Beers, 2005). Furthermore, long-term knowledge retention was found to be significantly higher for PBL students (Beers & Bowden, 2005). In addition to enhancing cognitive learning and critical thinking, PBL can provide a useful problem-solving framework that can carried forward into the student's clinical practice. An overview of the steps involved in implementing PBL is provided in Chapter 2.

Self-Reflection

Self-reflection is a useful way to facilitate affective learning, which is beneficial in learner development and socialization. Hydo, Marcyjanik, Zorn, and Hooper (2007) used a teaching strategy they referred to as "art as scaffolding" to provide self-reflection and self-exploration about nursing. As part of a first semester nursing course students were asked to use an art form of their choice (for example, music, poetry, drawing, dance, sculpture, story telling) to express what nursing was for them. They responded to a series of reflective questions and shared their art and responses in small groups. At the conclusion of the presentations, students identified things they learned about themselves in creating their presentation and things they learned from other students' presentations. The authors concluded that the process provided self-reflective learning that help students make mental links to different ideas.

The ANE can easily generate other types of reflective assignments that provide opportunities for learner development and socialization. For example, the ANE can identify topics for the student to use to explore personal learning experiences and future learning needs. Or the ANE can compose specific questions for students to respond to, related to learning and socialization to the role of nursing. Poirrier (1997) suggests the use of a dialectic format for writing. On one side of a page the student takes notes on readings or lecture material and on the other side provides comments on the notes in the form of analysis, further questions, or insights (p. 45). This activity can focus on a specific topic area or on an area of the student's choice and can be completed in class or as a homework assignment. Poirrier emphasizes that students should be familiarized with the benefits of written activities on learning including helping them understand "content, enhance their critical thinking, communication skills, and problem solving in practice settings" (p. 46). Furthermore, knowledge and insights from reflective writing can provide useful feedback that facilitates the student's personal growth.

Service Learning

Service learning is a teaching strategy that provides opportunities for application of classroom knowledge to real world settings. Bailey, Carpenter, & Harrington defined service learning as "a structured, reciprocal learning experience that combines and connects the service experience to academic coursework" (2002, p. 434). Although similar in some respects to student clinical practicums, Bailey and colleagues emphasize that service learning requires student reflection and reciprocity of learning between the student and agency partners. Components of service learning are summarized in Box 3-4.

Service learning is not a new pedagogy. In 1916, Dewey in his classic text, *Democracy and Education*, discussed the value of connecting service and education. Since then, service-learning experiences have been successfully implemented in a wide range of community settings such as a homeless shelter (Hunt, 2007), a community clinic (Carter & Dunn, 2002), a college campus (White, 1999), a Head Start program (Kulewicz, 2001), and faith-based community organizations (Herman & Sassatelli, 2002). Service learning has been implemented in all levels of higher education from community colleges (Holloway, 2002) through graduate level programs (Logsdon & Ford, 1998; Narsavage, Lindell, Chen, Savrin, & Duffy, 2002). Furthermore, implementation of service learning in nursing is not limited to service or clinical-related courses. Rash (2005) reports on the successful implementation of service learning in an undergraduate nursing research course. Throughout the

---

BOX 3-4   Components of Service Learning

Service learning:

1. Is experiential.

2. Addresses human and community needs.

3. Incorporates student reflection.

4. Is based on reciprocity between student and service-learning provider.

Data from Bailey, P. A., Carpenter, D. R., & Harrington, P. (2002). Theoretical foundations of service-learning in nursing education. *Journal of Nursing Education, 41*, 433–436.

course students collaborated with a community agency and completed written assignments, which culminated in a research project for the assigned community agency.

A large body of research in the late 1990s supports the positive effects of service-learning on students (Astin & Sax, 1998; Astin, Vogelgesang, Ikeda, & Yee, 2000; Gelmon, Holland, & Shinnamon, 1998; and Greene, 1998). In 2002, an entire issue of the *Journal of Nursing Education* was devoted to service learning. In the report of a faith-based service learning project, Herman & Sassatelli (2002) found that the students' critical thinking and insight increased and they developed an "expanded sense of self and community" (p. 444). In a service-learning partnership with a community health center, students focused on enhancing diabetes services to the community. As a result of the project, Carter & Dunn noted improved communication and collaboration between the students and health center staff (2002, para. 13). Other effects of service learning such as emotional learning, cross-cultural learning, and transformative learning have been reported (Hunt, 2007). Hunt conducted a service-learning project with undergraduate students and a homeless shelter. Interviews with students revealed that the service-learning component helped them establish relationships with persons outside the traditional scope of practice and broadened their perspective of nursing. As noted by these studies, service learning has a strong record of enhancing student knowledge and skills, and engaging them in diverse, yet real-world learning situations.

THEORY AND RESEARCH RELATED TO THE LEARNING ENVIRONMENT

One of the tasks of the ANE is to actively create positive learning environments and assist students in reframing their experiences in a positive light. The learning environment consists of physical and psychosocial aspects important when providing learning and developmental experiences for students. Environments that are too stressful, hostile, or do not provide positive learning experiences can be mitigated in numerous ways. In this section, the development and piloting of two innovative programs that created positive learning environments are highlighted. These initiatives may provide guidance or insights for the ANE who is seeking to modify the learning environment.

Partners in Practice

Educators at Ohio State University developed, implemented, and evaluated a program that met the needs of two different levels of nursing students (Daley, Menke,

Kirkpatrick & Sheets, 2008). The Partners in Practice program involved partnering senior nursing students in a leadership-management course with a faculty teaching a clinical group of first-year students. The leadership-management student was involved in overseeing patient care, assisting students with problem solving and prioritizing care through communication and sharing of their thinking processes. This partnership provided the opportunity for senior students to gain skills in organization, prioritization, troubleshooting, documenting, chart review, reporting, and addressing family needs. The seniors also gained experience in leadership-management skills such as mentoring the first-year students, dealing with role conflict, delegation, boundary issues, and following the chain of command. First-year students reported that the senior partners helped them focus on critical thinking about their patients, helped them refine their communication with patients, family, and staff, and gain more confidence in nursing knowledge and skills. The researchers found that the partners in practice program helped both levels of students to develop and refine clinical practice skills that can be carried forward into clinical practice after graduation.

Mindfulness-Based Stress Reduction Program

Another approach to creating a positive learning environment is the implementation of a mindfulness-based stress reduction (MBSR) program. The MBSR approach uses meditation and mindfulness techniques that enhance the student's ability to self-reflect, engage in self-care activities, and face difficult situations with less avoidance. In a meta-analysis of 20 studies on MBSR, participants improved their coping skills in both clinical and nonclinical situations (Grossman, Niemann, Schmidt, & Walsh, 2004). Improvement in ability to cope with clinical stressors can go a long way toward facilitating socialization to the profession. According to Shirey (2007), faculty who teach students an evidence-based strategy such as mindfulness early in their nursing program may "instill the necessary personal coping skills required for creating healthy learning and practice environments" (p. 570).

CONCLUSION

Facilitating learner development and socialization involves preparing students for the demands of nursing practice and easing the transition from student to nurse. This competency is also concerned with fostering the effective application of knowledge and skills acquired during the nursing program to nursing practice. Facilitating the development of affective dispositions needed to ease the student's transition from student to nurse and facilitation of ongoing professional development is emphasized. The ANE realizes the importance of blending of the student's cognitive, psychomotor, and affective knowledge and skills. To achieve this the ANE attends to attributes within the learner and teacher that influence development and socialization. The ANE also considers the influence of teaching strategies, subject matter content, and learning environment when developing and implementing a program of study.

SUMMARY

- Facilitating learner development and socialization involves helping the student acquire knowledge and skills needed to effectively transition to the role of professional nursing.
- A variety of theories and models are useful in facilitating learner development and socialization including andragogy, Bandura's Social Learning Theory, Benner's Novice to Expert Theory, and moral development theories.
- In teaching from an andragogical perspective, the ANE uses the processes of role modeling, questioning, and self-reflection.
- Social Learning Theory identifies factors important in determining whether or not a student will repeat an observed behavior.
- Benner's Novice to Expert Theory identifies 5 progressive stages of development in nursing including novice, advanced beginner, competent, proficient, and expert.
- Theories of moral development can be useful for understanding student's behavior and for planning ways to assist students' moral development.
- According to Kohlberg's (1981) theory of moral development, individuals progress through three levels of moral development: (1) preconventional, (2) conventional, and (3) postconventional. Each level is characterized by specific patterns of thinking and behaving.
- Gilligan's Theory of Moral Development emphasizes how moral development of women is achieved.
- According to Rest's Theory of Morality, moral judgment is fostered by awareness of the broader social context and the individual's relationship within society.
- Reflective learning opportunities broaden the students' awareness of their interrelationships with society and enhance their professional development and socialization into nursing.
- Characteristics that the student brings to the learning situation such as communication skills and cultural background can affect the student's development and socialization to the profession.

- The Joint Commission recommends teaching students the SBAR communication framework to enhance effective communication in practice. SBAR stands for Situation, Background, Assessment, and Recommendations.
- Aspects of Giger-Davidhizar's Model of Transcultural Assessment can be used to assess students and adapt teaching approaches. The model considers (1) communication, (2) time orientation, (3) space or distance preferences during interactions, (4) values and beliefs of influential social organizations, and (5) the amount of personal control the individual feels over the environment.
- Facilitating learner development and socialization of the RN to BSN student centers around expanding and enriching his or her professional roles and values.
- Mezirow's Transformative Learning Theory emphasizes understanding prior experiences and determining the meaning of those experiences.
- Teacher attributes that are helpful in facilitating learner development and socialization to nursing include teaching styles, skills in academic advising, counseling, mentoring, and role modeling.
- Providing developmental academic advising and counseling for students has great potential to impact the student's growth and development.
- Sharing knowledge of role expectations with students can help prepare them for clinical practice and facilitate socialization nursing.
- Role modeling and mentoring are effective teaching practices to enhance learner development and socialization.
- As the healthcare environment and patient demographics change, the learning needs and competencies for nursing practice have also evolved.
- Facilitating students' development of knowledge and skills in each competency area will help ensure students develop the skill sets needed for socialization to the role functions of today's practicing nurses.
- By incorporating learning objectives, assignments, and experiences that address progressively higher-order affective knowledge and skills, the ANE can facilitate the student's development and socialization into nursing.
- A major aspect of affective learning is reflected in professional and ethical behavior of students.
- Teaching strategies that expose the learner to real-world situations, build on foundational knowledge, utilize problem-solving skills, and emphasize affective or learning will help prepare the student to function in nursing practice.
- Teaching strategies that facilitate learner development and socialization to the profession include problem-based learning, self-reflection, peer review, and service learning.
- Problem-based learning is equally as effective as lecture in terms of student learning.

- The learning environment consists of physical and psychosocial aspects important when providing learning and developmental experiences for students.
- Two program initiatives designed to enhance the learning environment for students include the Partners in Practice program and the Mindfulness-Based Stress Reduction Program.

RECOMMENDED RESOURCES

Academic Advising

- The National Academic Advising Association (NACADA) is a membership organization focused on promoting quality advising in higher education. Visit the Web site at http://www.nacada.ksu.edu/index.htm for more information and to access the free online newsletter *Academic Advising Today*.
- Penn State publishes a free online journal entitled *The Mentor: An Academic Advising Journal*. Available at http://www.psu.edu/dus/mentor/.
- Learn and Serve America's National Service Learning Clearinghouse provides a newsletter, listserv discussion, full text e-library of resources on service learning, and more. Available at http://www.servicelearning.org/index.php.

Ethics in Education

- Explore the Center for the Study of Ethics in the Professions at the Illinois Institute of Technology Web site at http://ethics.iit.edu/index.html to learn about ethics across the curriculum, access publications, and conference presentations.
- The Society for Values in Higher Education at http://www.svhe.org/ focuses on ethical issues in higher education and promotes the study of these issues though its publications and events. Click publications to view and download the SHVE publications, member publications, and access a monthly newsletter.

Teaching Strategies

- The National Center for Case Study Teaching in Science at http://ublib.buffalo.edu/libraries/projects/cases/case.html contains numerous case studies with teacher's notes that can be used to foster learner development, and articles to help faculty design and implement case studies.

- Learn more about problem-based learning as a strategy to promote student development. The Interdisciplinary Journal of Problem-Based Learning at http://www.ijpbl.org/ provides free, full-text articles on theory, research, and implementation of PLB.
- Learn more about the SBAR communication framework for healthcare providers. An SBAR Tool Kit is available through the Arizona Hospital and Healthcare Association Web site at http://www.azhha.org/patient_safety/documents/SBARtoolkit_000.pdf.
- A variety of active learning and assessment strategies that can be used to enhance learner development and socialization may be found in the book, *Classroom Assessment Techniques* by Angelo and Cross (1993) and Silberman's (1996) *Active Learning: 101 Strategies to Teach Any Subject.*

REFERENCES

1. Allen, J. (2003). Fostering ethical competence in nursing education. *Clinical Research and Regulatory Affairs, 20*(4), 373–377.
2. American Association of Colleges of Nursing. (2008, October). *Essentials of baccalaureate education for professional nursing practice.* Retrieved March 30, 2009 from http://www.aacn.nche.edu/education/pdf/BaccEssentials08.pdf
3. Angelo, T. A., & Cross, K. P. (1993). *Classroom assessment techniques: A handbook for college teachers.* San Francisco, CA: Jossey-Bass Publishing.
4. Astin, A. W., & Sax, L. J. (1998). How undergraduates are affected by service participation. *Journal of College Student Development, 39,* 251–263.
5. Astin, A. W., Vogelgesang, L. J., Ikeda, E. K. & Yee, J. A. (2000). *How service learning affects students.* Higher Education Research Institute, University of California. Retrieved on March 9, 2009 from http://www.gseis.ucla.edu/heri/PDFs/HSLAS/HSLAS.PDF
6. Bailey, P. A., Carpenter, D. R., & Harrington, P. (2002). Theoretical foundations of service-learning in nursing education. *Journal of Nursing Education, 41,* 433–436.
7. Bandura, A. (1977). *Social learning theory.* Englewood Cliffs, NJ: Prentice Hall.
8. Baxter, P., & Boblin, S. (2007). The moral development of baccalaureate nursing students: Understanding unethical behavior in classroom and clinical settings. *Journal of Nursing Education, 46*(1), 20–27.
9. Begley, A. (2006). Facilitating the development of moral insight in practice: Teaching ethics and teaching virtue. *Nursing Philosophy, 7,* 257–265.
10. Benner, P. (1984). *From novice to expert. Excellence and power in clinical nursing practice.* Menlo Park, CA: Addison-Wesley.
11. Beers, G. (2005). The effect of teaching method on objective test scores: Problem-based learning versus lecture. *Journal of Nursing Education, 44*(7), 305–309.
12. Beers, G., & Bowen, S. (2005). The effect of teaching method on long-term knowledge retention. *Journal of Nursing Education, 44*(11), 511–514.

13. Bland, S. (2004). Advising adults: Telling or coaching? *Adult Learning, 14*(2), 6–9.

14. Brown, B., Matthew-Maich, N., & Royle, J. (2001). Fostering reflection and reflective practice. In E. Rideout (Ed.), *Transform nursing education through problem-based learning* (pp. 119–164). Sudbury, MA: Jones and Bartlett.

15. Carter, J., & Dunn, B. (2002). A service-learning partnership for enhanced diabetes management. *Journal of Nursing Education, 41*(10), 450–452.

16. Cruess, R., & Cruess, S. (2006). Teaching professionalism: General principles. *Medical Teacher, 28*(3), 205–208.

17. Daley, L. K., Menke, E., Kirkpatrick, B., & Sheets, D. (2008). Partners in practice: A win-win model of clinical education. *Journal of Nursing Education, 47*(1), 30–32.

18. Davidhizar, R., & Shearer, R. (2005). When your nursing student is culturally diverse. *The Health Care Manager, 24*(4), 356–363.

19. Dewey, J. (1916). *Democracy and education.* New York: Macmillan.

20. Duckett, L. J., & Ryden, M. B. (1994). Education for ethical nursing practice. In J. Rest, & D. Narvaez (Eds.), *Moral development in the profession,* (pp. 51–69). Hillside, NJ: Erlbaum.

21. Freeman, L. (2008, Winter). Establishing effective advising practices to influence student learning and success. *Peer Review, 10*(1), 12–14.

22. Gelmon, S., Holland, B., & Shinnamon, A. (1998). *Health professions schools in service to the nation: 1996–1998 final evaluation report.* San Francisco: Pew Health Professions Commission.

23. Gilligan, C. (1982). *In a different voice: Psychological theory and women's development.* London: Harvard University Press.

24. Ginsberg, M. B. (2005). Cultural diversity, motivation, and differentiation. *Theory Into Practice, 44*(3), 218–225.

25. Grasha, A. (2003, July/August). The dynamics of one-on-one teaching. *The Social Studies,* 179–187.

26. Greene, D. (1998). Student perceptions of aging and disability as influenced by service learning. *Physical and Occupational Therapy in Geriatrics, 15*(3), 39–55.

27. Grossman, P., Niemann, L., Schmidt, S., & Walsh, H. (2004). Mindfulness based stress reduction and health benefits: A meta-analysis. *Journal of Psychosomatic Research, 57*(1), 35–43.

28. Herman, C., & Sassatelli, J. (2002). DARING to reach the heartland: A collaborative faith-based partnership in nursing education. *Journal of Nursing Education, 41*(10), 443–445.

29. Hmelo-Silver, C. (2004). Problem-based learning: What and how do students learn? *Educational Psychology Review, 16*(3), 235–266.

30. Holloway, A. S. (2002). Service-learning in community college nursing education. *Journal of Nursing Education, 41*(10), 440–442.

31. Hunt, R. (2007). Service-learning: An eye-opening experience that provokes emotion and challenges stereotypes. *Journal of Nursing Education, 46*(6), 277–281.

32. Hydo, S. K., Marcyjanik, D. L., Zorn, C. R., & Hooper, N. M. (2007). Art as a scaffolding teaching strategy in baccalaureate nursing education. *International Journal of Nursing Education Scholarship, 4*(1), 1–13.

33. Johnson, S., & Finucane, P. (2000). The emergence of problem-based learning in medical education. *Journal of Evaluation in Clinical Practice, 6,* 281–291.

34. Johnson, S. A., & Martin, M. (2005). Academic dishonesty: A new twist to and old problem. *Athletic Therapy Today, 10*(4), 48–50.

35. The Joint Commission on Accreditation of Healthcare Organizations. (2006). *Meeting the joint commission's 2007 national patient safety goals* Oakbrook Terrace, IL: Joint Commission Resources.

36. Knowles, M. (1990). *The adult learner: A neglected species.* Houston, TX: Gulf Publishing Co.

37. Kohlberg, L. (1981). *Essays on moral development: Vol 1. The philosophy of moral development: Moral stages and the idea of justice.* San Francisco: Harper & Row.

38. Kohlberg, L., & Hersh, R. H. (1977). Moral development: A review of the theory. *Theory into Practice, 16*(2), 53–59.

39. Kolanko, K. M., Clark, C., Heinrich, K. T., Olive, D., Serembus, J. F., & Sifford, K. S. (2006). Academic dishonesty, bullying, incivility, and violence: Difficult challenges facing nurse educators. *Nursing Education Perspectives, 27*(1), 34–43.

40. Krathwohl, D. R., Bloom, B., & Masia, B. B. (1964). *Taxonomy of educational objectives. The classification of educational goals handbook II: Affective domain.* New York: David McKay Co.

41. Kulewicz, S. J. (2001). Service-learning: Head start and a baccalaureate nursing curriculum working together. *Pediatric Nursing, 27*(1), 34–37.

42. LEAP. (2008). *College learning for the new global century: A report from the national leadership council for liberal education & America's promise.* Executive summary. Washington, DC: Association of American Colleges and Universities. Retrieved Dec 16, 2008 from https://www.aacu.org/leap/documents/GlobalCentury_ExecSum_3.pdf.

43. Logsdon, M., & Ford, D. (1998). Service learning for graduate students. *Nurse Educator, 23*(2), 27–34.

44. Lyons, E. (2008). Examining the effects of problem-based learning and NCLEX-RN scores on the critical thinking skills of associate degree nursing students in a southeastern community college. *International Journal of Nursing Education Scholarship, 5*(1), art.21. Available at: http://www.bepress.com/ijnes/vol5/iss1/art21.

45. McKinley, M. G. (2004). Mentoring matters: Creating, connecting, empowering. *AACN Clinical Issues, 15,* 205–214.

46. Mezirow, J. (1991). *Transformative dimensions of adult learning.* San Francisco: Jossey-Bass.

47. Mezirow, J. (2000). *Learning as transformation: Critical perspectives on a theory in progress.* San Francisco: Jossey Bass.

48. Morris, A., & Faulk, D. (2007). Perspective transformation: Enhancing the development of professionalism in RN-to-BSN students. *Journal of Nursing Education, 46*(10), 445–451.

49. Narsavage, G. L., Lindell, D., Chen, Y., Savrin, C., & Duffy E. (2002). A community engagement initiative: Service-learning in graduate nursing education. *Journal of Nursing Education, 41*(10), 457–461.

50. National Council of State Boards of Nursing. (2006). *NCLEX-RN test plan for the national council licensure examination for registered nurses.* Retrieved April 4, 2009 from https://www.ncsbn.org/RN_Test_Plan_2007_Web.pdf.

51. National League for Nursing, Task Group on Nurse Educator Competencies. (2005). *Core competencies of nurse educators with task statements.* Retrieved September 10, 2008 from http://www.nln.org/facultydevelopment/pdf/corecompetencies.pdf.

52. Paul, R. (1993). Ethics without indoctrination. Retrieved April 4, 2009, from http://www.criticalthinking.org/articles/ethics-wo-indoctrination.cfm.

53. Poirrier, G. P. (1997). *Writing to learn. Curricular strategies for nursing and other disciplines.* New York: NLN Press.

54. Rash, E. M. (2005). Educational innovations. A service learning research methods course. *Journal of Nursing Education, 44*(10), 477–478.

55. Rest, J. R. (1979). *Development in judging moral issues.* Minneapolis, MN: University of Minnesota Press.

56. Rest, J. R. (1982). A psychologist looks at the teaching of ethics. *The Hastings Center Report, 12*(1), 29–36.

57. Rest, J. R. (1984). The major components of morality. In W. M. Kurtines, & J. L. Gewirtz (Eds.), *Morality, moral behavior, and moral development.* New York: John Wiley & Sons.

58. Rest, J. R. (1986). *Moral development: Advances in research and theory.* New York: Praeger Publisher.

59. Rest, J. (1994). Background: Theory and research. In J. Rest, & D. Narvaez (Eds.), *Moral development in the profession* (pp. 1–26). Hillside, NJ: Erlbaum.

60. Rollant, P. (2007). "How can I fail the NCLEX-RN with a 3.5 GPA?" Approaches to help this unexpected high risk group. In M. Oermann, & K. Heinrich. (Eds.), *Annual review of nursing education volume 5, 2007: Challenges and new directions in nursing education* (pp. 25–51).

61. Ruth-Sahd, L. (2003). Intuition: A critical way of knowing in multicultural nursing curriculum. *Perspectives in Nursing Education, 24*(3), 129–134.

62. Shirey, M. (2007). An evidence-based solution for minimizing stress and anger in nursing students. *Journal of Nursing Education, 46*(12), 568–571.

63. Shugart, S., & Romano, J. (2006). LifeMap: A learning-centered system. *Community College Journal of Research and Practice, 30*, 141–143.

64. Silberman, M. (1996). *Active learning 101 strategies to teach any subject.* Boston: Allyn and Bacon.

65. Utley-Smith, Q. (2004). Five competencies needed by new baccalaureate graduates. *Nursing Education Perspectives, 25*, 166–170.

66. Van Valkenburg, J., & Holden, L. (2004). Teaching methods in the affective domain. *Radiologic Technology, 75*(5), 347–354.

67. White, J. L. (1999). Wellness Wednesdays: Health promotion and service learning on campus. *Journal of Nursing Education, 38*, 69–73.

68. Williams, B. (2001). Developing critical reflection for professional practice through problem-based learning. *Journal of Advanced Nursing, 34*(1), 27–34.

69. Zubaidah, S. (2005). Problem-based learning: Literature review. *Singapore Nursing Journal, 32*(4), 50–55.

CHAPTER 4

Use Assessment and Evaluation Strategies—Competency 3

OBJECTIVES

1. Explore evidence-based assessment and evaluation strategies.
2. Compare strategies for assessment and evaluation of learners.
3. Identify best practices for providing feedback for learners.
4. Identify theories, principles, and guidelines used in educational assessment and measurement.
5. Examine frameworks for enhancing performance and learning.

KEY TERMS

Affective domain
Affective taxonomy
Assessment
Authentic assessment
Bloom's cognitive taxonomy
Classical Test Theory
Classroom Assessment Techniques (CATs)
Cognitive domain
Cognitive taxonomy
Computerized adaptive testing
Concept maps
Confidence-based marking
Criterion-referenced grading
Dave's psychomotor taxonomy
Formative evaluation

Gagné's cognitive taxonomy
Item Response Theory
Norm-referenced grading
Peer review
Portfolios
Primary Trait Analysis Scale
Psychomotor domain
Simpson's psychomotor taxonomy
Rubric
Summative evaluation
Structured objective clinical evaluation
Test blue print
Test item difficulty
Test item discrimination

DEFINITION AND DESCRIPTION OF COMPETENCY

One of the major activities of a nurse educator—whether in the classroom, clinical, skills laboratory, or online setting—involves assessment and evaluation of learners. Competency 3 is concerned with using assessment and evaluation processes in teaching effectively. Six task statements describe the competency in terms of knowledge of assessment and evaluation strategies, and the ability to develop and implement a variety of evidence-based strategies in each of the learning domains. The importance of providing effective feedback and creating and using clinical assessment tools is also addressed.

OVERVIEW OF ASSESSMENT AND EVALUATION _____

The terms assessment and evaluation refer to processes used with individuals, groups of students in specific courses, and groups of students in a program of study. Although the terms assessment and evaluation share similarities and are sometimes used interchangeably, the terms are distinctly different. A comparison of assessment and evaluation in terms of scope, purpose, uses, timing, types of data collected, and types of strategies used are provided in Table 4-1.

Assessment of Learning

Assessment is a "broad and comprehensive process of collecting quantitative and or qualitative data to make informed educational decisions about students" (McDonald, 2008, p. 9). Assessment also describes the process of determining the learners' attributes, (such as learning styles and preferences), and attributes of the environment that can facilitate or detract from learning. Assessment may also refer to determining whether students have achieved specific learning outcomes. In this chapter, the focus is on assessment of learning outcomes achieved by individuals and groups. Please see Chapter 2 for assessment of learners' attributes.

Types of Evaluation

Evaluation occurs at several levels. First, at the individual level, evaluation is concerned with determining if the student learned and the degree of learning that occurred. Faculty, students, and student peers can contribute to evaluation of an individual's learning. Evaluation involves the instructor's use of judgment to interpret the meaning of the student's performance (McDonald, 2008). For example, a student's responses on a multiple choice examination can be compared with the answer key, the percentage of correct responses can be calculated, and based upon a predetermined grading scale, the student's level of mastery of the content can be established to correspond with a letter grade (A, B, C, etc.). Similar processes are applied in evaluating presentations, essays, formal papers, and clinical performance. However, evaluation using these materials is more subjective than multiple-choice examinations, which have explicit correct and incorrect responses. Therefore, it is important

TABLE 4-1	Comparison of Assessment and Evaluation	
	Assessment	**Evaluation**
Scope	• Broad, comprehensive • Subsumes the term evaluation.	• Narrow scope
Purpose	• Provide support and feedback to enhance ongoing learning. • Determine strengths and learning needs. • Information may be mutually beneficial.	• Determine the degree and type of learning that has occurred because of teaching. • Evaluation findings are compared with quantitative or qualitative performance standard. • Findings are linked to course outcomes or course grade.
Uses	• Assessment information is used to modify teaching approaches, content, and learning environment. • Students use assessment feedback to guide learning.	• Determine if learning objectives have been met and quantify the student's achievement level. • Determine if program outcomes have been achieved.
Timing	• May be conducted before learning, or early in the learning process to provide formative feedback.	• Formative evaluation may be intermittent or ongoing during the learning session. • Summative evaluation is conducted at the conclusion of the learning experience.
Type of data collected	• May be qualitative or quantitative. • May reflect subjective commentary.	• Typically quantitative, objective, and measurable
Types of strategies used	• Games, individual and group activities, verbal questioning, show of hands, written assignments, performance checklists, pretests	• Written assignments, tests, performance checklists, return demonstrations, student presentations, clinical evaluation tools

that the grading criteria are made clear by differentiating characteristics of assignments that are A, B, C, and D level.

On another level, the learning of entire groups of students enrolled in a program of study can be evaluated. Program evaluation, which deals with curriculum, program design, and evaluation is discussed in Chapter 5.

Formative Evaluation

Formative evaluations are designed to provide information about the learner that will facilitate further learning and promote the achievement of learning objectives. Formative evaluation is conducted well before the end of a course of study to provide diagnostic information that can be used guide further study and help the student improve his or her performance (McDonald, 2008). Formative evaluation methods need to delineate what the learner has achieved in terms of learning and identify learning goals that remain unmet. Both the academic nurse educator (ANE) and the student can use the data from a formative evaluation to guide future learning activities. The ANE can summarize formative evaluation data from the entire class and determine which topics or processes students found easy or difficult. Analysis of formative evaluation data can help determine if the topic was poorly understood, or if certain types of information about the topic were unclear, such as pathophysiology or problem solving. McDonald cautions that "Because formative evaluation is a method that shapes the process of teaching and learning while it is in progress, it should not be used for assigning class grades" (p. 12).

Summative Evaluation

The purpose of summative evaluation is to determine how well the student learned after the instruction has been completed. Summative evaluation data may be collected periodically throughout the course after specific units of content have been covered, as well as at the end of the course to obtain a comprehensive view of the student's learning. As with formative evaluation, summative evaluation can provide feedback to the learner and the instructor in terms of the type of content mastered and degree to which the content was mastered.

Both assessment and evaluation processes may involve testing, writing papers, and instructor observation. The teacher uses evaluation strategies to determine the degree to which individual students have met the course objectives and ultimately the program outcomes.

Validity and Reliability of Assessment and Evaluation Data

Valid and reliable assessment and evaluation require that valid and reliable data are collected, measured, and interpreted appropriately. Oermann and Gaberson (2006) note that "validity is not an either/or judgment; there are degrees of validity depending upon the purpose of the test and how the scores are to be used" (p. 24).

Validity

Validity evidence is typically reported as face, content, criterion-related, or construct validity (Box 4-1). Validity is enhanced by assuring that the data collected reflect the course objectives in terms of content, taxonomy, and domain level. A test blueprint is used to identify the content, objectives, learning domain, and domain level measured by specific test questions. In a test blueprint, a grid or matrix is developed to classify test questions in terms of the type of content or subject matter being tested, the specific course objective, and domain level being evaluated (Figure 4-1). The test blueprint can be used to guide the "selection of a representative sample of the content and objectives of the course," which will enhance the validity and reliability of the test results (McDonald, 2008, p. 13).

Reliability

Definitions of reliability have evolved over the years. Reliability is commonly defined as the degree of consistency in test scores and is a necessary condition for establishing validity (Traub & Rowley, 1991). There are several types of reliability, including "stability, equivalent forms, internal consistency, and interrater reliability" (Oermann & Gaberson, 2006, p. 28). Stability reliability refers to the consistency of student scores over time. The use of test-retest procedures can establish stability provided the length of time between tests is neither too short nor too long. The equivalent forms of reliability involve administering two different forms of the same test to the same group of students and comparing the results. Both forms of the exam need to use the same test

---

BOX 4-1   Types of Validity

- Face validity—obtained by expert judgment, answers the question: Do the test items appear to be testing appropriate content?

- Content validity—based on expert review of test blueprint for content distribution and domain

- Criterion-related validity—"when test scores are related to scores from other measures of an associated trait" (Slavin, 2006, p. 518)

- Construct validity—subsumes all types of validity. "The extent to which score-based inferences about the construct of interest are accurate and meaningful" (Oermann & Gaberson, 2006, p. 36)

Some data from Oermann, M., & Gaberson, K. (2006). *Evaluation and testing in nursing education* (2nd ed.) New York: Springer; and Slavin, R. E. (2006). *Educational psychology: Theory and practice*. New York: Pearson.

	Objective or Content Area	Objective or Content Area	Objective or Content Area	
Taxonomy Level	Test Question Number	Test Question Number	Test Question Number	Number of questions at taxonomy level
Taxonomy Level	Test Question Number	Test Question Number	Test Question Number	Number of questions at taxonomy level
	Total number of questions in content area	Total number of questions in content area	Total number of questions in content area	

FIGURE 4-1 Test Blueprint Template.

blueprint to assure accurate results. Unlike equivalent forms and stability reliability, which require two separate administrations of the examination, internal consistency can be determined with one round of testing. To determine internal constancy the test is divided into two equal parts and the score for each part is determined. A high correlation between the two scores indicates that the exam is internally consistent.

Oermann and Gaberson (2006) identify three broad conditions that influence reliability: the student, the administration conditions, and the test itself. Student-related factors influencing test reliability include heterogeneity, motivation, and test-taking skills. Reliability is enhanced in student groups that are heterogeneous in age, background, and ability. Likewise, students with a high degree of test-taking skill may perform with greater reliability than those with weaker test-taking skills. Administrative conditions that can enhance reliability include informing students about the number of items in the test, the amount of time they will have to complete the test, and giving directions for dealing with questions that they are uncertain about answering. Several test factors can enhance or detract from reliability, including the number of test items, how homogenous or interrelated the items are, and the quality of the test items.

Guidelines for Assessment and Evaluation

Stassen, Doherty, and Poe (2001) have developed a comprehensive set of guidelines for developing an effective approach to assessment (Box 4-2). First, to enhance consistency of the findings the assessment process should be planned and follow a systematic process. A systemic process will assure that the data are obtained using similar methods and that all steps in the assessment process are followed. Second, the use of multidimensional assessments throughout the duration of the course can enhance reliability

BOX 4-2 Guidelines for Conducting Assessments

1. Use a planned and systematic assessment process.

2. Use multidimensional assessment methods throughout the course.

3. Assure that the assessment tool is aligned with the learning objectives.

4. Assure that the assessment tool is aligned with the emphasis given to the content and the appropriate level of complexity.

Data from Stassen, M. L., Doherty, K., & Poe, M. (2001, Fall). *Program based review and assessment: Tools and techniques for program improvement.* University of Massachusetts-Amherst, Office of Academic Planning and Assessment. http://www.umass.edu/oapa/oapa/publications/online_handbooks/program_based.pdf.

of the outcome measures and help to ensure that the student did indeed learn the material. Using diverse ways to gather measurable assessment data, such as reaction papers, formal term papers, clinical case studies presented verbally or in writing, performance testing, and written examinations are some of the many options. The third guideline is to ensure that the assessment methods are aligned with the course objectives, fit with the type of learning outcome expected, and fit with the learning experiences provided during the course. For example, a course objective calling for the student to prioritize patient care needs can be assessed using several different methods such as multiple choice test questions, a clinical case presentation, or a reaction paper.

The second part of the guideline requires that there be a link between the assessment approaches used, what was taught, and how it was taught. In the previous example, using assessments that ask the student to prioritize patient care needs would be a fit only if prioritization was covered during the course and preferably after students had opportunities to practice prioritizing skills in the classroom setting.

In the next section, theory and research that underlie data collection instruments, test administration practices, analysis of test items, and selected evidence-based assessment and strategies are discussed.

THEORY AND RESEARCH RELATED TO COMPETENCY

Knowledge and skills in conducting assessment and evaluation activities are essential for nursing faculty. Nursing education has been and continues to be built on assessment and evaluation. For example, course examinations and skills performance tests are used to evaluate student performance in specific courses, and standardized specialty and comprehensive examinations are used to assess content knowledge and readiness for successful completion of the NCLEX. Clearly, effective and accurate assessment and evaluation are integral to nursing education, and have far-reaching implications for nursing students and the nursing profession as a whole.

Developing valid and reliable test items takes knowledge, skill, and practice. Following general guidelines for developing specific test items will help ensure consistent, well-designed items that require higher-order thinking skills. Item writers also improve the test item quality by using peer review. In the following section, evaluation competencies and guidelines for multiple choice test items are presented, along with relevant research support when available.

Assessment and Evaluation Competencies for Educators

Awareness of the need for competence in assessment and evaluation has increased over the years, resulting in many professional organizations establishing standards and competencies for educators who are involved in assessment and evaluation. The National League for Nursing (NLN) has addressed assessment and evaluation tasks in ANE competency 3 (uses assessment and evaluation strategies); and in competency 4 (participate in curriculum design and program evaluation) (NLN, 2005). In addition, non-nursing organizations have developed standards and guidelines for assessment and evaluation that can be useful for teaching practice. In 1990, the American Federation of Teachers joined with the National Council on Measurement in Education (NCME) and the National Education Association to create the *Standards for Teacher Competence in Educational Assessment of Students*. The document identifies seven competencies for K–12 educators that can be easily adapted to provide useful guidelines for the ANE who seeks to develop greater knowledge and skills in assessment and evaluation (Box 4-3). The competencies cover practical aspects of assessment and evaluation, including: selection, development, administration, scoring, and interpreting data. Using data in decision making, communicating assessment findings, and recognizing inappropriate/unethical uses of assessments are also covered.

To further address the appropriate and ethical use of educational assessments, the NCME published the *Code of Professional Responsibilities in Educational Measurement* (1995), which elaborates on the responsibilities inherent in each of the competencies. The code identifies professional responsibilities for individuals who

> 1) develop assessments, 2) market and sell assessments, 3) select assessments, 4) administer assessments, 5) score assessments, 6) interpret, use, and communicate assessment results, 7) educate others about assessment, and 8) evaluate programs and conduct research on assessments (para. 6).

BOX 4-3   Assessment and Evaluation Competencies for Educators

Teachers should be skilled in the following areas:

1. Choosing assessment methods appropriate for instructional decisions

2. Developing assessment methods appropriate for instructional decisions

3. Administering, scoring, and interpreting the results of both externally produced and teacher-produced assessment methods

4. Using assessment results when making decisions about individual students, planning teaching, developing curriculum, and school improvement

5. Developing valid grading procedures that use student assessments

6. Communicating assessment results to students

7. Recognizing unethical, illegal, and otherwise inappropriate assessment methods and uses of assessment information

Data from American Federation of Teachers, National Council on Measurement in Education & National Education Association (1990) *Standards for teacher competence in educational assessment of students* (pp. 4–6). Available at http://www.unl.edu/buros/bimm/html/article3.html.

Although the NCME developed the code for its members it, "strongly encourages other organizations and individuals who engage in educational assessment activities, to endorse and abide by the responsibilities relevant to their professions" (1995, para. 4). A link to the complete document is provided in the Resource section.

Standards for educational and psychological testing have been jointly developed and published by the NCME, the American Educational Research Association (AERA), and the American Psychological Association (APA). The standards guide educators in the areas of test construction, evaluation, test administration practices, and specific testing applications such as program evaluation testing, and credentialing (AERA, APA, & AEA, 1999). The standards are useful for ensuring that best practices are implemented for all aspects of educational testing.

Developing an Assessment Plan

The development of an assessment plan begins with clarifying the expected learning outcomes. Typically, this is done by formulating written learning objectives using taxonomies to describe the learning activity and how the learner is expected to demonstrate that learning has occurred. Once formalized, the learning objectives provide the framework for course content and guide the ANE in the use of specific teaching and evaluation approaches.

Cognitive Learning Taxonomies

The development of learning taxonomies has provided structure for learning objectives and direction for formal education. Several prominent taxonomies, including Bloom's original and revised taxonomies and Gagne's Learning Taxonomy, are reviewed in this section.

Bloom's Cognitive Taxonomies

Bloom's original cognitive taxonomy, published in 1956, outlined the hierarchical structure of the cognitive domain into six levels: knowledge, comprehension, application, analysis, evaluation, and synthesis (Bloom, 1956). In 2001, Anderson *et al.* revised Bloom's original taxonomy, creating a two-dimensional framework consisting of six cognitive process dimensions: remember, understand, apply, analyze, evaluate, and create, and a knowledge dimension. The knowledge dimension is conceptualized as consisting of four subtypes of knowledge (factual, conceptual, procedural, and metacognitive). These four types of knowledge are subsumed within each of the six cognitive dimensions. In other words, within each of these cognitive process dimensions there are four levels or dimensions of knowledge, factual knowledge, conceptual knowledge, procedural knowledge, and metacognitive knowledge (Table 4-2). The first three knowledge dimensions (factual, conceptual, and procedural) were reflected in Bloom's original taxonomy subcategories. Metacognitive knowledge is a new addition that acknowledges the importance of being aware of one's own thinking and self-knowledge. Thus, when writing objectives for one of the six cognitive process levels, the ANE is able to further distinguish the objective in terms of the knowledge dimension that the objective requires (i.e., factual, conceptual, procedural, or metacognitive).

Developing cognitive learning objectives using Bloom's revised taxonomy involves determining the appropriate cognitive level for the subject, and selecting a corresponding verb to describe what the learner is expected to do. After the cognitive process dimension is determined by the choice of verb, the knowledge dimension is determined by the noun used or implied in the objective (Duan, 2006). Factual knowledge objectives involve knowing terminology or specific details such as laboratory values. Conceptual knowledge objectives address knowing classifications, categories, principles, or theories. Procedural knowledge involves determining actions to take and knowing when specific procedures are warranted. Metacognitive knowledge

TABLE 4-2 Categories of Knowledge	
Knowledge Dimension	**Description/Subcategories**
Factual	Knowledge of basic elements such as terminology
Conceptual	Knowledge of interrelationships among basic elements including classifications, generalizations, and theoretical knowledge
Procedural	Knowledge of techniques, skills, and algorithms; includes knowledge of criteria for determining when a skill should be performed
Metacognitive	General knowledge of cognition and cognitive tasks; includes self-awareness of one's thinking
Data from Krathwohl, D. (2002). A revision of Bloom's taxonomy: An overview. *Theory into Practice, 31*(4), 214.	

involves awareness of cognition in general and self-knowledge. Development of learning skills, test-taking skills, and self-reflection skills are examples of metacognitive knowledge.

Gagné's Learning Taxonomy

Gagné (1985) developed an instructional theory that includes three components, a taxonomy of learning outcomes, a description of internal and external conditions needed to achieve the outcomes, and a list of nine instructional events necessary for designing lessons. In comparing the five learning outcome categories to Bloom' revised cognitive taxonomy, several differences and similarities are noted. Gagné describes the first category of verbal information as recalling and presenting. The second category, intellectual skills, includes five subskills, which are discrimination, concrete concept, defined concept, rule-using, and problem-solving. Problem-solving skill is similar to several levels of Bloom's revised taxonomy (i.e., analyze, evaluate, and create). The final three learning outcome terms in Gagné's taxonomy include cognitive strategies, attitude, and motor skills. Thus, Gagné's learning taxonomy incorporates not only the cognitive domain, but also the affective and psychomotor domains.

In 2005, Gagné, Wagner, Golas, and Keller revised Gagné's original taxonomy. They described the learning outcome taxonomy as human capabilities and identified a "capability verb" that corresponds to each capability. The capability verbs are used to classify learning outcomes and are intended to reduce ambiguity when describing expected student behaviors. Nine capability verbs are depicted in Table 4-3. Each capability verb relates to one of five capabilities (i.e., intellectual, cognitive, verbal, motor, or attitude).

Similar to Bloom's cognitive domain taxonomy, Gagné and colleagues incorporate factual knowledge and intellectual aspects. Within the intellectual skills category, tasks such as discrimination, classifying concrete concepts, defining concepts, using rules that affirm a specific relationship between concepts, and problem-solving actions, are described. However, Gagné's taxonomy also includes attitudinal (affective) outcomes and a motor skills category, thus making it a more comprehensive classification system.

TABLE 4-3 Gagné's Learning Capabilities with Capability and Action Verbs

Human Capability	Capability Verb	Example of Objectives with Action *Verb*
Intellectual Skill		
• Discrimination	Discriminates	Discriminates by *selecting* the appropriate nursing interventions for a client with asthma
• Concrete concept	Identifies	Identifies the anatomical structures of the heart by *naming* the valves of the heart on a diagram
• Defined concept	Classifies	Classifies information by *drawing* a concept map of relevant factors
• Rule use	Demonstrates	Demonstrates accurate *calculation* of drug dosages, showing all work
• Higher-order rule (problem solving)	Generates	Generates a *written* care plan for promoting wound healing
Cognitive Strategy	Adopts	Adopts strategies for *self-reflection* for clinical journaling
Verbal Information	States	States in *writing* the responsibilities of proper medication administration
Motor Skill	Executes	Executes the *injection* of intramuscular and subcutaneous medications
Attitude	Chooses	The student will choose to *join* a professional nursing organization.

Adapted with permission from Gagné, R. M., Wager, W. W., Golas, K.C., & Keller, J. M. (2005). *Principles of instructional design* (5th ed., p. 136). Belmont, CA: Wadsworth/Thomson.

In formulating learning objectives using Gagné's taxonomy, the human capability is identified along with an action verb describing how the capability is to be carried out. Gagné also emphasizes that it is important to identify the conditions of learning and the constraints or special conditions that are expected of the performance. A five-part objective is recommended that describes: (1) the situation or context of the learning, (2) the learned capability, (3) the subject or content, (4) the action verb describing the observable behavior, and (5) constraints or conditions that describe acceptable performance (Gagné et al., 2005). Although not all five components are required, using them creates a more specific learning objective. The most essential components according to Gagné et al. are the capability verb and the subject.

The hierarchical structure of Gagné and Bloom's taxonomies is helpful in leveling objectives from simple cognitive processes to higher-level processes. Furthermore, the linking of specific verbs with each taxonomy level makes it relatively easy for the ANE to formulate learning objectives and outcomes.

Affective Learning Taxonomy

The affective domain is believed by most educators to be the most difficult and elusive to capture with behavioral objectives. Krathwohl, Bloom, and Masia's (1964) affective taxonomy is concerned with a person's emotions, feelings, attitude about a topic, and/or the degree of acceptance or rejection a person has toward a topic. The taxonomy describes behaviors ranging from merely focusing attention or being aware, to internalizing "consistent qualities of character and conscience" (p. 7). In this section key aspects of Krathwohl's affective taxonomy are reviewed. Additional discussion of the affective domain and taxonomy is presented in Chapters 2 and 3.

Krathwohl's Affective Taxonomy

Krathwohl *et al.* (1964) present a detailed affective taxonomy that views affective learning on a continuum. The affective taxonomy consists of five levels, each with two to three subcategories. The first affective level, receiving, begins with awareness or ability to perceive an event or situation, and being willing to attend and respond to phenomena. This level is focused on the student's sensitization to a situation or phenomenon; therefore, it is foundational to achievement of other affective levels. Receiving includes three subconcepts—awareness, willingness to receive versus avoiding exposure to the phenomenon, and controlled or selective attention to the phenomenon. The remaining four levels represent a personal, inner shift, in which the student's perceptions and responses become progressively internalized, organized, and reconceptualized (Krathwohl *et al.*, 1964).

The second affective category, responding, also includes three subcategories. The learner may respond at the acquiescence level, which is motivated by a sense of obligation, the willingness level, which indicates an inner drive, or the satisfaction level, which is characterized by a positive emotion or feeling associated with the response (Krathwohl *et al.*, 1964). At the willingness to respond level, there is a shift from passive obligatory responding to willingly choosing to respond. At this level, there is no longer a sense of resistance to the phenomenon or situation. As the student moves to the next level, satisfaction in response, an emotional component is brought to the process.

The valuing level of the affective domain is characterized by fairly stable and consistent internalized behavior. At this level the individual moves from accepting a value to preferring a value, and finally to commitment to the value. Underlying valuing is a commitment to the core value, a belief that "a thing, phenomena, or behavior has worth" (Krathwohl *et al.*, 1964, p. 180).

As a student integrates and internalizes a value, there comes a point at which situations invoke the consideration of multiple values. At the organization level, the individual "encounters situations for which more than one value is relevant" (p. 35). The learner must conceptualize the values and organize them into a value system. According to Krathwohl *et al.* (1964), this is when organization of values will be necessary. Two processes occur during this organization level. First, the student needs to conceptualize or think abstractly about the values to determine relationships between values. Then, the student needs to determine the dominant values and create a system in which dominant values are prioritized. Krathwohl and colleagues point out that those demonstrating the organization level of the affective domain may synthesize values to form a new value.

The final level of the affective domain is labeled "characterization by a value or value complex" (Krathwohl *et al.*, 1964, p. 184). This means that the student's values are internalized to the extent that others describe or characterize the individual by those values. At this affective level the beliefs, ideas, and attitudes have become incorporated into the student's world view. Two subprocesses at this level include forming a "generalized set," which is a tendency or predisposition to respond in a certain way and "characterization," which represents the highest degree of internalization at which time the student's responses become automatic or habitual. At the characterization level, the values are internalized further until they become consistent to such a degree that they influence the student's philosophy of life and are said to characterize the individual. Please see Chapter 3 for further details and examples of affective objectives in Table 3-9.

Psychomotor Taxonomies

Merritt (2008) notes that the three domains are not mutually exclusive, and almost all learning involves more than one domain. In nursing, psychomotor behaviors "contain elements of cognitive and affective behaviors within them" (p. 2). The inclusion of cognitive and affective aspects is apparent in Simpson's psychomotor taxonomy, which is reviewed in this section. In contrast, Dave's psychomotor taxonomy addresses the cognitive and affective domains indirectly. For the ANE, these taxonomies are useful in several ways. They enhance our understanding of how learners acquire psychomotor skills; enable leveling of skill performance; and assist in the identification of psychomotor learning objectives.

Simpson's Psychomotor Taxonomy

One of the earlier attempts to classify skill performance was developed by Simpson (1966). Her initial efforts culminated in a five-level taxonomy (Box 4-4). The first level is perception, which represents the person's use of sensory data to become aware of the objects, qualities, and characteristics needed to perform the skill. At the "set" level, the learner becomes physically, mentally, and emotionally ready to perform the skill. The guided response level describes the earliest attempts to perform the skill under guidance. Prerequisites for guided response are perception and set (readiness). In the mechanism stage, the learner has gained confidence in performing the skill through repeated practice. The final stage, called complex overt response, represents a higher level of performance of the skill. At this stage, the learner performs the skill smoothly, efficiently, and effectively. Simpson's original taxonomy was later revised to include two additional processes. Adaptation describes the ability to adapt parts of the

---

BOX 4-4   Simpson's Psychomotor Taxonomy

1. Perception

2. Set

3. Guided Response

4. Mechanism

5. Complex Overt Response

Data from Simpson, E. J. (1966). *The classification of educational objectives, psychomotor domain* (pp. 26–29). Vocational and Technical Education Grant Contract Report, US Department of Health, Education, and Welfare.

skill to meet the needs of a special situation. Origination involves creating new movements for special situations.

Dave's Psychomotor Taxonomy

Dave (1970) developed a five-level taxonomy for psychomotor skills, which outlines the refinement that occurs in the actual performance of a skill (Box 4-5). The first level is imitation, which involves observing the skill and copying the performance. Manipulation involves performing the skill with guided instruction, which results in a more detailed and exacting performance. At these earlier levels, the smoothness of the performance is strongly influenced by the complexity of the skill and the learner's familiarity with the parts of the skill. The third level is precision, which is characterized by greater accuracy in the skill performance. At this level, the learner is able to perform without the need to refer to notes and without the need for coaching or guidance. At the next level, referred to as articulation, the learner is able to combine two or more skills and perform them at a consistent level. Naturalization is the final level, which describes further refinement in skill performance. At the naturalization level, the learner is able to perform two or more skills in sequence, with little mental effort. The actions inherent in the skill have become automatic and no longer require deliberate focus.

Performance of a skill at Dave's naturalization level or at Simpson's complex overt response level (or higher) is most desirable. At these levels of performance, the knowledge and skills needed are now ingrained. The student no longer needs to focus on doing the task or remembering the steps in performing the task. This frees the student to be able to focus on important observations other than the skill, such as the patient's response to the procedure or other environmental cues.

BOX 4-5   Dave's Psychomotor Taxonomy

1. Imitation

2. Manipulation

3. Precision

4. Articulation

5. Naturalization

Dave, R. (1970). Psychomotor levels. In R. J Armstrong, (Ed.). *Developing and writing behavioral objectives.* Tucson: Educational Innovators Press.

Clinical Assessment and Evaluation

Clinical evaluation is a subjective process that relies on observation of the student's performance and interactions. Safe and effective clinical practice is essential in nursing, yet challenging to validate. This section reviews several strategies for evaluating clinical skills and performance, including clinical evaluation tools, objective structured clinical evaluation, and virtual clinical evaluation tools. The importance of conducting authentic assessments is addressed. In addition, reflective journaling and concept mapping are reviewed as methods of demonstrating critical thinking in nursing practice.

Authentic Assessment

Authentic assessment involves performing a task that is perceived as authentic by the learners, meaning it is similar in complexity to what would be expected in practice. As an assessment strategy, authentic assessment determines the students' abilities in "real-world" contexts by asking students to demonstrate skills and concepts they have learned. Authentic assessment requires the "student to use the same competencies, or combinations of knowledge, skills, and attitudes that they need to apply . . . in professional life" (Guliker, Bastiaens, & Kirschner, 2004, p. 69).

Based on a review of the literature, Guliker and colleagues (2004) identified five dimensions of authentic assessment. These include (1) the assessment task, (2) the physical context of the assessment, (3) the social context, (4) the results of the assessment, and (5) the criteria for assessment. In authentic assessment, the physical context is realistic and provides a situation in which resources, time, and available information are similar to what would be experienced in professional practice. The social context is authentic if it provides realistic opportunities for interaction and collaboration with others, yet supports individual accountability. Authentic assessment results are demonstrated by the end product or performance which can be shared or witnessed by others and can provide multiple indicators of learning. The authentic assessment criteria should be based on actual criteria used in clinical practice and be made explicit to the students before the task is undertaken. Each of these dimensions can vary in level of authenticity and importance in the assessment process.

Guliker and colleagues (2004) explored the dimensions of authentic assessment using scenarios that emphasized the dimensions in various combinations. For each scenario, teachers and nursing students were asked about the importance of each dimension and whether the five-dimension model was complete. Overall, the teachers, sophomores, and senior students agreed that the five-dimension framework represented elements that should be considered in conducting authentic assessments.

However, sophomores differed from senior students and teachers in their perception of the importance of the task, physical context, results, and criteria dimensions. Sophomores perceived the task, physical context, and criteria as most important, in that order. The seniors were in closer alignment to the teacher's perception, rating the results, task, and physical context as most important. All groups agreed that social context was a valid dimension, yet they perceived it as least important of the five dimensions. With the exception of social context, which was rated the lowest in importance by all groups, the students differed markedly in their perception of the results. Seniors rated this as most important, whereas sophomores rated it least important. The researchers speculated that inexperienced students might not have the knowledge or experience need to appreciate full-scale assessments that emphasize all dimensions. Because of the time and expense in conducting simulations, the researchers suggest that less attention to the social context of authentic assessments may be an alternative. In addition, exploring virtual simulations, which require less faculty time than mannequin-based simulations, may be a viable alternative for experienced students, because they rated physical context as less important.

Clinical Evaluation Tools

Most nursing programs have developed clinical evaluation tools (CET) which reflect the specific and unique expectations of each clinical course. CETs typically consist of the desired clinical outcomes for the course and either a two- or a multi-dimensional rating scale (Ignatavicius & Caputi, 2004). Examples of rating scales range from the simple satisfactory/unsatisfactory to leveled descriptive behaviors such as consistently, usually, occasionally, or rarely (Ignatavicius & Caputi, 2004). Clinical evaluation tools are typically program specific and designed to determine the student's performance level.

CETs are criterion-referenced grading tools, meaning students are expected to meet or exceed a predetermined level of performance to pass the course and achieve a certain grade. Developing a CET that accurately and reliably reflects the student's clinical performance is essential for ensuring that graduates have achieved a minimal level of proficiency in practice. Content validity of the CET is obtained by determining that the clinical outcomes are addressed in the CET and that the focus of the course and clinical experiences provide opportunities to meet the clinical outcomes. In terms of reliability, it is important to determine that consistent findings would be obtained even with different evaluators. One way to establish interrater reliability is for two or more instructors to evaluate the same group of students and compare ratings. Ignatavicius and Caputi (2004) recommend comparing observations of at least

30 students. Differences in ratings are then discussed and the CET can be revised for greater clarity and consistency.

In addition to the instructor's observations of student performance, assessment of clinical knowledge and skills is supported through a variety of other evaluation strategies. Bonnel (2009) identifies several categories of evaluation strategies, including observation, simulations, oral and written assignments, and self-evaluation. Selected strategies which reflect these categories are reviewed in the following sections.

Objective Structured Clinical Evaluation

Over the years, a process called objective structured clinical evaluation (OSCE) originally used in medical school instruction in Scotland, has spread to other countries and other disciplines (Rentschler, Eaton, Cappiello, McNally, & McWilliam, 2007). According to Rentschler *et al.*, OSCE involves "the use of a simulated and standardized format to measure synthesis of knowledge and clinical skills" (p. 135). In OSCE, individuals are trained to be standardized patients (SPs) who present themselves to the student as a real patient with a controlled yet realistic medical scenario. Benefits of using OSCE are multiple, and according to Rentschler *et al.*, are well validated. These benefits include:

1. Control and uniformity of the simulation
2. Realistic nature of the interactions
3. Reduced stress
4. The ability of SPs to provide immediate and formative feedback (2007, p. 135)

A pilot study by Rentschler *et al.* (2007) explored the feasibility of implementing the OSCE model in a senior undergraduate course. Students' evaluations of the OSCE were very favorable. The majority report that the experience helped them feel confident in their nursing and communication skills. Students also considered the OSCE to be good preparation for their final clinical experience.

Virtual Clinical Evaluation Tool

Development and implementation of a virtual clinical evaluation tool has been reported by Sander and Trible (2008). The impetus for the virtual tool stemmed from the need for students and faculty to have access to the tool for formative and summative evaluations and the need to provide timely evaluation feedback. The researchers developed the tool using a spreadsheet and created a Likert scoring system for each evaluation outcome. The clinical evaluation form was posted on Blackboard, where each student could download the form, enter a self-evaluation rating, add comments, and upload the form to Blackboard for the instructor's comments. Although the implementation process and tool needed refinement, at the conclusion of the project, the researchers reported that evaluation feedback was timely and objectivity of the reported comments improved.

Concept Maps

A concept map is a graphic representation of concepts and the relationships among them. Thus, students can develop concept maps that demonstrate their personal knowledge and understanding. Concept maps depict the "organization of an explicit set of concepts that allows visualization of concept relationships" (Hicks-Moore & Pastirik, 2006, p. 1). Researchers have found that the use of concept mapping helps students to clarify knowledge and understanding of relationships and helps them incorporate new knowledge into the conceptualization structure (Baugh & Mellott, 1998; Conceição & Taylor, 2007; Hicks-Moore & Pastirik 2006; Wheeler & Collins, 2003).

The literature generally supports a link between concept mapping and critical thinking. However, Hicks-Moore and Pastirik (2006) point out that there are inconsistencies in how concept mapping enhances critical thinking, and the methods used to evaluate critical thinking. To address these gaps, they used the Holistic Critical Thinking Scoring Rubric (HCTSR) developed by Facione and Facione (1994), as a tool for evaluating critical thinking in 18 concept maps. Results from this pilot study indicated that developing concept maps in the clinical setting fostered critical thinking and improved clinical preparedness.

Although concept maps were relatively unheard of in nursing education circles before the 1980s, they are now widely used in clinical education (Hicks-Moore & Pastirik, 2006; Hinck *et al.*, 2006; Schuster, 2000; Wheeler & Collins, 2003); and in skills laboratories, face-to-face classrooms, and online courses (Conceição & Taylor, 2007). To create a concept map requires the student to collect information, categorize it, and graphically depict how the information categories are related to one another. Concept maps allow the learner to create a visual representation of the interrelationships between concepts which is consistent with the constructivist model of learning.

Some authors have extended the use of concept mapping from specific course assignments to a means of course evaluation. In an undergraduate wellness course, MacNeil (2007) asked students to create concept maps at the beginning of lectures and again at the conclusion of the lectures. The maps were compared on the degree of complexity of the diagram and the relationships between the parameters. The initial maps were largely circular representations of physical parameters with a few descriptive terms and details indicated for other wellness parameters and relationships. In contrast, the maps created after the content was covered were more clearly organized, more detailed, and included more relationships between concepts. Although the study was limited to students in one course, the approach could be easily applied to other courses. Completing one concept map at the beginning of a course could be similar to a course pretest, and completing a new map at the end of a course would be similar to a course post-test. A major difference is that the concept mapping would allow the student to demonstrate his or her personal construction of the new knowledge, rather than using instructor-selected test questions.

Reflective Writing

Reflective writing is "the purposeful contemplation of thoughts, feelings and happenings that pertain to recent experiences" (Kennison & Misselwitz, 2002, p. 239). The use of reflective writing in nursing education is a process that allows the student to explore subject matter on a personal level and can serve to demonstrate critical thinking skills. It is not merely the recording of knowledge, but a way to explore what is known and not known, so that a clearer understanding is reached.

Achieving consistency and fairness in grading reflective writing can be difficult. However, the use of written guidelines and defined terms may be helpful. For example, Baker (1996) recommends asking the student to include: (1) identification, (2) description, (3) significance, and (4) implications of the subject in their reflective writing. Based upon a review of literature, Craft (2005) recommends that instructors initially provide a structure for writing such as, what topics would be appropriate, and what aspects could be explored about the topic. Students should be provided guidelines for writing until they feel comfortable with the introspective process. Also, emphasis should be placed on the process rather than the content. Thus, feedback on reflective writings should provide probing commentary about the processes the student is describing. Pass/fail grading of the assignment can be based on the student meeting the guidelines.

Kuiper (1999) has delineated a model that helps nursing students structure their reflection activities. Kuiper's reflective Self-Regulated Learning Model (SRL) incorporates behavioral, metacognitive, and environmental self-monitoring. In the behavioral component, the self-observation of performance and self-judgment of competency are explored. The metacognitive component involves use of knowledge and thinking strategies. The environmental component is involved with skills, activities, and the physical context. Kuiper used the three components of the SRL model to generate questions for student self-reflection. Instead of journaling each week about their clinical experiences, students provided an audio recording of their responses. A comparison of the audio recorded responses and written journals of students from the previous semester revealed longer narratives by the audio group, more frequent use of higher-order, causal types of statements, and more statements demonstrating self-monitoring behaviors. Kuiper concludes that the prescriptive use of the SRL model to guide reflection may prompt greater cognitive and metacognitive development. This in turn helps students develop clinical reasoning skills that will be needed as graduate nurses.

A study by Kautz, Kuiper, Pesut, Knight-Brown, and Daneker (2005) used the SRL model and the Outcome of Present State Model to explore the development of clinical reasoning skills in nursing students. The students reported significant qualitative gains in the use of self-monitoring behaviors such as self-observation, self-judgment, and metacognitive self-evaluation. They were able to use the tools and worksheets developed from the models to document their learning.

Classroom Assessment and Evaluation Strategies

Educational scholars agree that using multiple assessment and evaluation strategies provides more valid and reliable results than single strategies. In this section, a diverse array of strategies and tools are described for use in online and face-to-face classroom settings. These may be used in conjunction with faculty-developed tests to enhance the instructor's confidence that the learning outcomes have been achieved.

Classroom Assessment Techniques

Classroom assessment techniques (CATs) may be described as a diverse group of creative and interactive processes that can be used in formative evaluation in many diverse learning settings. According to Angelo and Cross (1993), a CAT should address five criteria:

1. Provide information about what the student is learning
2. Identify aspects that can be modified to enhance learning
3. Be used formatively
4. Be easy to develop and use
5. Provide findings that are quick and easy to examine.

In their book, *Classroom Assessment Techniques: A Handbook for College Teachers*, Angelo and Cross provide specific examples of CATs that can be used in a variety of settings and disciplines. They describe the purpose of each technique, followed by instructions for implementing and evaluating the findings. To further guide the instructor in selecting a useful technique, an estimate of the difficulty level and time commitment for using each strategy is identified.

An example of a commonly used CAT is the one-minute paper in which students respond to two questions at the conclusion of class. The first question asks them to identify the most important thing they learned in class. This requires students to review and reflect on the learning experience. In the second question, students are asked to identify anything that is still unclear, referred to as the muddiest point. This helps to determine how well students are learning and can provide information that can guide the ANE in modifying teaching strategies. Chizmar and Ostrosky (1998) studied the effectiveness of the one-minute paper on a sample of more than 300 students from four different courses. Examination scores were compared with a control group of more than 250 students who did not write the one-minute paper. Those students who participated in the one-minute paper demonstrated scores that were 6.6% higher. Furthermore, this increase did not vary with student or instructor ability level. The authors conclude that for the time invested in using the one-minute paper, the effect on learning was significant and worthwhile.

Another strategy the ANE can use is to pose a question to students at the end of class, such as, "What were the most important points in this lecture?" or "What are the nurse's responsibilities in caring for patient with this condition?" This one-minute paper can provide valuable feedback to the teacher about the students' thinking and learning. The CATs discussed by Angelo and Cross are not subject specific and can be easily adapted to a variety of classroom settings.

In addition to providing the teacher with feedback on student learning, the CATs have an additional advantage of helping students think about what they are learning and further develop their meta cognitive skills. Silberman (1996) suggests an assessment technique called reconsidering to determine students' views before and after a topic is presented. The instructor poses questions such as, "How would you deal with a specific problem?" and "What is the value of a specific event or observation?" Alternatively, the instructor may ask students to write down a situation that they did not handle as well as they would have liked. Responses can be obtained using discussion, a questionnaire, or a written statement. At the end of the lesson, the instructor asks the students if their view has shifted. Both Silberman (1996) and Angelo Cross (1993) offer a variety of engaging and interactive activities for assessing student learning. The ANE will find the activities clearly explained and easily adapted to various courses. CATs can provide meaningful formative data about the quality of student learning.

Evaluating Students' Writing

Development of written communication skills is highly valued in nursing. Narrative charting, developing educational materials, and clinical policies are common expectations in nursing practice. Educators rely on research papers, clinical journals, reaction papers, care plans, and other varieties of written assignments, to facilitate learning and provide a means of assessing and evaluating learning. In this section, the writing across the curriculum initiative and the use of evaluation tools such as rubrics and Primary Trait Analysis Scales are discussed.

Writing Across the Curriculum Initiative

The importance of writing skills in the learning process has become evident in recent years through a curriculum reform movement called writing across the curriculum (WAC). Poirrier's (1997) text, *Writing to Learn* (WTL) supports the WAC approach and emphasizes the importance of writing as a skill needed by college graduates. Poirrier addresses the multitude of nursing endeavors that rely on writing skills, such as documentation, patient education materials, health policies, writing for publication, and research.

Poirrier notes that each type of writing in nursing involves communicating information to different audiences. Therefore, one of the principles of the WAC philosophy is that "writing embraces discourse with varying purposes and audiences" and consequently requires that students learn how to adapt their writing to meet the need of various groups (Hult, 1997, p. 179). The second principle emphasizes that "writing is a mode of learning" (p. 177). Hult acknowledges that writing is essential to learning, as it helps the student clarify and analyze ideas, understand the experiences they write about, and develop independent thinking skills. Writing also is viewed as "a complex developmental process" (p. 178). This principle requires a shift from exclusively emphasizing the finished written product to placing more emphasis on the writing process. According to this principle, writing improves with practice and with growth in cognitive, reading, and language skills.

Along with the increased emphasis on WAC and WTL is the need for assessment and evaluation practices that provide the student with accurate, fair, and consistent feedback on their writing processes and the quality of the final written product. A study of the writing experiences of preregistration student nurses by Whitehead (2002) found that a major theme concerned instructor feedback on writing. Student's expectation of equitable and consistent feedback was found to be a source of frustration for many students.

Despite the frequency of using written assignments in nursing education, Giddens and Lobo (2008) report a lack of research emphasis on evaluation strategies for writing assignments. To fill this research gap, Giddens and Lobo implemented a study of writing evaluation practices of graduate nurse educator students (n = 47) enrolled in a nurse educator course. As part of a course assignment, the students graded a mock paper with deliberate errors and inconsistencies. The students received the writing guidelines for the mock paper, grading criteria, and a scoring sheet. The students' written comments and corrections were made directly on the paper, and a scoring sheet was completed and analyzed.

The scoring of the mock paper was based on four attributes: the introduction of the problem, summary of issue, resolutions identified, and writing style (i.e., APA format). The scores awarded for each attribute and total score for the paper varied widely. Those with previous academic teaching experience scored the paper significantly lower in three out of the four attributes. Interestingly, the number of written comments on grammar, APA formatting, and substantive comments on the topic itself did not differ with teaching experience, nor with other demographic variables (Giddens & Lobo, 2008). Thus, those with academic experience tended to score the mock papers lower but did not differ significantly from the other scorers in terms of the number or type of evaluative comments provided on the papers. This study, though not conclusive, provides food for thought concerning interrater variability and the effect of academic experience on evaluation of written course work.

Rubrics

Varying expectations and grading criteria can add to student frustration with writing assignments. However, these frustrations may be minimized by using a rubric evaluation tool that provides a clear description of expectations for each level of performance. A useful tool to guide evaluation of papers, observed performances, and projects is a rubric, or a scoring tool that lists the grading criteria and levels of achievement for each criterion. Rubrics can be individualized for specific course assignments, yet they all share commonalities. All rubrics should focus on measuring a specific objective and rate the performance from low to high.

Several varieties of tools are available to assist in developing rubrics. An example of a template for developing a rubric is provided in Figure 4-2. In the far left column, the assignment objectives are listed. Across the top of the form the description of the performance levels and corresponding point values are listed. These levels and point values are tailored to the specific needs of the assignment. The cells in the center contain the descriptions of leveled behaviors that are specified by the instructor.

(Describe the task or performance that this rubric is designed to evaluate.)

	Beginning 1	Developing 2	Accomplished 3	Exemplary 4	Score
Stated Objective or Performance	Description of identifiable performance characteristics reflecting a beginning level of performance	Description of identifiable performance characteristics reflecting development and movement toward mastery of performance	Description of identifiable performance characteristics reflecting mastery of performance	Description of identifiable performance characteristics reflecting the highest level of performance	
Stated Objective or Performance	Description of identifiable performance characteristics reflecting a beginning level of performance	Description of identifiable performance characteristics reflecting development and movement toward mastery of performance	Description of identifiable performance characteristics reflecting mastery of performance	Description of identifiable performance characteristics reflecting the highest level of performance	
Stated Objective or Performance	Description of identifiable performance characteristics reflecting a beginning level of performance	Description of identifiable performance characteristics reflecting development and movement toward mastery of performance	Description of identifiable performance characteristics reflecting mastery of performance	Description of identifiable performance characteristics reflecting the highest level of performance	

FIGURE 4-2   Rubric Template (Reprinted with Permission B. Dodge, The WebQuest Page at http://webquest.sdsu.edu/rubrics/weblessons.htm.)

Primary Trait Analysis Scale

Walvoord and Anderson (1998) suggest a variation called a Primary Trait Analysis (PTA) scale for evaluating written assignments. They describe a PTA scale as a highly explicit, assignment specific, scoring rubric. To develop a PTA scale, the ANE adheres to the following steps:

1. Choose the assignment to be evaluated.
2. Clarify objectives for the assignment.
3. Identify traits or criterion that will be measured.
4. Describe the traits as brief noun phrases.
5. Identify a continuum of two to five descriptive statements that depict the trait.
6. Test the PTA scale with a sample paper, if available.

According to Walvoord and Anderson (1998), instructors who used PTA scales found them helpful on several levels. The explicit nature of the PTA scale helped the instructor capture the true criteria that differentiates excellent student papers from others. PTA scales also are helpful for increasing consistency when teaching assistants are caught up in grading papers, or when multiple instructors are involved in teaching multiple sections of a course. They also noted that the PTA scale can save time in the grading process and provides clear identification of student's strengths and weakness.

Critical Thinking Scale

Kennison (2006) describes the development and testing of the Critical Thinking Scale (CTS), designed to evaluate critical thinking components in student's written assignments. The scale was developed using data from the American Philosophical Association Delphi study on critical thinking (Facione, 1990) and a nursing Delphi study by Scheffer and Rubenfield (2000). Kennison (2006) found moderate interrater reliability between all three experts who used the tool to evaluate more than 50 written assignments. Higher interrater reliability was found between the raters who were most familiar with the CTS, indicating that instruction may further improve interrater reliability.

Portfolios

A portfolio is a flexible, creative, means of facilitating student learning through self-reflection, as well as a means for assessing student learning in a specific course or program of study. Many definitions of portfolios have been documented in the literature. McMullen *et al.* (2003) characterize a portfolio as "a collection of evidence, usually in written form, of both the products and processes of learning. It attests to achievement and personal and professional development by providing critical analysis of its contents" (p. 288).

The use of portfolios in student assessment is supported by several theoretical perspectives. The recognition of past learning experiences is the foundation of portfolio development and is consistent with Knowles' Theory of Adult Learning. Most experts acknowledge that portfolios should include a reflective component in which the student reviews what was accomplished and the learning outcomes achieved. This reflection process is congruent with Kolb's Experiential Learning Model, in which the learner reflects and analyzes experiences to clarify concepts and generalizations (McMullen *et al.*, 2003). An outcome of the self-assessment and reflection process is acknowledgment of the student's personal and professional development. The student who is able to see how much he or she has grown throughout the course or program of study is likely to enrich his or her sense of self-esteem. These outcomes correspond with the humanism perspective, which values the learner's growth and development.

Contents of a portfolio are highly individual. According to McMullen *et al.* (2003), "It is important that a portfolio is not just a collection of items in a folder, but that it shows how reflection by the student on these items demonstrates learning" (p. 290). McMullen *et al.* emphasize that the student should provide a rationale for why he or she selected each example and an evaluation of what was learned or how the assignment influenced professional development. To facilitate development of a portfolio assignment, the instructor should provide clear criteria and guidelines for content selection. Exemplars of well-crafted narratives which describe the rationale for selection, reflection on, and evaluation of learning components also can be provided. As a learning tool, the value of portfolios is supported by multiple theoretical perspectives, making it a very rich, versatile, and valuable learning tool.

Peer Evaluation

The growing emphasis on critical thinking, self-regulation, collaboration, and learner-center learning has resulted in an interest in peer evaluation. Peer evaluation, also called peer review and peer assessment, is a type of collaborative activity in which students, guided by evaluation criteria, provide their peers with feedback on their work (van den Berg, Admiraal, & Pilot, 2006). The goals of peer evaluation activities are to provide benefits to the student who receives the feedback and to assist the peer evaluator in developing skills and knowledge relevant to the assignment.

A review of research on peer evaluation by Topping (1998) found that students do learn from reviewing and evaluating their classmates' written assignments. However, research on the optimal designs for peer review activities is relatively new. Specific peer evaluation designs used in seven different history classes were studied by van den Berg *et al.* (2006). The researchers found three specific design features associated with optimal peer review processes. First, for peer feedback to be useful the student needs adequate time to the make revisions suggested by peers before submitting the assignment to the faculty for grading. Because the amount of time needed to accomplish peer review varies depending on the nature of the assignment, no specific time recommendations were provided. The second design factor related to the directionality of the review. Assigning peer reviewers in a reciprocal two-way fashion was easiest to organize and streamlined the process. With this arrangement, the two students are paired, each one reviewing the other's work. The third design feature related to size of peer review groups. Having only reviewer dyads was problematic because it reduced the amount of feedback; the quality of feedback could be inferior if weak students were paired together. Optimal group size was three to four students, which allowed each student to receive feedback from two to three classmates, compare comments, and evaluate the relevance of the comments.

Developing and Using Multiple Choice Tests

Faculty-developed test items are perhaps the most commonly used objective method of evaluation. Because the student's ability to progress in the nursing program and ultimately sit for the licensure examination are based on the testing experiences during the program, it is essential that students are exposed to high-quality, relevant test items. Instructor-developed test questions should be designed to measure the students' learning and achievement of course outcomes. To help assure that high-quality, fair, and unbiased questions are created, guidelines for writing items are discussed in this section.

Guidelines for Developing Multiple Choice Test Items

According to a recent review of guidelines for multiple choice (MC) test item writing, "The science of MC item writing is advancing, but item writing is still largely a creative act that we inexorably link to content standards and instruction" (Haladyna, Downing & Rodriguez, 2002, p. 329). A review by Masters *et al.* (2001) found little support for many commonly accepted guidelines. Most undergraduate nursing programs rely heavily on objective MC test items to assess student learning and critical thinking skills. Therefore, generating test items that are accurate and reliable indicators of the student's knowledge and skills, and items that can tap into the student's critical thinking abilities is essential. In this section, the general principles for writing test items are reviewed, followed by recommendations for enhancing critical thinking skills involved in choosing test time responses.

Masters *et al.* (2001) present several examples of commonly accepted guidelines that are not supported by the literature. For example, one belief is that the stems of a test item should be in a question format instead of in a sentence completion format. Masters *et al.* reported that several studies found no significant difference in discrimination or difficulty level between test item stems worded as a question or in a sentence completion format. Another practice not supported in the review is the use of four or five distractors instead of only three. The use of four or more response options may actually increase the probability of including a poor or weak distractor. Providing high quality distractors requires students to think and rationalize when selecting an answer. Therefore, three good distractors serve just as well as four or five distractors in which one or two are weak choices.

A review by Haladyna *et al.* (2002) validated 32 test-item writing guidelines using a review of text book recommendations and research studies. They found the guidelines most commonly represented in the literature related to content, the structure of the stems, structure of the response choices, formatting, and style concerns. In reviewing the guidelines many may seem self-evident, yet in practice implementing these guidelines is not an easy task.

BOX 4-6   Content Related Guidelines for Writing Test Items

1. Reflect a single specific piece of content.

2. Test important content.

3. Use novel material to test higher-level learning.

4. Keep items independent from other items.

5. Avoid over-specific and over-general content.

6. Avoid opinion-based items.

7. Avoid trick items.

8. Keep vocabulary simple.

Some data from Haladyna, T., Downing, S., & Rodriguez, M. (2002). A review of multiple choice item-writing guidelines for classroom assessment. *Applied Measurement in Education, 15*(3), 312; and Masters, J. C., Hulsmeyer, B. S., Pike, M. E., Leichty, K., Miller, M. T., & Verst, A. L. (2001). Assessment of multiple choice questions in selected test banks accompanying text books used in nursing education. *Journal of Nursing Education, 40*, 25–31.

Content-related guidelines for writing test items are summarized in Box 4-6. The first two guidelines concern writing items with a singular focus and testing important content. Although these guidelines seem obvious, both are easy to violate. Often in an attempt to write high-level questions, the item writer may present stems with more than one focus or multiple pieces of extraneous information. It is also common to believe that writing test items about specific details is a way to test advanced or higher-ordered learning, but that is not the case. The ANE should strive to test key concepts over details. Another guideline is to use novel material that paraphrases content presented in the text or lecture. Using a test item drawn word for word from the textbook tends to test a student's recall more than his or her ability to generalize the information. Keeping test items independent from one another may seem like an obvious guideline, but in practice can be difficult to implement. This requires that information in the stem or response items of one question should not provide clues to the answer of another question. Furthermore, the correct response to one item should not be required to determine the correct response to another item. The fifth guideline suggested by Haladyna and colleagues involves avoiding being over-specific and over-general in the question stem. Over-specific questions tend to test knowledge of details versus higher-order thinking ability. Questions that are too general leave room for speculation, and students will tend to need more clarity to respond to the question.

The final guidelines Haladyna et al. (2002) recommend relate to format and style. A variety of format options are possible, including sentence completion, and best answer versions of the conventional MC, true-false (TF), matching, complex MC, alternate choice, and the multiple true-false (MTF) format. Instructors are most likely familiar with the conventional MC, true-false, and matching formats that are commonly used in testing. In the complex MC format, the responses are listed and the student selects from various combinations of those responses. For example, if the responses are listed as:

1. Change the dressing
2. Have the patient ambulate
3. Notify the doctor
4. Administer the prescribed antibiotic,

the response choices would be various combinations of those listed, such as:

A. 1 and 3
B. 2 and 3
C. 1 and 4
D. 2 and 4

According to Haladyna et al. (2002), the complex MC format is the only format not supported by research. In fact, they note that most test-writing experts agree that the use of complex MC format should be avoided. Making the response items more complex in terms of combinations does not translate to making questions that use the student's higher-order thinking.

Style guidelines for writing test items refer to editing and proofing items for correct grammar, punctuation, capitalization, spelling, and excessive wordiness. If the examination score is used to evaluate content knowledge and thinking skills, it is crucial that the questions do not inadvertently include clues to the correct response. Test questions may provide clues in many ways. For example, Haladyna *et al.* (2002) list the use of terms that can indicate that the response is incorrect, such as using "always," "never," "completely," and "absolutely" in the response choices. Using word choices in the responses that resemble words in the stem can also be a clue to the correct response. Another clue to identifying the incorrect response is grammatical inconsistency in tense or pluralization. Using two or three similar response choices and only one item that is dissimilar may also provide a clue to the correct or incorrect response. For example, in the list of responses:

A. Check blood pressure every 4 hours
B. Check blood pressure every 8 hours
C. Check capillary refill every 2 hours

item C is different from the other choices. If item C were the intended correct response, a better option would be to make responses A and B dissimilar to each other or make all items homogeneous by including a reference to capillary refill.

Making all distractors plausible may seem like an obvious guideline; however, in practice it is often difficult to create distractors that are plausible yet incorrect. Haladyna *et al.* (2002) suggest using commonly observed errors and misconceptions as a basis for writing distractors. For example, student questions and misconceptions noted in the classroom or clinical setting can serve as plausible distractors. Guidelines for writing multiple choice stems and response choices are summarized in Box 4-7.

Confidence-Based Marking

Confidence-based marking (CBM) is a modified version of multiple choice questions. In CBM examinations, the student indicates the answer selected and rates his or her degree of confidence that the answer selected is correct. The points earned for each question reflect a combination of the answer and the student's level of confidence or certainty that the answer is correct. For example, a correct response selected with

BOX 4-7   Guidelines for Writing Multiple Choice Stems and Response Choices

Stem Guidelines:

1. Provide clear directions.

2. Include the central idea.

3. Avoid excessive verbiage.

4. Phrase stem positively.

Response Choice Guidelines:

1. Three response choices are adequate.

2. Include only one correct response.

3. Vary the location of the right answer (A, B, or C).

4. Sequence choices in logical order.

5. Keep response choices independent.

6. Keep response choices homogeneous.

7. Keep response choices similar in length.

8. Use "None-of-the-above" carefully.

9. Avoid using "All-of-the-above."

10. Phrase choices positively.

11. Avoid giving clues to the correct response.

12. Use plausible distractors.

13. Use common errors of students as distractors.

14. Use humor carefully.

Some data from Haladyna, T., Downing, S., & Rodriguez, M. (2002). A review of multiple choice item-writing guidelines for classroom assessment. *Applied Measurement in Education, 15*(3), 309–334; and King, K. V., Gardner, D. A., Zucker, S., & Jorgensen, M. A. (2004). *The assessment report. The distractor rationale taxonomy: Enhancing multiple choice items in reading and mathematics.* Pearson Education, pp. 1–14. http://pearsonassess.com/NR/rdonlyres/D7E62EC6-CC3F-47B6-B1CB-A83F341AD768/0/Distractor_Rationales.pdf.

high certainty would earn the highest point value, whereas an incorrect response selected with high certainty would earn the lowest point value. Gardner-Medwin (2006) report on the use of CBM examinations during the first 2 years of medical school. One of the benefits of having the student rate his or her confidence in the answer selected was that it required the student to reflect and self-assess his or her understanding of the material.

In summary, written tests are a common way to evaluate learners' knowledge. However, it is not practical to test students' knowledge of the entire subject matter domain. Instead, tests and other assessments should provide an adequate sampling of the subject matter (Gronlund, 2004; Gronlund & Brookhart, 2009; Nitko, 2004). McDonald (2008) cautions that "using a single test or type of measurement instrument is not a satisfactory assessment strategy. Most course objectives require a variety of measurement and evaluation strategies to determine student competency in a particular course" (p. 14).

Criteria for Developing Critical Thinking Test Items

Morrison and Free (2001) discuss the use of four criteria for creating multiple choice test items to test critical thinking (Box 4-8). The first criterion is to include a rationale for each response item. This is based on the awareness that testing is both a learning opportunity and an evaluative process. Test item rationales should include why the distractors are incorrect and explain why the correct item is the best response. Morrison and Free (2001) recommend that test reviews allow students the opportunity to review the test and see the rationales given for each item. This encourages the student to engage in critical thinking by thinking about the reasons he or she chose a particular response.

The second criterion for developing critical thinking test items is to write questions at the cognitive level of application or higher. The use of verbs associated with Bloom's taxonomy of educational objectives can be helpful in this regard. The explicit use of specific verbs in a test question can be a guide to the cognitive level. However, sometimes verbs are not explicitly identified. In those cases, the ANE needs to look at the underlying nature of what the student is being asked. For example, is the student expected to compare normal to abnormal or distinguish a significant finding from a nonsignificant finding to answer the question correctly? If so, the question is written at the analysis level.

Developing test items that require multilogical thinking is the third criteria. Morrison, Smith, and Britt (1996), define multilogical thinking test items as those "requir-

---

BOX 4-8   Criteria for Developing Critical Thinking Test Items

- Write a rationale for the correct and incorrect responses.

- Write at the application level or higher.

- Require the use of multilogical thinking.

- Require a high level of discrimination.

Data from Morrison, S., & Free, K. W. (2001). Writing multiple-choice test items that promote and measure critical thinking. *Journal of Nursing Education, 40,* 17–24.

---

ing knowledge of more than one fact (or concept)" (p. 20). For example, a test item that requires the student to distinguish which assessment finding is most significant for a particular medical condition requires knowledge of the condition, knowledge of the signs and symptoms of the condition, and the ability to determine which symptom is most important in the given situation.

Creating test items with a high level of discrimination is the fourth criterion described by Morrison and Free (2001). Discriminating items ask the student to prioritize, select the most important item, or select an answer that requires calculation. However, Morrison and Free emphasize that to be truly discriminating, all choices must be plausible options, with one item being the best. These types of questions, in which all responses are correct, but one is the better choice, are perhaps the most difficult for students to master. Implementing the four criteria for developing critical thinking test items can help ensure that the items are testing students' higher cognitive skills.

Providing Feedback to Learners

Providing feedback to learners is a component of both formative and summative evaluation. Feedback is essentially "communication of information to the student . . . that helps the student reflect on the information, construct self-knowledge relevant to learning, and set further learning goals" (Bonnel, 2008, p. 290). Nicol and Macfarlane-Dick (2006) synthesized the research on assessment and feedback and generated a model to depict the feedback processes.

According to the model, learning tasks or assignments serve as a stimulus for students to initiate self-regulatory processes. Self-regulation is defined as "the degree to which students can regulate aspects of their thinking, motivation, and behavior during learning" (Nicol & Macfarlane-Dick, 2006, p. 199). They point out that although it is assumed that students can self-regulate internal states and behaviors as well as some aspects of the environment, this [self-regulation] does not mean that the student always has full control. Learning tasks set by teachers, marking regime, and other course requirements are not under students' control, even though students still have the latitude to self-regulate with such constraints (p. 205).

According to researchers, even students who are academically at risk can learn self-regulation. The benefits of encouraging self-regulation of students are many. Students who are self-regulated tend to be high achievers who are confident in their learning. They are more persistent and resourceful in their learning efforts (Pintrich, 1995; Zimmerman & Schunk, 2001). The ANE can help students develop self-regulation skills by teaching about meta cognition, self-monitoring, meta cognitive skills, and by providing an environment in which students can practice those skills (Nicol & Macfarlane-Dick, 2006).

The student uses related knowledge and personal beliefs about the learning activity to give personal meaning to the assignment. Personal goals and strategies are then selected to accomplish the goals. As the learner interacts with the learning task, internal (self) feedback as well as external feedback from peers and teachers is received and interpreted. When interpreting the feedback, the learner compares the current progress with the desired goals and determines if any adjustments are needed. According to Nicol and Macfarlane-Dick, the self-regulation that occurs may involve, "reinterpreting the task . . . an adjustment of internal goals, tactics, or strategies . . . (or) the student might even revise his or her domain knowledge or motivational beliefs" (p. 202).

Principles of Good Feedback

Within the model, Nicol and Macfarlane-Dick (2006) have identified seven principles of good feedback practice (Box 4-9). The first principle is foundational to the others and is simply that the feedback identifies or clarifies what is expected for good performance. This involves establishing goals and criteria, and identifying the standards that the student is expected to achieve. The feedback should relate back to goals, criteria, and or standards so that it is clear to the student what aspects were or were not achieved. Nicol and Macfarlane-Dick (2006) cite several studies that report a discrepancy between student and teacher in the interpretation of grading standards. Poor student performance was found to correlate with the amount of discrepancy. They recommend that teachers share exemplars of written assignments that students can see and use as a comparison. They also recommend using carefully designed grading criteria that define the performance levels for each letter grade. Then discuss the

---

BOX 4-9   Seven Principles of Good Feedback

1. Clarify what good performance is.

2. Facilitate self-assessment.

3. Deliver high-quality feedback information.

4. Encourage teacher and peer dialogue.

5. Encourage positive motivation and self-esteem.

6. Provide opportunities to close the gap.

7. Use feedback to improve teaching.

Data from Nicol, D., & Macfarlane-Dick, D. (2006). Formative assessment and self-regulated learning: A model and seven principles of good feedback practice. *Studies in Higher Education, 31*(2), 203.

---

criteria in class and allow opportunities for peer review in which students can apply the criteria to other students' papers.

The second principle is that good feedback should facilitate self-assessment. This can involve using structured self-assessment tasks, peer evaluation, or asking students to use the established assignment criteria to identify the strengths and weakness of their work. To apply the second principle "facilitates the development of self-assessment in learning" the ANE needs to create structured opportunities for feedback during classroom activities and for written assignments (Nicol & Macfarlane-Dick, 2006, p. 208). Strategies such as asking students to identify the type of feedback they prefer on written assignments and having students identify the strengths and weakness of their work before turning it in may be helpful.

The third principle is that good feedback should "deliver high quality information to students about their learning" (Nicol & Macfarlane-Dick, 2006, p. 208). Feedback should not only relate to strengths and weaknesses of the student's work, but to corrective actions and trouble shooting that would be helpful for the student in future assignments. Some suggestions are to: (1) provide corrective advice in addition to comments on strengths and weaknesses, (2) prioritize the areas needing improvement, (3) provide timely feedback, and (4) limit the amount of corrective feedback so that it is more likely to be used.

It is important that feedback is understood and internalized by the student. One way Nicol and Macfarlane-Dick suggest increasing the student's understanding and internalizing of feedback is to encourage dialog about the feedback with peers and faculty. Thus, the fourth principle of good feedback is to, "encourage teacher and peer dialog around learning" (p. 210). Feedback needs to be more than just telling students or conveying information. Posing written questions or providing a time for students to meet in small groups and discuss feedback may be helpful. To encourage teacher and peer dialog around learning (principle four), Nicol and Macfarlane-Dick (2006) emphasizes that students need to understand the feedback given. Dialog about the feedback is one way for students to gain this understanding. Rather than thinking of feedback as "telling" students, they recommend thinking of feedback as dialog with students that can incorporate peer feedback as well. When class size prohibits direct dialog with individual students, the instructor may engage in small group discussions about the instructor and peer feedback received. The group sessions may serve to clarify the feedback and provide students with suggestions for implementing the feedback in future assignments. In addition, technology, such as electronic student response systems, may be used to collect in-class responses to the feedback received. The responses can be tallied and displayed to the class and can serve as a basis for further discussion.

There is evidence that motivation to learn and self-esteem (principle five) are affected by the quality and type of feedback received. For example, praising students in terms of achievement of learning goals has been found to be more effective in motivating students than praising their ability to do the work, or making positive comments about their intelligence (Black & William, 1998). A feedback strategy that may enhance student motivation and self-esteem involves providing frequent opportunities for formative assessment. Both serial writing assignments in which students can submit a draft for feedback before grading and using frequent online practice tests can provide formative feedback.

Principle 6, referred to as closing "the gap between current and desired performance" (Nicol and Macfarlane-Dick, 2006, p. 5), requires that students demonstrate what they have learned from the feedback received. Strategies that can help students apply the feedback received include: (1) designing two-stage assignments in which the feedback from the first stage can be useful for completing the second stage, (2) demonstrating strategies to the class, and (3) small group activities in which students generate suggestions about how to implement written feedback. Submission of drafts or outlines of projects for feedback will provide additional opportunities to demonstrate learning from the feedback received.

Unlike the other principles of good feedback that are student focused, the final principle is teacher focused. The goal of this principle is for the teacher to use the feedback information to identify areas in which students are having difficulty and take actions to remedy the difficulty. The key is in observing student behavior and using frequent, brief assessments to collect information about how well students understand the material.

Another example Nicol (2007) provides is offering an MC examination before the final exam and using the results of the testing to guide further class discussion. In this case, the teacher uses several principles of good feedback. If the teacher discovers a specific content area that students did not do well on, the teacher can use that information to guide discussion. Class discussion on the subject matter encourages dialog between students and teacher, which uses principle four—encourage dialog around learning.

Multiple Choice Items Development Assignment

Another way to assess and evaluate learning is to have students write test items on the content covered in class. Fellenz (2004) formalized the student's writing of test questions into an assignment called the multiple choice items development assignment (MCIDA). Students were provided instruction on writing MC questions and how to classify them using Bloom's taxonomy. Throughout the course, students wrote MC test items, including the response choices and rationale for each answer. They also worked in groups to give each other feedback on the questions and rationale. The final test questions submitted by the students were worth a portion of the final course grade.

Using the MCIDA provided a mechanism for applying all seven principles of good feedback (Nicol, 2007). Principle one (clarify goals, criteria, and standards) was established by having the students use their knowledge of MC test item writing and subject matter knowledge to write questions geared to specific criteria. The process of developing questions, rationale, and evaluating the level of Bloom's taxonomy required the students to self-reflect and assess what they had written (principle two). In Fellenz's study, quality feedback was provided by a trained tutor (Fellenz, 2004). Dialog and discussion was encouraged during the group feedback process (principle four). Principle five, (feedback and motivation), was activated by making the MCIDA a formative process and using selected MC questions in the final examination. This served to motivate students during the process. Using the MC questions in a formative manner and allowing students to answer until they reached a specific level of performance helped to close the gap, thereby meeting principle six. The final principle, using feedback to shape teaching, can be easily implemented by using the results of the student's testing to identify areas in which students showed a need for greater understanding and then using that information to guide further class sessions.

In evaluating the MCIDA, Fellenz (2004) found several positive outcomes. Students commented that providing a rationale for their answers deepened their understanding of the subject matter. The process of peer reviewing the MC test items and receiving feedback enhanced collaboration. Fellenz also reported that students became more vested in the assessment process because of their participation. Through this example and others, Nicol (2007) points out that MC questions can be an effective means of testing higher-order thinking, especially when the seven principles of good feedback are applied.

Feedback in Technology-Based Classrooms

Providing feedback to students enrolled in-off campus interactive television (ITV) courses represents a unique set of challenges. Clow (1999) found that off-campus ITV students rate the adequacy of feedback lower than do their on-campus counterparts. Graduate and undergraduate students also differed in their evaluation of ITV and on-campus courses. Undergraduate students tended to find the ITV courses less valuable, and they tended to be less engaged in the subject matter. In addition, they perceived the instructor as being less prepared and less responsive to student needs. To counter the students' negative perceptions, Clow recommends that faculty receive comprehensive preparation and practice in the use of educational technology. Such training will enable the instructor to be more student focused, and able to readily address student questions and provide feedback. In addition, the instructor can incorporate teaching strategies that provide opportunities to connect and interact with other students as well as the instructor, which will increase opportunities for students to connect and give and receive feedback.

Feedback is valuable to combat the sense of isolation that students enrolled in ITV and online courses may experience. According to Bonnel (2008), it is important that multiple feedback mechanisms be built into the design of online courses. Bonnel (2008) summarizes evidence-based feedback strategies for online courses into three categories; those related to course design, teacher roles, and student participation (Box 4-10). Although intended for use in online and other distance learning formats, these feedback strategies may be adapted to other course formats in which opportunities for feedback are limited.

Bonnel (2008) emphasizes that building feedback opportunities into the design of online courses is the foundation for providing good feedback. Bonnel's research on more than 70 students supports the notion that students view feedback as more than comments from the instructor. Self-reflection activities, peer feedback, and automated feedback from case studies and quizzes are also mechanisms for feedback that should be planned into the course design.

Faculty feedback can be provided to individual students, student groups working

---

BOX 4-10   Evidence-Based Online Feedback Strategies

Course Design Strategies:

1. Specify in course welcome letter, course announcements, or an introductory module, the expectations, responsibilities, type, and amount of feedback that will be provided.

2. Use several forms of feedback, such as online practice questions, case studies, survey responses, and self-reflection.

3. Develop mini-assignments that are part of a larger project.

Faculty Roles:

1. Provide a weekly bulleted summary of what has been covered.

2. Clearly identify e-mail comments as feedback on a specific assignment.

3. Use positive conversational tone in written feedback.

4. Include questions as feedback to stimulate student self-reflection.

5. Use rubrics to guide feedback.

6. Inform students about online discussion strategies and responsibilities.

7. Facilitate student peer review and group projects.

Data from Bonnel, W. (2008). Improving feedback to students in online courses. *Nursing Education Perspectives, 29*(5), 291.

---

online course delivery systems involves providing students with information about examination score ranges and averages. Faculty can enhance this form of automated feedback by briefly discussing and interpreting the meaning of the examination statistics. In addition, the instructor can provide feedback to the entire group about the subject matter, types of questions that the majority of students did well with, or areas that could use further study.

The third component of online feedback involves the students' active role. Students need to be informed and reminded about their role in seeking feedback and the use of feedback rubrics when needed. The ANE can provide assignments in which students can give, receive, and use feedback and engage in self-reflection about the learning activity. If peer evaluation is used, students can be guided in how to give peer feedback. According to Bonnel, "good feedback helps students reflect on information, construct self-knowledge, and set further learning goals" (2008, p. 293). Some additional strategies for feedback suggested by Nicol and Macfarlane-Dick (2006) include asking each student to indicate on his or her papers and other assignments, areas in which he or she had trouble. Students working in groups can identify questions or scenarios and ask the class to respond. Whichever strategies are used, if one or more of the principles of good feedback are incorporated, cognitive and motivational aspects associated with self-regulation of learning will be enhanced.

Test Administration

Oermann and Gaberson (2006) emphasize the need to control testing conditions to enhance the reliability of test scores. One factor that can be helpful in this regard is providing consistent and complete instructions and reminders for students before the exam. Apprising students of the total number of questions, how much time they will have to complete the exam, what to do if a question is unclear, and any special instructions for completing the exam, may be helpful. They also recommend providing sufficient time for completing the test, pointing out that reliability will be lower if students who know the material do not have sufficient time to complete the test. Measures to reduce cheating are also important for establishing valid as well as reliable test scores. Students who cheat are likely to "respond correctly to items to which they actually do not know the answer . . . thus contributing to inaccurate and less meaningful interpretations of test scores" (p. 34).

Analyzing Test Items

There are two statistical models commonly used in educational measurement and test item analysis, Classical Test Theory (CTT) and Item Response Theory (IRT). CTT is commonly used for course-specific, teacher-developed tests, whereas IRT more commonly is used for computerized adaptive testing for credentialing and licensure examinations. A comparison of CTT an IRT is provided in Table 4-4.

Classical Test Theory

CTT is widely used for analyzing instructor-generated test items. Within CTT, factors that influence reliability of test scores can be categorized as student, test item, and/or test administration factors (Frisbie, 1988). Student factors such as the diversity of the group, the student's level of motivation or indifference about their test performance, and their test-taking skills can affect reliability, item difficulty, and discrimination indices. Test item factors such as the test length, test content, item difficulty, and discrimination can also affect the consistency of test scores. Factors related to test administration such as enforcing time limits and methods to control cheating also affect error rates and the reliability of the test.

TABLE 4-4   **Comparison of Classical Test Theory and Item Response Theory**

	Classical Test Theory	Item Response Theory
Focus	• Test level	• Item level
Key concepts	• True score • Error score • Observed score	• Probability of getting an item correct is a function of a latent trait or ability. • Inferences made are concerned with the instrument rather than the test scores.
Statistical assumptions	• Weaker, easier to meet with test data	• Strong, more difficult to meet with test data • Test measures one trait and item responses are independent of other responses
Statistical measures	• Test item difficulty and discrimination commonly used • Reliability determined for the entire test	• Numerous statistical approaches • Reliability is related to individual test items
Limitations	• Statistical measures are group dependent (i.e., vary with the test takers)	• Requires larger more heterogeneous sample
Strengths	• Easier to detect poor-quality items • Underlying concepts are easier to understand • Can be used for smaller student groups	• Interpretations that are more flexible are possible • Useful for computerized adaptive testing

Some data from Fan, X. (1998). Item response theory and classical test theory: An empirical comparison of their item/person statistics. *Educational and Psychological Measurement, 58*(3), 1–7; Hambleton, R., & Jones, R. (1993). An NCME instructional module on comparison of classical test theory and item response theory and their applications to test development. *Educational Measurement: Issues and Practice, 12*(3), 38–47; Yu, C. H., Jannasch-Pennell, A., & DiGangi, S. (2008, February 21). A non-technical approach for illustrating item response theory. *Journal of Applied Testing Technology, 9*(2), 1–32.

Central concepts in CTT are the students' observed or measured test score, the error score, which includes both random and systematic error, and the true score. The relationship between these concepts is commonly depicted as an equation in which the student's true score = observed score + error score. Ideally, the true score represents the student's ability, and variations in observed scores are caused by random errors such as omissions, guessing, reading errors, and fatigue. In the end, these

> **BOX 4-11   Formulas for Test Item Analysis Statistics**
>
> 1. Difficulty index = number of students choosing the correct response (divided by) total number of students answering the question
>
> 2. Discrimination index = the fraction of highest scoring students who answered correctly (minus) the fraction of lowest scoring students who answered correctly
>
> Data from Davis, B. (2009). *Tools for teaching* (2nd ed., pp. 398–399). San Francisco: Jossey Bass.

random errors are assumed to cancel each other out. Statistical analysis performed under the CTT umbrella includes test item difficulty and item discrimination. In addition, analyzing test item distractors is important for determining validity of the item.

Applying the guidelines for developing MC questions and developing critical thinking items will provide a good foundation for developing quality test items. After the test is administered, the test items can be analyzed statistically for difficulty and discrimination. These indices are useful for confirming or in some cases refuting the quality of specific test items. Many computerized item analysis programs automatically report the difficulty index and discrimination index; however, they may be calculated manually using the formulas in Box 4-11.

Difficulty Index

The difficulty index of a test item refers to the percentage of students who answer the item correctly. It is commonly reported as a p value ranging from zero to 1.00 (Oermann & Gaberson, 2006, p. 174). Items that all students answered correctly are reported as a value of 1.00 and items that all students missed have a value of 0.00. The desirable range for the difficulty index statistic is typically between 0.30 and 0.70. Higher difficulty index values tend to be obtained by test takers with higher ability; conversely, lower difficulty index values by test takers with below average ability (Hambleton & Jones, 1993). Oermann & Gaberson caution that the difficulty index for a specific test item needs to consider the student's ability and the teacher's effectiveness. Both factors can influence the reliability of the index scores.

Discrimination Index

The discrimination index identifies how well a test item discriminated between those who scored high on the examination overall and those who scored low on the examination overall (Oermann & Gaberson, 2006). The value of the discrimination index

(D) statistic ranges from −1.00 to +1.00. A positive discrimination index is desirable as it indicates that the item was answered correctly more often by students who did well on the test than by those who did not do well. Generally a D value of +0.40 or higher is considered a strong discriminator between students who did well and those who did not do well, and D values between +0.30 and +0.39 indicate a good level of discrimination (Oermann & Gaberson, 2006). D index values less than +0.29 and into the negative range represent poor discrimination and most likely should be revised or not used again (Nitko, 2004). Hambleton and Jones emphasize that discrimination indices are most meaningful when test takers have similar test item knowledge or skill. Higher values tend to be obtained from groups who are heterogeneous, and lower values from groups who are homogeneous (1999). Thus, student groups with a narrow grade point average (GPA) range may produce lower discrimination index values and those with a wider GPA range.

Oermann & Gaberson (2006) caution that test items deemed weak or of poor quality based on the difficulty and discrimination index should also be analyzed for the quality of the distractors before deciding to eliminate or revise the item. Criteria for good distractors are summarized in Box 4-12. Poor test item distractors can be identified by the number and type of students who select the distractor. Red flags for poor quality distractors include a distractor that is not selected by any of the lower-scoring students or a distractor that is selected by high-scoring students with approximately the same frequency as the correct response. A good distractor will be selected by at least one lower-scoring student.

Item Response Theory

Compared with CTT, IRT is a robust, complex theory based on stringent statistical assumptions. Fagerlund and McShane defined IRT as "a family of mathematical models used to determine the difficulty of test questions and estimate the ability of candidates" (2005, p. 22). IRT is used hand-in-hand with computerized adaptive

---

BOX 4-12   Criteria for Good Distractors

1. Each distractor is selected at least once.

2. Each distractor is selected by a greater number of lower scoring students than higher scoring students.

Data from Oermann, M., & Gaberson, K. (2006). *Evaluation and testing in nursing education* (2nd ed., pp. 176–177). New York: Springer.

testing to select test items from a test bank. Selection of specific test items is adjusted or adapted to meet the student's ability level. With adaptive testing, the test is dynamically created based on the student's response to each successive question. Myer (2008) notes that "for simple test items such as right or wrong answers, item response theory specifies that the probability of answering an item correctly should increase in a predictable manner as the level of the student's ability increases" (p. 2).

IRT is used to develop computerized adaptive examinations that are unique for each individual test taker. "A computerized adaptive test begins with administration of an item of medium difficulty, and the examinee's response to that item determines which level of item difficulty is administered next" (Reid *et al.*, 2007, p. 180). Professional examinations such as the NCLEX-RN and the Self-Evaluation Examination (SEE) for nurse anesthetists (Fagerlund & McShane, 2005); and large standardized examinations such as the GRE and SAT use computerized adaptive testing (Lawson, 2006). An advantage of using IRT for adaptive testing is that a smaller number of representative test items need to be completed to ensure that test takers have an adequate knowledge base. Another advantage is that computerized adaptive testing is able to measure the test taker's abilities without the need to impose time restrains that could negatively influence reliability (Reid *et al.*, 2007).

Grading Students' Test Performance

Grading schemes can be categorized as norm- and criterion-referenced, depending on the purpose of testing and the process used to determine test grades. "These two tests differ in their intended purposes, the way in which content is selected, and the scoring process which defines how the test results must be interpreted" (Bond, 1996, para. 1). Each approach has advantages and disadvantages that are outlined in Table 4-5.

Criterion-Referenced Grading

In criterion-referenced grading (also called standards-referenced testing), "a letter grade reflects a student's level of achievement against a specific standard or benchmark, independent of how other students in the class have performed" (Davis, 2009, p. 419). A major advantage of criterion-referenced grading is that students are aware of the level of performance expected for each grade level before testing. In addition, one student's grade will not be affected by other student's grade and there is no limit to the number of students who can achieve each specific grade level (Davis, 2009,

p. 420). A disadvantage includes the need to establish fair cutoffs, which accurately reflect A, B, C, D, and F level performance. This is especially important in nursing programs that rely on course examinations to determine whether students have gained sufficient knowledge and are ready to progress to the next course and eventually graduate.

TABLE 4-5 Comparison of Norm and Criterion-Referenced Grading		
	Criterion-Referenced Grading	**Norm-Referenced Grading**
Purpose	• To determine how well the student is learning the course content • To determine how well the content was taught	• To produce a rank ordering of students • To classify students
How content is selected	• Content determined by significance to the curriculum and emphasis given during the instruction	• Content is determined by how well it discriminates among strong and weak students.
How the test results are interpreted	• Reported as the number or percent of correct responses and compared to a pre-established criterion	• Reported as percentile rank scores distributed along a bell curve • Majority of scores fall in the center of the curve, which corresponds, to average or C-level performance.
Advantages	• Student grade is compared to preestablished criterion or benchmark. • Students know the level of performance expected for a specific grade. • No limit to the number of students who can earn a specific grade • Low scores provide feedback on student difficulty with material or teacher's lack of effectiveness in teaching or evaluating.	• A flexible approach • Rewards students who perform well compared with their classmates • Assures some students will receive A's no matter how difficult the material or how few items were answered correctly

(continues)

TABLE 4-5 Comparison of Norm and Criterion-Referenced Grading *(continued)*		
	Criterion-Referenced Grading	**Norm-Referenced Grading**
Disadvantages	• Instructor may need guidance in establishing standards and cutoffs, which reflect the desired level of knowledge and skills.	• Grades do not necessarily indicate achievement of learning outcomes. • Grading "standards" are student performance based rather than learning outcome based. • Grading "standards' are not consistent from term to term. Weak students may receive passing grades. • Grades do not reflect student difficulty in learning, nor the teacher's difficulty in teaching and evaluating learning. • There is no predetermined level of performance; thus, students do not know what or how much is expected of them.

Data from Bond, L. A. (1996). Norm- and criterion-referenced testing. *Practical Assessment, Research & Evaluation, 5*(2), available at http://PAREonline.net/getvn.asp?v=5&n=2; and Davis, B. (2009). *Tools for teaching* (2nd ed., pp. 420–423). San Francisco: Jossey Bass.

Norm-Referenced Grading

In norm-referenced grading, the student's test grade is determined by comparing the student's test score to other students' scores. Commonly referred to as grading on a curve, norm-referenced grading does not use pre-established raw scores cutoffs. Instead, the instructor may determine who has earned a specific grade by using preset percent allocations for each letter grade, or by converting the raw score to a percentile. Using preset percent allocations, Gronlund and Waugh (2008) suggest that the greatest number of students—40% to 50%—should be awarded C's followed by 20% to 30% awarded B's. Ten to twenty percent would earn A's and D's, and 0% to 10% would earn F's.

An advantage of using norm-referenced grading is that it rewards students who perform exceptionally well in comparison with others (Davis, 2009). However, criticisms of using norm-referenced grading are numerous. Most of the criticisms relate to underlying concerns regarding the reliability and validity of the process and the type of learning atmosphere that is perpetuated. Davis points out that the grade achieved when grading on a curve does not indicate how much the student has learned. It is quite possible for a student who receives an A on a norm-referenced test to be equated with a much lower grade if the test was criterion-referenced, because grading on the curve mandates that the highest scoring student receive an A no matter how low the score. In essence, the norm-referenced approach is based on the assumption that "classes are large enough and diverse enough to generate a full range of grades" (Davis, 2009, p. 422). Thus, no matter how exceptional a particular student group is, some will earn C's, D's, and possibly F's, and likewise extremely weak students could earn A's and B's. However, in nursing courses that tend to be smaller and homogenous, the assumption that classes are large and students are diverse enough to generate a wide range of scores may not be applicable.

Another issue is that in norm-referenced grading the majority of students will pass a course with a C or higher, whether or not they have actually mastered the material. Thus, norm-referenced grading tends to mask any difficulty students may be having in learning, whether resulting from the student's lack of ability or motivation, or the instructor's difficulty in teaching and evaluating the material. In terms of consistency, grading standards may fluctuate from term to term with norm-referenced grading. Depending on the composition of a class, a student could earn one grade one semester but an entirely different grade for the same performance if enrolled in a different semester. For professions that demand that graduates achieve a minimal competency level, norm-referenced grading is counterproductive and not recommended.

CONCLUSION

Assessment and evaluation are integral components of teaching practice. Reliability and validity of assessment and evaluation data is crucial for determining the degree to which learning objectives have been met. The accuracy of data hinges on the ANE's knowledge and skill in developing and implementing assessments, and interpreting findings. Effective evaluation of cognitive, affective, and psychomotor learning is enhanced by using multiple methods and data sources.

SUMMARY

- Competency four involves the use of effective assessment and evaluation practices in teaching.
- Assessment and evaluation strategies can be used in all learning environments for all learning domains.

- The terms assessment and evaluation refer to processes used with individuals, groups of students in specific courses, and groups of students in a program of study.
- The term assessment is broader in scope and subsumes the term evaluation.
- Evaluation refers to determining the degree to which individual students have met the course objectives and program outcomes.
- Formative evaluation is conducted early and/or ongoing throughout a course, to provide feedback to the instructor and student concerning learning needs.
- Summative evaluation is used to determine how well the student has learned after the instruction has been completed.
- Both assessment and evaluation processes may involve testing, writing papers, and instructor observation.
- Validity of assessment and evaluation data involves determining if the test items are an accurate reflection of what was taught and if they correspond to the learning objectives of the course.
- Types of validity include face, content, criterion, and construct validity (see Box 4-1).
- A test blueprint identifies the content area, objectives, learning domain, and domain level being measured by specific exam questions and supports the validity of the examination (see Figure 4-1).
- Three conditions influence reliability of assessment data, the student, the administration conditions, and the test itself.
- Student-related factors influencing test reliability include heterogeneity of the student group, motivation, and test-taking skills.
- Students with a high degree of test-taking skill may perform with greater reliability than those with weaker test-taking skills.
- Administration factors that influence test reliability include timing, providing consistent instructions, and enforcing measures to control cheating.
- Several test factors can enhance or detract from reliability, including the number of test items, how homogenous or interrelated the items are, and the quality of the test items.
- Guidelines for conducting an assessment include: (1) using a systematic assessment process, (2) using multidimensional assessment methods throughout the course, (3) aligning assessments with the learning objectives, and (4) aligning assessment with the type and complexity of content taught.
- Assessment and evaluation competencies for educators provide guidance in issues related to: (1) test item development, (2) evaluation of scores, (3) docu-

mentation, (4) responsibilities of test takers, and (5) specific testing applications (see Box 4-3).

- Developing an assessment plan involves forming learning objectives, and determining teaching and evaluation strategies.
- Leveled learning objectives can be written for the three learning domains, cognitive, affective, and psychomotor.
- Cognitive learning domain is concerned with acquiring and using knowledge and thinking skills.
- Bloom's original cognitive taxonomy describes a hierarchy of cognitive learning complexity (i.e., knowledge, comprehension, application, analysis, evaluation, and synthesis).
- Bloom's revised cognitive taxonomy is a two-dimensional model, which consists of six cognitive process dimensions and four levels of knowledge.
- The cognitive process dimensions of Bloom's revised cognitive taxonomy include remember, understand, apply, analyze, evaluate, and create.
- The knowledge levels of Bloom's revised cognitive taxonomy include factual, conceptual, procedural, and metacognitive knowledge.
- Gagné's learning taxonomy incorporates human capabilities categorized as intellectual, cognitive, verbal, motor, and attitude.
- The affective learning taxonomy developed by Krathwohl, Bloom, and Masia is concerned with feelings and attitudes about a topic and the degree of acceptance and internalization the person displays concerning the topic.
- The affective taxonomy developed by Krathwohl, Bloom, and Masia is a five level hierarchy, which includes receiving, responding, valuing, organization, and culminates in characterization by a value complex.
- The psychomotor domain includes learning to perform motor skills and physical tasks.
- Simpson's Psychomotor Taxonomy identifies a hierarchy of skill mastery that includes the cognitive and affective aspects needed to perform a skill.
- Dave's Psychomotor Taxonomy describes a five-level hierarchy emphasizing progressive mastery of skill performance.
- Following general guidelines for developing test items will help ensure consistency and provide well-designed items that require higher-order thinking skills (see Boxes 4-7, 4-8, and 4-9).
- Four criteria for creating multiple choice test items that test critical thinking are: (1) write a rationale for correct and incorrect response items, (2) write questions at the application level or higher, (3) develop multilogical thinking test items, and (4) create highly discriminating test items.

- Classical Test Theory (CTT) and Item Response theory (IRT) are used in objective multiple choice examinations.
- CTT uses test item difficulty and item discrimination indices to determine appropriate test items.
- Control of testing conditions enhances the reliability of test scores.
- Test item factors such as the test length, test content, item difficulty, and discrimination can also affect the consistency of test scores.
- The difficulty index for each test question is reported as a value of 1.00 to 0.00. Easier questions are closer to 1.00 and difficult items closer to 0.00.
- Item discrimination refers to the ability of the test items to discriminate between high- and low-scoring students.
- Difficulty index for a specific test item may be influenced by the student's ability and the teacher's effectiveness.
- Poor test item distractors can be identified by the number of type of students who select the distractor.
- IRT is used with computerized adaptive testing. The test is dynamically created based on the student's response to each successive question.
- Development of skills in learning, test taking, and self-reflection are examples of metacognitive knowledge.
- Feedback is essentially communication of information about performance that helps the student achieve learning goals.
- Benefits of engaging in self-regulation include higher achievement and confidence in one's knowledge base.
- Kuiper's Self-Regulated Learning Model outlines behaviors, metacognitive, and environmental factors, that can be used to guide students in self-reflection.
- The principles of good feedback include: (1) clarifying requirements of good performance, (2) facilitating student self-assessment, (3) providing information to students about their learning, (4) encouraging dialog around learning, and (5) using feedback to shape learning, (6) encouraging application of feedback to new learning situations, and (7) using feedback from students to modify teaching approaches.
- Feedback is valuable to combat the sense of isolation that students enrolled in interactive TV and online courses may experience.
- Evidence-based feedback strategies effective for online courses are related to course design, teacher roles, and student participation (see Box 4-11).
- Good and effective feedback helps students construct self-knowledge and determine personal learning goals.

- Useful evaluation strategies include the use of rubrics, Primary Trail Analysis Scale, clinical evaluation tools, virtual evaluation tools, concept maps, reflective writing, scholarly papers, portfolios, and peer evaluation.
- Objective structured clinical evaluation involves the use of simulated standardized scenarios to evaluate clinical knowledge and skills.
- Authentic assessment strategies involve the application of knowledge and skills to situations, which closely resemble the "real-world."
- A portfolio is a flexible, creative, means of facilitating student learning through self-reflection, as well as a means of assessing student learning in a specific course or program of study.
- In peer evaluation, students use instructor identified evaluation criteria to provide their peers with feedback about assignments. Students learn from evaluating their classmates written assignments and from the feedback received on their own assignments.
- Writing across the curriculum is an initiative that values the writing skills needed by professionals and acknowledges writing as a learning process.

RECOMMENDED RESOURCES

General Resources

- American Association for the Advancement of Curriculum Studies (AAACS) Web site at http://calvin.ednet.lsu.edu/~aaacs/index.html houses a link to the annual online *Journal of the American Association for the Advancement of Curriculum Studies* and a link to the Professional Ethics and Standards for Scholars of Curriculum Studies document.
- The National Council on Measurement in Education Web site features a quarterly newsletter available at http://www.ncme.org/pubs/ncmenews.cfm and houses a series of articles on educational measurement called Instructional Topics in Educational Measurement Series (ITEMS). These may be downloaded at http://www.ncme.org/pubs/items.cfm.
- The Assessment in Higher Education Web site at http://ahe.cqu.edu.au/index.htm is a resource designed for researchers and others involved in student assessment in higher education. The site contains links to online articles, books, journals, and more.

- Practical Assessment, Research, and Evaluation (PARE) is a free, online, peer-reviewed journal available at http://pareonline.net.
- The Harvard Educational Review is available online at http://www.hepg.org/main/her/Index.html.
- The National Education Association is a professional employee organization concerned with public education from preschool through graduate level. The higher education page can be accessed at http://www2.nea.org/he/ and features access to several free publications including the *NEA Almanac of Higher Education* and the peer reviewed journal, *Thought and Action*.

Assessment and Evaluation Strategies

- Angelo and Cross have written a text describing numerous classroom assessment techniques and the implementation process for each. See Angelo, T. & Cross, K. (1993). *Classroom Assessment Techniques: A Handbook for College Teachers*. Hoboken, NJ: John Wiley and Sons.
- Silberman's 1996 text *Active Learning:101 Strategies to Teach Any Subject*, includes assessment and evaluation activities that enhance learning. Each strategy is clearly described and variations are suggested.
- For information and resources on rubrics, visit Rubrics for Web Lessons Web site at http://webquest.sdsu.edu/rubrics/weblessons.htm.
- Inter/National Coalition for Electronic Portfolio Research Web site at http://ncepr.org/index.html houses reports, presentations, and publications by coalition members, and a link to the *Connections* newsletter, published since 2005, available at http://ncepr.org/connections.html.

Multiple Choice Tests

- A PDF manual titled, *Constructing Written Test Questions for the Basic and Clinical Sciences*, published by the AMA can be downloaded at http://www.nbme.org/PDF/ItemWriting_2003/2003IWGwhole.pdf.
- Michigan State University publishes a Web site on test item writing available at https://www.msu.edu/dept/soweb/writitem.html.
- A tutorial on item response theory is available at http://www.creative-wisdom.com/multimedia/IRTT.htm.

REFERENCES

1. American Educational Research Association, American Psychological Association, American Educational Association. (1999). *Standards for educational and psychological testing*. Washington, DC: American Educational Research Association Publishers.
2. American Federation of Teachers, National Council on Measurement in Education & National Education Association (1990). *Standards for teacher competence in educational assessment of students*. Retrieved January 29, 2009 from http://www.unl.edu/buros/bimm/html/article3.html.
3. Anderson, L., Krathwohl, D., Airasian, P., Cruikshank, K., Mayer, R., Pintrich, P., *et al.* (2001). *A taxonomy for learning teaching and assessing: A revision of Bloom's taxonomy of objectives*. New York: Addison Wesley Longman.
4. Angelo, T., & Cross, K. (1993). *Classroom assessment techniques: A handbook for college teachers*. Hoboken, NJ: John Wiley and Sons.
5. Baker, C. (1996). Reflective learning: A teaching strategy for critical thinking. *Journal of Nursing Education, 35*, 19–22.
6. Baugh, N. G., & Mellott, K. G. (1998). Clinical concept mapping as preparation for student nurses' clinical experiences. *Journal of Nursing Education, 37*, 253–256.
7. Black, P., & William, D. (1998). Assessment and classroom learning. *Assessment in Education, 5*(1), 7–74.
8. Bloom, B. S. (Ed.). (1956). *Taxonomy of educational objectives: The classification of educational goals, handbook 1. The cognitive domain*. New York: David McKay.
9. Bond, L. A. (1996). Norm- and criterion-referenced testing. *Practical Assessment, Research & Evaluation, 5*(2). Retrieved March 2, 2009 from http://PAREonline.net/getvn.asp?v=5&n=2.
10. Bonnel, W. (2008). Improving feedback to students in online courses. *Nursing Education Perspectives, 29*(5), 290–294.
11. Bonnel, W. (2009). Clinical performance evaluation. In D. M. Billings, & J. A. Halstead, (Eds.), *Teaching in nursing: A guide for faculty* (3rd ed.). St. Louis: Saunders Elsevier.
12. Chizmar, J. F., & Ostrosky, A. L. (1998, Winter). The one-minute paper: Some empirical findings. *Journal of Economic Education, 29*(1), 3–10.
13. Clow, K. E. (1999). Interactive distance learning: Impact on student course evaluations. *Journal of Marketing Education, 21*, 97–105.
14. Conceição, S. C. O., & Taylor, L. D. (2007). Using a constructivist approach with online concept maps: Relationship between theory and nursing education. *Nursing Education Perspectives, 28*, 268–275.
15. Craft, M. (2005). Reflective writing and nursing education. *Journal of Nursing Education, 44*(2), 53–57.
16. Dave, R. (1970). Psychomotor levels. In R. J. Armstrong, (Ed.), *Developing and writing behavioral objectives*. Tucson, AZ: Educational Innovators Press.
17. Davis, B. (2009). *Tools for teaching* (2nd ed.). San Francisco: Jossey Bass.
18. Duan, Y. (2006). Selecting and applying taxonomies for learning outcomes: A nursing example. *International Journal of Nursing Education Scholarship, 3*(1),10.
19. Facione, P. (1990). *Critical thinking: A statement of expert consensus for purposes of educational assessment and instruction. Executive summary. "The delphi report."* Millbrae, CA: The California Academic Press.

20. Facione, P., & Facione, N. (1994). *The holistic critical thinking score rubric.* Milbrae, CA: California Academic Press. Retrieved October 31, 2008 from http://www.insightassessment.com/hctsr.html.

21. Fagerlund, K., & McShane, F. (2005). The self-evaluation examination: Past, present and future. *AANA Journal, 73*(1), 21–23.

22. Fan, X. (1998). Item response theory and classical test theory: an empirical comparison of their item/person statistics. *Educational and Psychological Measurement, 58*(3), 1–7.

23. Fellenz, M. R. (2004). Using assessment to support higher-level learning: The multiple choice item development assignment. *Assessment & Evaluation in Higher Education, 29*(6), 703–719.

24. Frisbie, D. A. (1988, Spring). NCME instructional module on reliability of scores from teacher-made tests. *Instructional Topics in Education, 55–65.*

25. Gagné, R. M. (1985).*The conditions of learning and theory of instruction* (4th ed.). New York: Holt, Rinehart, and Winston.

26. Gagné, R. M., Wager, W. W., Golas, K. C., & Keller, J. M. (2005). *Principles of instructional design* (5th ed.). Belmont, CA: Wadsworth/Thomson.

27. Gardner-Medwin, A. R. (2006). Confidence-based marking: Towards deeper learning and better exams. In C. Brian, & K. Clegg (Eds.), *Innovative assessment in higher education.* London: Taylor & Francis.

28. Giddens, J. F., & Lobo, M. (2008). Analyzing graduate student trends in written paper evaluation. *Journal of Nursing Education, 47*(10), 480–483.

29. Gronlund, N. E. (2004). *Writing instructional objectives for teaching and assessment.* Englewood Cliffs, NJ: Prentice-Hall.

30. Gronlund, N. E., & Brookhart, S. M. (2009). *Gronlund's writing instructional objectives* (8th ed.). Upper Saddle River, NJ: Pearson Education.

31. Gronlund, N. E., & Waugh, C. K. (2008). *Assessment of student achievement.* Boston: Allyn and Bacon.

32. Guliker, J. T., Bastiaens, T. J., & Kirschner, P. A. (2004). A five-dimensional framework for authentic assessment. *ETR & D, 52*(3), 67–86.

33. Haladyna, T., Downing, S., & Rodriguez, M. (2002). A review of multiple choice item-writing guidelines for classroom assessment. *Applied Measurement in Education, 15*(3), 309–334.

34. Hambleton, R., & Jones, R. (1993). An NCME instructional module on comparison of classical test theory and item response theory and their applications to test development. *Educational Measurement: Issues and Practice, 12*(3) 38–47.

35. Hicks-Moore, S. L., & Pastirik, P. J. (2006). Evaluating critical thinking in clinical concept maps: A pilot study. *International Journal of Nursing Education Scholarship, 3*(1), 1–15.

36. Hinck, S. M., Webb, P., Sims-Giddens, S., Helton, C., Hope, K. L., Utley, R., *et al.* (2006). Student learning with concept mapping of care plans in community-based education. *Journal of Professional Nursing, 22*(1), 23–29.

37. Hult, C. (1997). What is WAC and how do we get it at our university? In G. L. Poirrier (Ed.), *Writing to learn: Curricular strategies for nursing and other disciplines* (pp 173–186). New York: NLN Press.

38. Ignatavicius, D., & Caputi, L. (2004) Evaluating students in the clinical setting. In L. Caputi, & L. Engelmann (Eds.), *Teaching nursing: The art and science, volume 1.* Glen Ellyn, IL: College of DuPage.

39. Kautz, D. D., Kuiper, R. A., Pesut, D. J., Knight-Brown, P., & Daneker, D. (2005). Promoting clinical reasoning in undergraduate nursing students: Application and evaluation of the outcome present state test (OPT) model of clinical reasoning. *International Journal of Nursing Education, 2*(1), 1–19.

40. Kennison, M. (2006). The evaluation of students' reflective writing for evidence of critical thinking. *Nursing Education Perspectives, 27*(5), 269–273.

41. Kennison, M. M., & Misselwitz, S. (2002). Evaluating reflective writing for appropriateness, fairness, and consistency. *Nursing Education Perspectives, 23,* 238–242.

42. Krathwohl, D. R., Bloom, B., & Masia, B. B. (1964). *Taxonomy of educational objectives. The classification of educational goals handbook II: Affective domain.* New York: David McKay.

43. Kuiper, R. (1999). The effect of prompted self-regulated learning strategies in a clinical nursing preceptorship. *Dissertation Abstracts International, 60.* (University Microfilms No. 9928324).

44. Lawson, D. M. (2006). Applying the item response theory to classroom examinations. *Journal of Manipulative and Physiological Therapeutics, 29*(5), 393–397.

45. MacNeil, M. (2007). Concept mapping as a means of course evaluation. *Journal of Nursing Education, 46*(5), 232–234.

46. Masters, J. C., Hulsmeyer, B. S., Pike, M. E., Leichty, K., Miller, M. T., & Verst, A. L. (2001). Assessment of multiple choice questions in selected test banks accompanying text books used in nursing education. *Journal of Nursing Education, 40,* 25–31.

47. McDonald, M. (2008). *The nurse educators guide to assessing learning outcomes* (2nd ed.). Sudbury, MA: Jones and Bartlett.

48. McMullen, M., Endacott, R., Gray, M., Jasper, M., Miller, C., Scholes, J., *et al.* (2003). Portfolios and assessment of competence: A review of the literature. *Journal of Advanced Nursing, 41*(3), 283–294.

49. Merritt, R. D. (2008). The psychomotor domain. *EBSCO Research Starters,* 1–9.

50. Morrison, S., & Free, K. W. (2001). Writing multiple choice test items that promote and measure critical thinking. *Journal of Nursing Education, 40,* 17–24.

51. Morrison, S., Smith, P., & Britt, R. (1996). *Critical thinking and test items writing.* Houston: Health Education Systems.

52. Myer, S. (2008). Item response theory. *EBSCO Research Starters Education,* 1–5.

53. National League for Nursing, Task Group on Nurse Educator Competencies. (2005). *Core competencies of nurse educators with task statements.* Retrieved September 10, 2008 from http://www.nln.org/facultydevelopment/pdf/corecompetencies.pdf.

54. NCME Ad Hoc Committee on the Development of a Code of Ethics. (1995). *Code of professional responsibilities in educational measurement.* National Council on Measurement in Education. Retrieved January 29, 2009 from http://www.natd.org/Code_of_Professional_Responsibilities.html.

55. Nicol, D. (2007). E-assessment by design: Using multiple choice tests to good effect. *Journal of Further and Higher Education, 31*(1), 53–64.

56. Nicol, D., & Macfarlane-Dick, D. (2006). Formative assessment and self-regulated learning: A model and seven principles of good feedback practice. *Studies in Higher Education, 31*(2), 199–218.

57. Nitko, A. (2004). *Educational assessment of students.* Upper Saddle River, NJ: Prentice Hall.

58. Oermann, M., & Gaberson, K. (2006). *Evaluation and testing in nursing education* (2nd ed.). New York: Springer.

59. Pintrich, P. (1995). *Understanding self-regulated learning.* San Francisco: Jossey Bass.
60. Poirrier, G. L. (Ed.), (1997). *Writing to learn: Curricular strategies for nursing and other disciplines.* New York: NLN Press.
61. Reid, C., Kolakowsky-Hayner, S., Lewis, A. N., & Armstrong, A. J. (2007). Modern psychometric methodology: Applications of item response theory. *Rehabilitation Counseling Bulletin, 50*(3), 177–188.
62. Rentschler, D., Eaton, J., Cappiello, J., McNally, S., & McWilliam, P. (2007). Evaluation of undergraduate students using objective structured clinical evaluation. *Journal of Nursing Education, 46*(3), 135–140.
63. Sander, R., & Trible, K. (2008). The virtual clinical evaluation tool. *Journal of Nursing Education, 47*(1), 33–36.
64. Scheffer, B., & Rubenfeld, M. (2000). A consensus statement of critical thinking in nursing. *Journal of Nursing Education, 39,* 352–359.
65. Schuster, P. (2000). Concept mapping: Reducing clinical care plan paperwork and increasing learning. *Nurse Educator, 25*(2), 76–81.
66. Silberman, M. (1996). *Active learning:101 strategies to teach any subject.* Boston: Allyn & Bacon.
67. Simpson, E. J. (1966). *The classification of educational objectives, psychomotor domain.* Washington, DC: Vocational and Technical Education Grant Contract Report, US Department of Health, Education, and Welfare.
68. Stassen, M. L., Doherty, K., & Poe, M. (2001, Fall). *Program based review and assessment: Tools and techniques for program improvement.* University of Massachusetts-Amherst, Office of Academic Planning and Assessment. Retrieved Sept 10, 2008 at http://www.umass.edu/oapa/oapa/publications/online_handbooks/program_based.pdf.
69. Topping, K. (1998). Peer assessment between students in colleges and universities. *Review of Educational Research, 68,* 249–276.
70. Traub, R., & Rowley, G. (1991). An NCME instructional module on understanding reliability. *Educational Measurement: Issues and Practice, 10*(1), 37–45.
71. van den Berg, I., Admiraal, W., & Pilot, A. (2006). Design principles and outcomes of peer assessment in higher education. *Studies in Higher Education, 31*(3), 341–356.
72. Walvoord, B. E., & Anderson, V. J. (1998). *Effective grading: A tool for learning and assessment.* San Francisco: Jossey Bass.
73. Wheeler, L., & Collins, S. (2003). The influence of concept mapping on critical thinking in baccalaureate nursing students. *Journal of Professional Nursing, 19*(6), 339–346.
74. Whitehead, D. (2002). The academic writing experiences of a group of student nurses: A phenomenological study. *Journal of Advanced Nursing, 38*(5), 498–506.
75. Yu, C. H., Jannasch-Pennell, A., & DiGangi, S. (2008, February 21). A non-technical approach for illustrating item response theory. *Journal of Applied Testing Technology, 9*(2), 1–32.
76. Zimmerman, B. J., & Schunk, D. H. (2001). *Self-regulated learning and academic achievement: Theoretical perspectives.* Mahwah, NJ: Lawrence Erlbaum Associates.

CHAPTER 5

Participate in Curriculum Design and Evaluate Program Outcomes— Competency 4

OBJECTIVES

1. Discuss concepts, principles, and theories relevant to curriculum design implementation, evaluation, and revision.
2. Describe the processes used to develop learning objectives and correlate learning objectives with learning activities and evaluation.
3. Explore the relationship between institutional and program philosophy and mission statements.
4. Differentiate program and institutional outcomes and learning objectives.
5. Explore characteristics of successful program outcome and evaluation models.

KEY TERMS

ACE Star Model	Interactive Model of Program Planning
Affective domain	KATTS model
Affective taxonomy	Learning Evaluation and Program
Bloom's taxonomy	Effectiveness Model
Change theory	Learning objectives
Chen's program evaluation theory	Learning outcomes
CIPP Model	Mission statement
Clinical home community model	New taxonomy
Cognitive domain	Nursing Residency Model
Cognitive taxonomy	Philosophy statement
Continuous quality improvement process	Program outcomes
Curriculum	Psychomotor domain
Curriculum design	Psychomotor taxonomy
Educational Systems Analysis Model	Visual analog scale

DEFINITION AND DESCRIPTION OF COMPETENCY _____

Competency 4, "Participate in curriculum design and evaluation of program outcomes" (NLN, 2005, p. 4), involves all components of curriculum design, from assessment of program needs to planning the evaluation of program outcomes. The competency includes eight task statements that describe common activities within the competency. These include using educational theory, principles, and research to guide design and implementation. Demonstration of this competency involves using knowledge of curriculum processes such as a needs assessment and implementing the phases of curriculum planning. It involves designing curriculum to meet the needs of the learners and the community they will serve, and identifying measurable program outcomes.

The relationship among the institution, program, and individual course objectives along with factors that influence program and course outcomes are depicted in Figure 5-1. Implementation of new curriculum and revision of existing curriculum are guided by change theories and are supported by established educational partner-

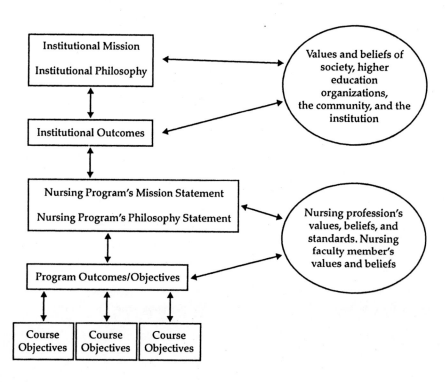

FIGURE 5-1 Factors Influencing Program Outcomes and Course Objectives

ships within the community. The academic nurse educator (ANE) integrates recommendations and requirements from regulatory organizations such as licensure boards and accreditation agencies and works with these organizations to assure program quality.

THEORY AND RESEARCH RELATED TO COMPETENCY

Several topics are discussed in this section, including change theories as applied to curriculum development and implementation, and frameworks outlining curriculum design processes. Formats for developing cognitive, affective, and psychomotor objectives are reviewed, as well as published reports of selected curriculum design, implementation, and evaluation projects.

Organizational Change

Designing curriculum and evaluating programs are processes that hinge on the ability of the institution and all of its players to accept change. Change may be in the form of a new or revised course or a more profound change to the entire curricular structure. Nurse educators who are familiar with organizational change theories will be armed with knowledge that can be applied to the curriculum change process. Successful utilization of change theories will facilitate the achievement of the best possible outcomes.

Review of Organizational Change Literature

A review of the literature by Shanley (2007) revealed seven themes concerning organizational change. First is the matter of power, specifically the power of financial conditions to stimulate or limit change, and the power of management to activate and regulate changes in the institution. Organizational power is concerned with identifying "whose agendas are being served and how openly" (p. 539).

The second theme reported by Shanley (2007) is the role of politics and the political environment in the process of change. According to Shanley, power and politics are closely linked, yet often the influence of politics in the change process are under-recognized. Shanley cites the works of Buchanan and Badham (1999) as well as Hardy (1996), who emphasizes that it is important to bring politics out into the open where it can not be easily ignored. When implementation of organizational change fails, part of the reason may be the lack of attention paid to the political influences (Shanley, 2007).

A third theme in the organizational change literature is the issue of planning and controlling change (Shanley, 2007). Lewin's (1947,1951,1958) work in the area of planned change has stimulated the development of many change-related theories. Lewin developed a three-stage model of organizational change that involves: (1) unfreezing the present situation, (2) moving into a new situation, and (3) refreezing the new situation (Lewin, 1951, 1958). This process has been widely embraced in organizations. Critics of Lewin's Theory of Planned Change note that it does not take into account the influences of power and politics, and that planned change paints a picture of change as an organized, linear process (Shanley, 2007).

The direction of the impetus for change is the fourth theme (Shanley, 2007). This refers to determining whether the direction for change is top down (coming from administration); bottom up (coming from the employees); or a lateral direction indicating mutual impetus from administrators and employees. Shanley (2007) points out advantages of each of these approaches. Top-down change, driven by administrators, is characterized by greater power and authority to fully implement the change. In addition, administrators, by virtue of their position the organization, may hold a broader view of the factors that can help or hinder the implementation of a specific change. In contrast, change initiated from the bottom up is typically backed by energy, enthusiasm, and conviction of the employees. In many cases change in the lateral direction represents a blend of the power, authority, and energy needed to accomplish change.

The fifth theme is an often overlooked aspect of the change process. According to Shanley's (2007) review, the role of personal aspects such as emotions and emotional reactions to organizational change have often gone unappreciated or discounted. Failing to consider personal reactions to a change can reduce morale and productivity (Iacovini, 1993), and create anxiety, insecurity, and dissatisfaction (Stuart, 1996). Shanley notes that the role of emotions in the change process, and the effect of the change on morale can have far-reaching effects on loyalty, commitment, and sense of trust (2007). When dealing with emotional issues related to change, it may be beneficial to use what Frost and Robinson (1999) call a toxic handler, someone who listens, provides emotional support, offers suggestions for improvement, and helps to reframe the worker's perception of the change.

Part of the change process should involve anticipating any adverse emotional reactions to the proposed change and introducing strategies to mitigate the reaction. Often piloting the change on a small scale will allow the ANE and administration to obtain feedback about the change and modify the plan as needed. In the case of a curricular change, piloting the change also allows a small subsample to become familiar with the new curriculum. Piloting a change project creates a sense of empowerment for students, faculty, and other stakeholders who will be able to give input before the change is finalized. Because change can have adverse effects, these effects need to be anticipated and included in the calculation of the costs and benefits of the new program. The underlying message in this theme is the importance of acknowledging the emotional impact of change and planning strategies to deal with those emotional responses.

Another theme in the change literature is the focus on prescriptive and analytical approaches to managing change. Shanley (2007) notes there are numerous prescriptive models of change that "take the reader through a series of steps to successfully manage the change process" (p. 543). These approaches are tempting to use because they are straightforward, relatively simple to use, and linear in nature. Prescriptive approaches to change suggest that if one "sticks to the script they can be confident of achieving the changes they want" (p. 543). Although there may be value in the prescriptive approaches as an overall framework, Shanley reports a lack of empirical research to support one approach over another. The downfall of many of the prescriptive approaches is that they do not recognize the "complexity and iterative nature of change" (p. 543). A contrast to the prescriptive step-by-step approaches are what Shanley (2007) calls the analytical approaches proposed by authors such as Collins (1998), Dawson (1994), Pettigrew (1990), and others. What the analytical approaches have in common is that they acknowledge that the process of change is complex and uncertain, and does not consist of a predetermined number of steps. The analytical approaches consider the complexity of change in terms of multiple internal and external influences and multiple stakeholders. Analytical approaches also support proactive discussion of the complexities of the environment. These discussions make it more likely that issues will be anticipated before they arise and thus handled more effectively. The analytical models acknowledge the uncertainty and confusion that occurs during change and the unpredictability of the change process. Analytical models also encourage discussion of the complexity to help decrease the emotional impact of the change and lead to a resolution of the problem.

A benefit of analytical change theories according to Shanley (2007) is that they promote a more comprehensive look at the environment in which the change will occur. Interestingly, an 8-year longitudinal study by Pettigrew (1990) supports that belief. Pettigrew found that planned change theory neither accounted for, nor explained the complexity of the change process as well as emergent or analytical change theories. In addition, planned change does not consider organizational history, the context in which the change occurred, or the processes used (Shanley, 2007, p. 541). Other strengths of analytical change theories are that they allow the incorporation of contingency plans and encourage continual review of the plans to consider unexpected influences and outcomes.

The final theme in the change literature is a common dilemma in theoretical knowledge, and that is relating change theory to practice. This theme is concerned with the question, "why do managers need to be aware of, and familiar with, theories surrounding the management of change?" (Shanley, 2007, p. 544). Scholars addressing this theme acknowledge that awareness of a variety of theoretical approaches to change allows the change agent to select approaches that fit the situation, and permits greater understanding of the rationale for specific actions. According to Shanley, "Every choice made about the management of change is based on the consideration of theory—if only at an implicit level" (p. 544). However, awareness of the theoretical basis of change makes our understanding explicit, which fosters greater responsibility and accountability.

As a curricular change agent, the ANE is responsible for the management and evaluation of curricular change. Being aware of the underlying theoretical basis for change within an organization can facilitate the process of change. Shanley also emphasizes that because each environment and circumstance is different and the complexities of change situations are unique, "there is not a single or best way to understand change management" (2007, p. 544).

Curriculum Development

Curriculum development involves planning and designing a program of study or curriculum. Curriculum can be further defined as a set of courses or set of lessons in a related field of study designed to achieve specific learning outcomes or objectives. Curriculum is shaped by various social, political, and economic forces and impacts the learning needs of students. Halstead (2007) concurs and describes curriculum as "needing to be flexible enough to change as needed, to meet discipline, community, and societal needs" (p. 100). Change is therefore an inherent ingredient in the curriculum development process.

Processes of Curriculum Development

Iwasiw, Goldenberg, and Andrusyszyn (2009) describe the process of curriculum development beginning with determining the need for curriculum change and ending with evaluation of the implemented curriculum (Figure 5-2). The model describes an iterative process in which decisions at one point have an influence on future decisions, as well as lead to a rethinking of past decisions.

In nursing education, many factors can stimulate the need for curriculum development, such as advances in healthcare practices, changes in population demographics, changes in disease, illness, and injury patterns, and standards of practice

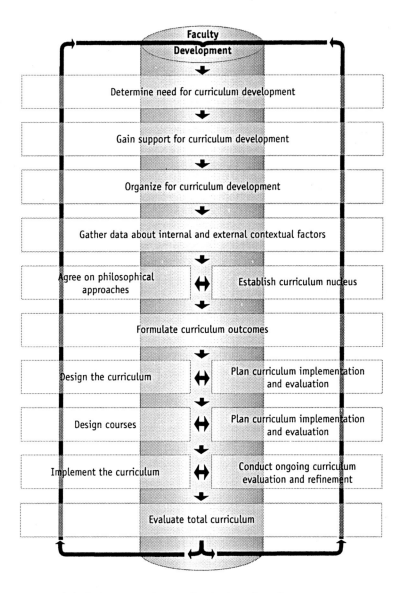

FIGURE 5-2 Model of Context Relevant Curriculum Development
Source: Data from Iwasiw, C., Goldenberg, D., & Andrusyszyn, M. (2009). Curriculum development in nursing education. (2nd ed.) Sudbury, MA: Jones and Bartlett, p. 8.

developed by professional organizations. In addition, feedback from faculty, students, and preceptors may serve as a stimulus for curriculum development.

Several strategies have been identified by Warner and Misener (2009) for identifying issues and trends that can influence curriculum development. One strategy involves a process called environmental scanning, which entails monitoring and evaluating information from a variety of sources in the external environment. Data can be collected via networking, conference attendance, and review of scholarly and lay literature. Forecasting is a strategy that allows the ANE to develop a curriculum that will prepare students for future nursing practice. Using knowledge of current data and deductive, inductive, and or retroductive reasoning processes, the ANE makes predictions and judgments about future educational and healthcare trends. Epidemiologic data on specific populations, illnesses, and environmental factors can be studied to determine trends that can influence healthcare needs as well as curricular needs and planning. Finally, the use of survey research and consensus building processes such as the Delphi technique can be used to gather data from a variety of individuals who are knowledgeable about educational and healthcare influences.

Once information supporting a need has been collected, the data are evaluated to determine if curricular action is warranted at the current time. Factors such as the scope, magnitude, and persistence of healthcare trends can be considered, as well as the alignment of the learning need with the mission and philosophy of the institution and nursing program. Limitations in type and amount of physical and personnel resources may inhibit the ability to undertake a specific curriculum revision. Consideration of these factors enables decision makers to determine the likelihood that the identified need can be addressed effectively and in a timely manner through curriculum development.

Once the need for curriculum change has been determined, it is important to gain support of faculty and administrators who have not been directly involved in the needs assessment process. The process of gaining support involves communication with faculty, administration, and other community stakeholders about the rationale underlying the need for change, and explaining how the proposed change is in alignment with the goals and values of the institution, program, and community.

The next step described in the curriculum development model involves "organizing for curriculum change" (Iwasiw et al., 2009, p. 3). This involves establishing the infrastructure in terms of committee members and leadership. In addition, the committee should agree on the general processes and approaches that will be used to make decisions and develop the curriculum. During this part of the development process, the committee identifies major milestones that will need to be accomplished and outlines a realistic timetable for working through the process (p. 3).

The next two processes involve agreeing on a philosophical approach and determining curriculum directions and outcomes. These are operationalized hand-in-hand, one influencing the other. A philosophy statement for the nursing program should reflect the values and beliefs of the faculty, who in turn reflect values and beliefs of nursing, the institution, and the community at large. According to Iwasiw *et al.* (2009), "Reaching resolution about the philosophical approaches is a critical milestone . . . since all aspects of the finalized curriculum should be congruent with the espoused values and beliefs" (p. 5). When determining the direction and outcomes of the curriculum, committee members must consider the ways in which the philosophy statement can be realized by identifying "important concepts, competencies, potential designs, and possible learning activities" (p. 5). The integration of philosophy with curriculum outcomes provides the foundation for developing explicit program goals, which comprises the next steps of the process.

Based on the information collected during all of the preceding processes, the curriculum goals or program goals are formulated. These are more general than learning objectives for specific courses, as they must reflect the cumulative knowledge and skills that the graduates will demonstrate after completion of the entire program. Unlike learning objectives, which are made known to the individual students enrolled in a specific course, curricular goals are often made known to a wider audience using program marketing materials and program Web sites. Therefore, the curricular goals should describe the graduate in terms of broad abilities.

The next process in the curriculum development model involves designing the curriculum structure and individual courses. The overall curriculum design for an entire nursing program includes setting goals for each level (freshman, sophomore, junior, and senior); determining the required nursing courses, support courses, and electives; and the sequencing for each level (Iwasiw *et al.*, 2009). The design of individual courses includes developing the course description, learning objectives, determining content, teaching, and evaluation methods. The components of individual courses needs to be congruent with the overall curriculum plan identified previously.

Curriculum Philosophies

A curriculum philosophy is an extension of the overall philosophy of the program. It is defined as "the beliefs held by faculty about the purpose of education, learners, learning, and teaching" (Iwasiw *et al.*, 2009, p. 172). Figure 5-1 identifies the influence of values and beliefs on the formation of the mission, philosophy, and outcomes at the institutional and program levels. At the institutional level, the values and beliefs of higher education regulatory bodies and the community will be reflected in the institution's mission and philosophy statements. A well-defined mission statement will describe the institution and programs, why they exist, who they serve, and the purpose or goals of the institution. In addition, a strong mission statement will define the geographic location that the institution or program serves and the types of programs provided.

Educational and curricular philosophies permeate all aspects of teaching and curriculum development. According to Csokasy, "Every time a teacher makes a decision about curriculum, he or she is confronted with options. Decisions about content, course sequence, and evaluation strategies will reflect a teacher's belief system" (2009, p. 108). According to Csokasy, faculty who are aware of their personal teaching philosophy, as well as the philosophy of the program and institution, will be better equipped to develop a curriculum that provides consistent and appropriate learning experiences within a selected philosophical framework (2009, p. 108).

In nursing education programs, the articulation of a philosophy as a foundation for curriculum development is generally supported (Iwasiw *et al.*, 2009). However, Bevis (1989) states that "philosophy alone is a weak cornerstone for curricular development" (p. 35). Bevis also notes that identification of assumptions could be used in-

---

BOX 5-1   Types of Curriculum Philosophies

Traditional Philosophical Approaches:

- Idealism

- Realism

- Pragmatism

Learning Theory Philosophies:

- Behaviorism

- Cognitivism

- Humanism

Nursing Philosophical Approaches:

- Action-Sensitive Pedagogy

- Apprenticeship

- Collaborative Inquiry

- Critical Social Theory

- Life Skills

Data from Csokasy, J. (2009). Philosophical foundations of the curriculum. In D. Billings, & J. Halstead (Eds.), *Teaching in nursing: A guide for faculty* (pp. 105–118). St. Louis: Saunders Elsevier; Iwasiw, C., Goldenberg, D., & Andrusyszyn, M. (2009). *Curriculum development in nursing education.* Sudbury, MA: Jones and Bartlett.

stead of a formal philosophy (2000). Regardless of the curricular philosophy or assumptions adopted, it is important that the ideas expressed are congruent with the curriculum, the faculty, and institutional values and beliefs. Useful philosophies and assumptions should be realistic and should present concepts that are specific enough to be meaningful yet not too narrow.

Csokasy (2009) and Iwasiw and colleagues (2009) reviewed a variety of philosophies currently used in nursing programs (Box 5-1). The idealism curricular philosophy is described as one that values humanism, broad intellectual development, liberal arts education, personal growth of students, and role modeling of desired behaviors (Iwasiw *et al.*, 2009, p. 174). The idealism philosophy is often reflected in the mission and philosophy statements of religious-based colleges and universities (Csokasy, 2009). In contrast, a realism-based philosophy emphasizes the natural laws and provides concrete, structured, learning that reflects the real world. Csokasy (2009) notes that realists believe that the teacher is responsible for presenting new knowledge to the student in a well thought out, organized manner. Pragmatism is a more recent philosophy that was stimulated by the development of science and technology (Csokasy, 2009). Pragmatism represents a blend of idealism and realism that involves inquiry and use of the scientific method for learning.

In addition to the traditional philosophies, Csokasy (2009) and Iwasiw *et al.* (2009) note that any of the learning theories such as behaviorism, cognitivism, or humanism, could be used as a curriculum philosophy. However, many philosophies currently used in nursing programs reflect a synthesis of several learning theories, rather than one theory. A central issue when using a learning theory is to select a theory or theories that matches the values, assumptions, and perspectives held by the faculty and the institution. Please see Chapters 2 and 3 for an overview of learning theories.

The nursing philosophies highlighted in Box 5-1 represent some commonly used philosophical approaches to curriculum development. The action-sensitive pedagogy emphasizes ethical action in a caring manner and promotes holistic understanding through phenomenology. The apprenticeship philosophy values learning by doing and learning from experts. The students move through a curriculum structure that provides exposure to increasingly complex skills and cognitive learning experiences. The collaborative inquiry philosophy describes an approach to teaching and learning characterized by shared "power and responsibility for decision-making. . . . Learners use experiences to generate new knowledge by action and reflection" (Iwasiw *et al.*, 2009, p. 176). Critical social theory views the understanding of social history as essential for interpreting and giving meaning to experiences. Curriculums guided by social critical theory emphasize understanding social, cultural, and political practices and the development of human relation skills such as empathy and advocacy. The

ANE focuses on assisting the student to understand the perspectives of others by posing questions for self-reflection and facilitating the student's development of human skills. Finally, there is the life skills philosophy, which is based on acquiring basic skills that will endure through a changing environment. Communication, collaboration, and critical thinking skills are examples of life skills that can be applied to multiple situations. Additional examples of curricular philosophies and frameworks are discussed in the works of Csokasy (2009) and Iwasiw *et al.* (2009).

Outcomes and Objectives

Another key aspect of curriculum design involves establishing outcomes. Boland (2009) links curriculum frameworks and outcomes using the following analogy, "If curriculum frameworks are road maps to understanding the discipline of nursing, then outcomes can be equated with the trip's destination" (p. 143). However, program and institutional outcomes and course learning objectives differ in several vital respects (Table 5-1). Institutional outcomes are broad in scope, focusing on general learning, whereas program outcomes are discipline specific. Course objectives represent the learning outcomes for specific courses and are content specific. In a well-designed curriculum, the learner first demonstrates progressive achievement of course objectives. As the learner comes to the end of the program of study, the knowledge and skills accumulated enable the learner to demonstrate behaviors consistent with the program and institutional outcomes as well.

Glennon (2006) differentiates between program outcomes and program objectives and discusses a recent shift in the emphasis on using program outcomes instead of objectives to guide the curriculum. According to Glennon, objectives relate to instruction and student learning, whereas outcomes relate to professional practice and the results of the instruction. Glennon sees the shift as being driven by "societal forces such as economics, information technology, and external standards" (p. 55). The emphasis on the development of program outcomes should produce true outcomes as opposed to simply rewording program objectives. She cautions that differences between objectives and outcomes need to be understood to enable faculty to develop true outcomes. According to Glennon, "Outcomes can be thought of as more complete than objectives because outcomes take objectives to a more advanced level. Objectives are often specific, content-focused, and useful for instructors to plan courses or class modules, but are not broad enough to state the intended learning that results" (2006, p. 56). Although learning objectives and program outcomes are typically phrased using a similar verb and noun structure such as "The student will apply (verb) the nursing process (noun)" the difference is in the orientation. Outcomes

TABLE 5-1 Comparison of Program Outcomes and Course Level Objectives

	Program Outcomes	Course Objectives
Purpose	Describes attributes graduates will have or skills they will possess after completing the program of study	Describes content-specific knowledge or skills the individual student will learn after completing a specific course
Characteristics	Broad scope Not content specific Focuses on program graduates as a whole	Narrow scope Content specific Focuses on the individual's learning

Data from Boland, D. L. (2009). Developing curriculum: Frameworks, outcomes and competencies. In D. Billings, & J. Halstead (Eds.), *Teaching in nursing: A guide for faculty* (pp. 137–153). St. Louis: Saunders Elsevier; Glennon, C. (2006). Reconceptualizing program outcomes. *Journal of Nursing Education, 45*(2), 57.

identify what the student will do as a result of the academic activity versus objectives, which identify the academic activity.

At the course level, learning objectives are developed to clarify and facilitate achievement of content-related outcomes. Caffarella (2002) delineated five categories of learning outcomes that can be considered when developing learning objectives. These include: (1) knowledge, (2) cognitive skills, (3) psychomotor skills, (4) problem-solving and problem-finding capabilities, and (5) affective development (Box 5-2). Knowledge outcomes are concerned with acquiring information about factual subject matter that is commonly associated with the cognitive domain described in Bloom's

BOX 5-2 Types of Learning Outcomes

1. Knowledge
2. Cognitive skills
3. Psychomotor skills
4. Problem solving and problem finding capabilities
5. Affective development

Data from Caffarella, R. (2002). *Planning programs for adult learners: A practical guide for educators, trainers, & staff developers.* San Francisco: Jossey-Bass.

taxonomy (Bloom, 1956). Outcomes related to cognitive skill call for the learner to apply the knowledge to their personal or professional life (see cognitive taxonomies discussed in Chapter 4). Psychomotor skill outcomes concern the development of physical skills or performance of technical tasks. Psychomotor taxonomies have been developed to depict the progression in skill acquisition (see psychomotor taxonomies of Simpson and Dave discussed in Chapter 4). The ability to find and solve problems involves the development of a spirit of inquiry, questioning, and community involvement. This learning outcome category is integrated within aspects of the affective and cognitive taxonomies discussed in Chapters 3 and 4.

Format for Objectives

Developing learning objectives provides the foundation for developing course content as well as teaching and evaluation strategies. In this section, two formats for writing objectives for the cognitive, psychomotor, and affective learning domains are discussed, the general format and the five-component format. The general format for objectives includes three components in each objective; a statement of who (the learner, the student, the mentee); a verb to describe the action to be taken by the learner, such as demonstrate, analyze or identify; and a statement specifying what content will be learned. Mager (1984) also has suggested a five-component format that adds a statement of the conditions of learning and a statement of the level of acceptable performance.

Deciding which format to use depends on the purpose of the course and the degree of specificity required. Caffarella (2002) notes that in certain situations, using specific behaviors or performance criteria may not be appropriate, such as "when creativity, confidence, sensitivity, feelings, attitudes, and values are the focus of the learning activity" (p. 172). However, a curriculum that uses competency-based practices may want to assure that students have obtained a predetermined level of proficiency by wording objectives using the five-component format. Table 5-2 shows a comparison of written objectives using each format.

Program Planning and Design Models

Successful curriculum planning and design involves open communication with community stakeholders to determine the needs of the community, the resources, and the types of student learning experiences that are available in the community. This section reports on the use of innovative curricular planning and design models for nursing programs. Awareness of these programs may provide insights into the planning and design processes that the ANE can apply to his or her home institution.

TABLE 5-2	Comparison of Objectives Using General and Specific Formats	
	General Three-Part Format	**Specific Five-Part Format**
Components	Who, How (verb), What	Conditions, Who, How (verb), What, Criteria for Performance
Cognitive domain	The student (who) will differentiate (how) the stages of pressure ulcers (what).	Given images of pressure ulcers at various stages (conditions), the student (who) will differentiate (verb) the stages of pressure ulcers (what) with 100% accuracy (criteria).
Psychomotor	The learner (who) will demonstrate (how) how to obtain vital signs on an infant (what).	In the clinical setting (condition) the learner (who) will demonstrate (how) how to obtain vital signs on an infant (what) in less than 5 minutes (criteria).
Affective	The mentee (who) will advocate (how) for the client's rights (what).	When assigned to care for vulnerable clients (condition) the mentee (who) will advocate (how) for clients' rights (what) with all clients (criteria).

Interactive Model of Program Planning

The Interactive Model of Program Planning described by Caffarella (2002) integrates ideas from several other program planning models, such as Knowles (1980), Cervero and Wilson (1994,1996), and Sork (1997, 2000) into a 12-component model (Box 5-3). However, Caffarella distinguishes the model from others by four key aspects. First is the model's "interactive and comprehensive design" (p. 20). When planning education programs, Caffarella notes that several actions described in the 12 components may be conducted at the same time by several different people, yielding an interactive process. In addition, the starting point for the process may vary, depending on the situation. For example, for large educational conferences, the starting point may be driven by the environment such as facility and speaker availability; whereas for academic programs that have established facilities and teachers, the process may begin with sorting and prioritizing program ideas or determining program objectives. The program planning components are comprehensive enough to include processes needed for new and large educational programs. Depending on the nature, scope, and newness of the educational program, not all components will need to be addressed (Caffarella, 2002, p. 25).

Second, the model recognizes the importance of people and the environment in the planning process. According to Caffarella (2002), "Program planning becomes a negotiated activity between and among educators, learners, organizations, and other stakeholders, all of whom bring their own beliefs and contexts with them to the planning table" (p. 22). When planning for courses ranging from local clinical courses, to study away programs, educational planning calls for considering the interaction among the community, students, and teachers, and how the learning atmosphere and political relationships may be affected.

Third, the planning model considers cultural differences in the planning process and allows for flexible approaches that may be influenced by cultural preferences. For example, the model is flexible enough to allow linear program planning processes, which are appropriate for dealing with autocratic groups in the planning process. This flexibility is especially important as more and more courses and entire programs of study are offered to students from different geographic areas.

BOX 5-3   Components of the Interactive Model of Program Planning

1. Discern the context

2. Build a solid base of support

3. Identify program ideas

4. Sort and prioritize program ideas

5. Develop program objectives

6. Design instruction plans

7. Devise transfer of learning plans

8. Formulate evaluation plans

9. Make recommendations and communicate results

10. Select formats, schedules, and staffing needs

11. Prepare budget and marketing plans

12. Coordinate facilities and on-site events

Caffarella, R. (2002). *Planning programs for adult learners: A practical guide for educators, trainers, & staff developers* (p. 21). San Francisco: Jossey-Bass.

According to Caffarella, the fourth aspect that distinguishes the model from others is usefulness. She has developed a checklist outlining activities within each of the 12 components of the model. The checklist provides the ANE with specific recommendations and suggestions for implementing the model. Please see Caffarella (2002) for full details.

Educators and program planners who have used the model have identified factors that are most important when deciding which components to concentrate on. For large, comprehensive programs undergoing initial development, all components are useful. However, when decisions need to be made about which components to use, the planning context and parameters of the program are usually most important. This includes factors such as: the time frame and whether content, format, presenters, and location are mandated or predetermined. During the planning process, it is recommended that the ANE determine whether certain factors have been adequately addressed, including "discerning the context, identifying program ideas, developing clear objectives, designing instructional plans, designing transfer of learning plans, and formulating evaluation plans" (Caffarella, 2002, pp. 46–47). These components are essential for assuring quality and cohesiveness of the educational offering.

Nursing Residency Model

In 2003, the NLN position statement titled *Innovation in Nursing Education: A Call to Reform,* prompted ANEs to explore innovative curricular approaches, not only in terms of content and teaching strategies, but also in terms of curriculum delivery systems. Using a model originally outlined by Porter-O'Grady in 2001, faculty members from the University of Delaware School of Nursing describe the curriculum revision process undertaken to institute the Nurse Residency Model (Diefenbeck, Plowfield, & Herrman, 2006).

When instituting the Nurse Residency Model, accountability for learning moves from instructor-driven to student-driven as the curriculum progresses. The first 3 years of the program consist of largely instructor-driven learning experiences, such as didactic courses, laboratory practice, simulation, and field experiences (Diefenbeck *et al.,* 2006). During the first 2 years, the students learn about the role of the nurse, history of nursing, basic nursing skills, pharmacology, and health assessment in conjunction with liberal arts and science courses. During the third year, students complete the classroom portion of the traditional nursing specialty courses. In addition, students enroll in an internship course in which they receive course credit for working clinically. The senior year culminates in a clinical immersion experience in which the students complete supervised clinical experiences in the traditional specialties of medical-surgical, obstetrics, pediatrics, mental health, and community nursing.

According to Diefenbeck *et al.* (2006), implementation of the Nurse Residency Model was an adjustment for faculty, students, and clinical agencies. However, in terms of administrative outcomes they were able to reduce the overall number of faculty FTEs by approximately 20%. Benefits to the students included a smoother transition into practice as they were accustomed to clinical work patterns. In addition, students had the benefit of having a recent and concentrated experience in each clinical specialty during their final year of the program.

Clinical Home Community Model

Traditional models for nursing education have emphasized acute care of clients in the medicine-based specialties of pediatrics, obstetrics, mental health, and medical-surgical areas. However, over the past few decades, healthcare trends have changed. People with conditions that used to be treated in the hospital are now managing their conditions at home. Today hospitalized patients are much sicker than they used to be, and are being discharged from the hospital sooner than in the past. As a result, more people are living at home with higher levels of illness and injury acuity. Thus, the educational emphasis for some programs is shifting to caring for patients where they live, rather than exclusively relying on acute care settings. This movement toward community-based education (CBE) is more than "a collection of experiences that take place in a variety of settings. It also encompasses services that emerge from needs and assets of both the community and educational entities" (Williams-Barnard, Sweatt, Harkness, & DiNapoli, 2004).

An example of the development of an integrated CBE program is described by Williams-Barnard *et al.* (2004). For them, the process began by conducting an internal survey to identify the pros and cons for developing a CBE program. Faculty then conducted an asset mapping of the community. Asset mapping involves "cataloguing the skills and experiences of individual community members, as well as its local citizen organizations, associations, and institutions" (p. 107). This process provided faculty with a list of potential clinical sites for students, many of which had not been recognized previously. Next, the faculty used the information from the internal survey and asset mapping to identify goals for the CBE experiences. Two traditional courses were selected for piloting the CBE curriculum.

The CBE curriculum project was evaluated using objective measures such as test scores in critical thinking, NCLEX-RN pass rates, and qualitative data from student focus groups. The results indicated that this project achieved goals that sometimes can be difficult to obtain, such as being responsive to healthcare trends, preparing students for future practice, and providing knowledge and experiences that result in passing the NCLEX. Evaluation of the pilot project confirmed improvements in critical thinking and NCLEX-RN scores (Williams-Barnard *et al.*, 2004). Student focus groups reported an increased ability to "understand, connect, and empathize with the lived health-illness experiences of members of their clinical home community" (p. 109). Faculty reported stronger community partnerships, which also served as sources for additional scholarship and service activities. According to Williams-Barnard *et al.*, the CBE model was cost effective and offered "formalized mechanisms for faculty to maintain connection and provide services by engaging in community health promotion efforts" (2004, p. 110).

Curriculum and Program Evaluation

In conducting a program evaluation, the ANE engages in an ongoing process of data collection to determine compliance with professional and educational standards. Ideally the evaluation plan should be systematic, realistic, and guided by the program or curricular philosophy (Hamner & Bentley, 2003). In addition, data collected for evaluation should be meaningful to community stakeholders, the faculty, and students as a whole. According to Gard, Flannigan, and Cluskey (2004), "having an ongoing, systematic plan for evaluation will make it easier to plan and prepare for accreditation visits, address the need for timely curricular or other program changes, maintain consistency within the curriculum, and provide a mechanism to maintain currency with the trends in nursing education" (p. 176).

Gard and colleagues identify five purposes of program evaluation, which are summarized in Box 5-4. The purposes are achieved by using a systematic evaluation plan that considers the (1) evaluation framework, (2) existing program resources, (3) data, and (4) a timeline for evaluation (p. 176). The evaluation framework is based on the outcome measures selected for evaluation. Typically the outcomes are selected from accrediting agency standards and criteria. Additional outcome measures can be based on unique program or institutional outcomes that are not necessarily reflected in the accreditation standards. To determine which outcomes to select, Gard and colleagues (2004) suggest that the ANE answer two questions, "What do we want to know?" and "Why do we want to know it?" (p. 176).

After the outcomes have been selected, a plan for data collection, analysis, and storage needs to be developed. At this stage in the process, Gard *et al.* (2004) propose the ANE ask two additional questions, "What should we measure?" and "How should we measure it?" (p. 176). Multiple data sources are recommended for each outcome. Quantitative as well as qualitative data can be collected and compiled. For example,

---

BOX 5-4   Purposes of Program Evaluation

1. Maintain program quality

2. Evaluate curriculum and instruction as a whole

3. Identify issues and challenges within the program

4. Facilitate efforts in program improvement

5. Inform state, accrediting, and governing bodies about program quality

Data from Gard, C., Flannigan, P., & Cluskey, M. (2004). Program evaluation: An ongoing systematic process. *Nursing Education Perspectives, 25*, p. 179.

---

for the outcome of critical thinking, data may take the form of student test scores, student self-assessment of critical thinking skills, alumni survey responses about critical thinking, or samples of student papers and projects that demonstrate critical thinking. Data tables in self-study reports can provide a template for data collection.

A timeline for data collection, analysis, and reporting needs to be developed, as well as a timeline for the evaluation, curriculum, and bylaws committees to review and revise material. Before the program evaluation cycle is completed, it is important to close the cycle by documenting how the information is ultimately used to improve the program (Gard *et al.*, 2004).

Holaday and Buckley (2007) acknowledge that several factors account for difficulties in evaluation of clinical outcomes. In particular, the nature of the clinical settings, patient populations, clinical experiences, and difficulty in evaluating numerous subjective variables that are integral to the clinical environment, all contribute to evaluation difficulties.

To address the difficulties inherent in evaluating clinical outcomes, Holaday and Buckley (2007) developed and tested an evaluation toolkit based on the 1998 AACN Essentials document. The tool kit includes 11 consensus-based clinical outcomes that are leveled according to the student's educational preparation. A five-point criterion-referenced rating scale, adapted from the work of Bondy (1983), was used to evaluate performance and achievement of the outcomes. Rating scale categories ranged from dependent, novice, assisted, and supervised, to totally self-directed.

The quality of the student's performance was evaluated for safety, accuracy, skillfulness, and the amount of guidance needed to demonstrate the competency. The aim of the toolkit is to "assist with a fair and valid clinical assessment and evaluation across the broad spectrum of nursing roles, responsibilities, settings, and education levels"

(Holaday & Buckley, 2007, p. 146). Holaday and Buckley report that both 2- and 4-year nursing programs have adopted the toolkit and are evaluating the effectiveness of the toolkit in their programs.

Models for Program Evaluation

Many models for program evaluation have been developed and used by nursing programs. In this section, the use of six models for program evaluation are reviewed, including Iwasiw's Components of Curriculum Evaluation, Chen's Program Evaluation Theory, Learning Evaluation and Program Effectiveness Model, the Educational System Analysis Model, and the use of a visual analog scale for evaluation of graduate program outcomes. Although each teaching institution is unique, familiarity with the evaluation models in this section may be used to guide the ANE during the program evaluation process and provide insights that can be adapted to specific teaching settings.

Iwasiw's Components of Curriculum Evaluation

According to Iwasiw and colleagues (2009), curriculum evaluation should address several essential components (Box 5-5). First, the curricular philosophy should be evaluated for congruence and fit with other aspects of the curriculum, such as teaching methods and evaluation. Next, the goals of the curriculum should be evaluated for relevance to the mission and philosophy of the program and institution. It is also important to evaluate the curriculum design for its ability to meet current and emerging healthcare needs of the community and profession, and to prepare graduates for safe and effective practice. Specific aspects of curriculum design to consider include: (1) the type of program, such as generic baccalaureate or baccalaureate completion; (2) the type of curricular pattern, such as blocked and integrated (threaded) content; and (3) the type, amount, and sequence of nursing and supportive courses offered. Achievement of curriculum outcomes such as communication, critical thinking, and therapeutic nursing interventions are also evaluated.

The specific teaching and evaluation practices also need to be evaluated for effectiveness and congruence with the overall design and curriculum outcomes. This includes determining the effectiveness and appropriateness of general teaching approaches such as online, face-to-face, or use of blended formats. It also includes deciding on the content emphasis of the program, such as community or acute care nursing; and deciding on the use of a specific teaching modality, such as service learning or problem-based learning. The implementation and evaluation plans for clinical courses should consider administrative aspects such as establishing contracts with

BOX 5-5	Components of Curriculum Evaluation

1. Congruence of philosophical approaches

2. Curriculum outcomes/goals

3. Curriculum design

4. Courses

5. Teaching and evaluation strategies

6. Resources

7 Curriculum policies

8. Learning climate

Data from Iwasiw, C., Goldenberg, D., & Andrusyszyn, M. (2009). *Curriculum development in nursing education* (pp. 295–300). Sudbury, MA: Jones and Bartlett.

community agencies for clinical experiences, scheduling, space for clinical conferences, clinical orientation of faculty and students, and access to the agencies computerized record keeping. These clinical factors can directly affect opportunities for students to demonstrate achievement of course and program outcomes. In addition, clinical courses require on-campus classroom facilities, skills laboratory space, and equipment and supplies for skills practice and testing. When planning the implementation and evaluation of on-campus courses, factors such as classroom scheduling, classroom size, desired seating configuration, and availability of educational technology also must be considered. When administrative and classroom factors that cannot be changed (such as class size and seating configuration) are believed to adversely affect the achievement of program outcomes, learning assignments, teaching strategies, and possibly course delivery methods can be modified instead. For courses offered online or through other distance learning formats, it is important to evaluate the effectiveness of faculty development, ongoing technology support, and program marketing.

Evaluation of resources involves comparing assets with current and emerging needs. Resources such as library holdings, educational hardware, software, computerized mannequins for clinical simulation, availability of classroom space, and clinical sites need to be reevaluated periodically. Reviewing the availability of human resources and supportive services are also important. Questions to consider include: Are instructors and clinical preceptors with specific types of needed expertise available?

Are services that support the curriculum available? Do these services meet the needs of the students? For example, are training programs and help desk support accessible? Are services from the campus library, testing center, and computer labs available? And are these services meeting the needs of the learners?

Evaluating curriculum policies involves taking a broad look at the entire program and learning environment to determine areas in which policies are not being effective or additional policies may be indicated. The learning climate can be affected by each of the curriculum factors discussed previously. Some factors, such as teaching and evaluation practices, resources, and policies, have a more direct impact on learning climate than others. Evaluation of these curriculum factors can be integrated into aspects of the program evaluation, student evaluation feedback, alumni, and employer surveys.

Chen's Program Evaluation Theory

Sauter, Johnson, and Gillespie (2009) define program evaluation theory as "a framework that guides the practice of program evaluation" (p. 467). They describe the components of Chen's (1990) theory-driven approach to nursing program evaluation as emphasizing elements of the program and program interventions. The framework provides a comprehensive mechanism for determining the relationship between program elements and outcomes. Furthermore, the framework is useful for programs in various stages of development, ranging from the initial planning stage, to well-established programs.

Chen's framework identifies six types of evaluation which stem from the six domains of program evaluation theory. First, is normative outcome evaluation, which is concerned with determining the appropriateness of program goals and outcomes. Data collection methods include surveying employers and other stakeholders, conducting focus group interviews, or obtaining input from advisory council members. Normative treatment evaluation involves comparing the original treatment (curriculum and teaching strategies) with those implemented in the program. The second evaluation element is what Sauter *et al.* (2009) refer to as a normative treatment evaluation. Normative treatment evaluation simply refers to determining if the treatment (i.e., the curriculum) has been implemented as planned. Sauter and colleagues point out that when outcomes are not being met, conducting a normative treatment evaluation can determine whether the problem is a result of the curriculum or inaccurate implementation of the curriculum.

The third element of Chen's evaluation framework involves the implementation environment. This includes aspects that affect how the program is delivered such as the (1) participant (i.e., student), (2) implementer (i.e., faculty), (3) delivery mode, (4) organization, (5) interorganizational relationships, and (6) context. Evaluation of these aspects can involve collecting demographic data about students and faculty, standardized test scores of students, and teacher qualifications and effectiveness ratings. The evaluation of delivery modes is concerned with effectiveness, appropriateness, and determining whether the delivery mode agrees with stakeholder expectations. Evaluation of the organizational factor is concerned with the leadership structure, policies, and the organizational culture of the institution on achievement of program outcomes. A survey of faculty about their role in the development and implementation of curriculum policy may be helpful (Sauter et al., 2009). The nature of the interorganizational relationships between the institution and clinical agencies may influence collaboration, and sharing of resources and information, and thus affect achievement of program outcomes. The level of cooperation, collaboration, and types of relationships with community agencies can be evaluated through employer surveys, feedback from advisory committee members, or focus groups.

The final aspect of the implementation environment is concerned with the micro context. The micro context includes aspects of the immediate environmental that can support or detract from the learning experience. Evaluation of the micro context may involve determining the types of services available that support learning, such as the campus library, testing centers, computer centers, tutoring programs, online support staff, and opportunities for learning through noncredit campus events and student organizations. The macro context is concerned with the influences of broader societal influences on the implementation of the program, such as shifts in healthcare trends, job market demands, and political and cultural factors.

The fourth category of evaluation is perhaps the most familiar to the ANE. Impact or outcome evaluation involves determining if the program outcomes have been achieved. Common outcomes evaluated include graduation or retention rates, NCLEX pass rates, and employment rates. Failure to achieve a desired program outcome warrants determining the influence of one or more of the aspects of program evaluation on outcome achievement. Revisiting the original goals for appropriateness and comparing the actual and planned implementation processes used may provide insights into the reasons the outcomes were not achieved.

Chen refers to the fifth type of evaluation as the "intervening mechanism evaluation." In education, intervening mechanisms refers to the teaching strategies, program activities, and student conditions or variables that influence learning. This evaluation component provides a cause-and-effect link between teaching and the achievement of program outcomes. Determining the ANE's rationale for using certain teaching strategies and learning activities can support the link between teaching and the outcomes measured. Admission data from student transcripts, student surveys, and focus groups can be used to identify student factors that influenced student learning.

The final evaluation category is Chen's generalization evaluation. Conducting program evaluation as a research study enables the evaluation findings to be generalized to other situations. One component of this process involves establishing the validity and reliability of the assessment tools used. According to Sauter *et al.* (2009), "Evaluation of the effectiveness of the program evaluation plan in improving program outcomes is the final aspect of generalization evaluation" (p. 472).

Learning Evaluation and Program Effectiveness Model

Menix (2007) describes the Learning Evaluation and Program Effectiveness Model (LEPEM), which is adaptable to the evaluation of academic as well as continuing education programs. The central component of the model addresses the question, "What is happening within the program?" (p. 202). Evaluators explore four factors including: "a) the vision, mission, and goals of the program, b) the educational process and learning outcomes, c) the domains of learning, and d) the evaluation plan and effectiveness determinants" (p. 202). "These factors may be influenced by external elements such as professional standards, legislation, business ethics, and evidence based-practices" (p. 202).

The evaluation process described by the LEPEM involves establishing outcomes and criteria that are congruent with the four components of the educational program mentioned previously, and determining the external influences. The next step is to determine what data are needed to evaluate the program and what evaluation tools and processes can be used. Data are then collected and analyzed. Analysis is accomplished by comparing data to the established outcomes and criteria (Menix, 2007). The final aspects of the evaluation process involve making judgments about the value of the findings, then reviewing and revising the program and evaluation processes used. A plan for ongoing evaluation is then established by resetting the outcomes and criteria (p. 202). It is important that research on program evaluation be conducted to determine effective and efficient processes. Using evaluation models such as the LEPEM, which outline a systematic and comprehensive evaluation process, is essential to establishing a strong and well-designed program.

Educational System Analysis Model

Clark (2004) describes the Educational System Analysis Model (ESAM), which can be used by administrators and ANEs to guide the analysis of a nursing program. The

ESAM consists of external and internal elements that affect the operation of the nursing program. External elements are categorized as environmental, community of interest issues, and other factors that are not a part of the program or the institution but have an impact on the operation of the program. Environmental factors include: legal, regulatory, political, and ethical issues, societal values, technology, reputation of the institution and nursing program, demand for educational services, and competition with other institutions and nursing programs. The community of interest is what Clark calls the stakeholders of the program, those who have an interest in "the mission, goals, and expected outcomes of the nursing unit [and] its effectiveness in achieving them" (p. 5). The community of interest includes the pool of prospective students, employers of nursing graduates, program alumni and donors, and the members of the community served by the nursing graduates.

Clark (2004) recommends that the program evaluator ask questions and seek data related to the environment and community of interest factors. She identified four external factors as sources of critical information. First, the reputation of the program and institution are determined. The characteristics perceived as strengths and weaknesses by the public and the reputation of the graduates compared to other programs can provide useful information for guiding curriculum revisions. The second critical factor concerns the prospective students, who they are, and what they expect in terms of programs and services. Third is the information about employers of nursing graduates. The program evaluator needs to identify who the main employers are and what types of relationships exist between the nursing program and employers. In addition, information on employer expectations and whether nursing graduates are meeting these expectations is important. The final aspects to assess include the regulatory, legal, and political influences and what kinds of impact these influences have on the operation of the institution and nursing program. The environmental factors and characteristics of the community of interest are depicted in the model as influencing each other as well as the internal elements of the model.

The internal elements that affect the performance of the nursing program include factors within the nursing program itself and the institution (Clark, 2004). In analyzing internal factors, the content aspects (what was done and why), and process aspects (how and by whom) are addressed. Internal factors include:

- Mission and goals
- Institutional and program values and culture
- Expectations of employers and current students
- Organizational structure and relationships
- Programs, services, and resources offered, and
- Program outcomes.

Clark also recommends assessment of visible artifacts, defined as "observable signs and symbols that underlie a system's organizational culture." These visible artifacts include "physical structures, rituals, ceremonies, language, stories, and legends" (2004, p. 12). Of all of these internal aspects, Clark identifies five that are critical for any institution: the mission and goals, institutional culture, relationships, resources, and outcomes. However, Clark notes that the mission and goals are most important "since all else within the [educational] system should flow from and contribute to them" (p. 10).

Context, Inputs, Process, and Product Model

The Context, Inputs, Process, and Product (CIPP) model developed by Stuffelbeam (2000) uses context, inputs, process and product as indicators of accountability. Evaluation of the context component involves looking at the need and rationale for the program from the stakeholder's perspective, and determining organizational and program strength and weaknesses. The input component is concerned with evaluating human and physical resources. Policies, procedures, and program implementation are reviewed in the process component of the model. The product component involves looking at the program outcomes and comparing them with the needs of the stakeholders. Each of these indicators can be used separately or in combination to provide a comprehensive evaluation framework.

The use of the CIPP model for developing a comprehensive program evaluation framework was reported by Singh (2004). A matrix was developed for each evaluation component (context, inputs, process, and product). Each matrix consisted of a series of major overriding questions, specific subquestions, and indicators. A separate column identified specific sources of data for the indicators. The final column identified methods of data collection such as document review, surveys, interviews, focus groups, or observation.

When applying the CIPP model, the evaluation matrix developed by Singh (2004) can be individualized depending on specific program issues and outcomes of concern. The work of developing the CIPP evaluation matrix, gathering, and evaluating data can be the responsibility of a single internal evaluator or dispersed among members of the evaluation committee. For details about the development of the CIPP evaluation matrix and the processes used, please see the full report by Singh (2004).

Visual Analog Scale for Program Evaluation

Foley (2008) describes the development and use of a visual analog scale (VAS) for measuring program outcomes in a final masters capstone experience. Masters students had the option of completing one of three types of capstones: a thesis, a project such as implementing a change strategy, or a practicum. All capstone options required completion of a scholarly paper and oral presentation, which were designed to address two program outcomes, communication and critical thinking.

Evaluation of the scholarly paper for evidence of critical thinking involved rating the student's paper on clarity of thought, level of thought, scholarly merit, writing style, and format (Foley, 2008, p. 211). The students' oral presentations were used to evaluate the communication outcome. Factors such as organization, emphasis on important content, poise, and use of visual aids were evaluated. The faculty rated the individual items by placing a mark on a horizontal line that represented a continuum of poor to excellent. They provided an overall rating on critical thinking and communication in a similar fashion. Reliability of the instrument was between 0.93 and 0.98, indicating strong internal consistency. In addition to these promising findings, Foley reports that the evaluation tool was easy to complete and required little faculty time.

Continuous Quality Improvement

A final aspect to consider in relation to curriculum design and evaluation competency is the inclusion of mechanisms for continuous quality improvement (CQI). Nurses in clinical practice are familiar with CQI as a method to ensure quality patient care; however, the term has applications in nursing curriculum as well. According to Brown and Marshall (2008), CQI was originally applied to processes used in the manufacturing of goods in the 1930s. Since that time, the use of CQI principles and processes has spread to other areas, including nursing practice and nursing education. CQI basically describes a process of problem solving. Deming (1986) describes four phases or steps in the CQI process (Box 5-6). The first phase is planning, which involves articulation of a clear statement of the mission and philosophy of the institution and program. The progress in manifesting goals inherent in the mission and philosophy is also determined.

The second phase of the CQI process involves developing and implementing an action plan, or what Deming (1986) refers to as the "do" phase. Data are collected to define the problem area and obtain estimates of the costs, materials, and people that will be involved in addressing the problem (Brown & Marshall, 2008). What is unique about the CQI process is that it can be instituted to deal with a particular problem, and once the problem is remedied, CQI can serve as a proactive mechanism to monitor outputs and prevent reoccurrence.

Next is the "study" phase, which involves monitoring the effect of any actions taken by comparing the original data with data collected after the change was imple-

---

BOX 5-6 Phases of the Continuous Quality Improvement Process

Phase 1: Plan—Gather assessment data, align mission, philosophy, and outcomes.

Phase 2: Do—Develop and implement the plan.

Phase 3: Study—Compare data gathered pre- and post-implementation.

Phase 4: Act—Take action to integrate the changes into the organization.

Data from Deming, W. E. (1986). *Out of the crisis* (pp. 88–89). Cambridge, MA: Massachusetts Institute of Technology, Center for Advanced Engineering Study.

---

mented. During the study phase, data about the outcomes and the perception of the change are collected (Brown & Marshall, 2008). Timing of the data collection needs to be carefully considered to assure that the full effect of the change can be captured in the data.

After sufficient data have been collected to assure that the change is effective and is leading to desirable outcomes, the "act" phase is initiated. The act phase involves incorporating the changes into the organization's infrastructure and policies. Mechanisms for providing education about the change and ongoing CQI monitoring are integrated within the institution (Brown & Marshall, 2008).

Brown and Marshall discuss the implementation of a CQI program for their nursing program that explored four program outcomes: (1) NCLEX pass rates, (2) graduation rates, (3) student satisfaction, and (4) employer satisfaction (2008). They began the CQI process by identifying factors thought to influence the program outcomes and established goals for areas needing improvement. Eight factors were assessed for their effect on the program outcomes. These included:

1. Faculty
2. Students
3. Program of study
4. Resources
5. Policies and procedures
6. Standards
7. Environment, and
8. Assessment and evaluation practices.

The authors developed a quality enhancement plan (QEP) to address each area using a variety of strategies to effect changes in faculty and student engagement and professional involvement. For the faculty, professional development opportunities, online workshops, and consultant visits were offered. Faculty and student engagement was enhanced through the development of educational research projects that were related to the QEP.

Results of the project are promising. An initial review conducted 1 year later revealed improvement in the NCLEX pass rates (Brown & Marshall, 2008). Although the long-range outcome of employer satisfaction will take longer to show the full results, some progress has been noted already.

The phases of CQI have been successfully used in many studies in nursing education. In a review of CQI studies conducted between 2000 and 2002, Brown and Marshall found that CQI had been used to predict student's likelihood of success or failure and to develop and evaluate interventions for student success (Benefield, Walker, Halpin, Halpin, & Trentham, 1996). Others used the CQI process to develop an "annual report card" to measure NLN program outcomes (Yearwood, Singleton, Feldman, & Colombraro, 2001). More recently, Montano, Hunt, and Boudreaux (2005) applied the CQI process to academic advising to improve student outcomes. These studies support the application of CQI to a wide range of curricular and program outcomes. Although exact replication of evaluation research is often not practical because of variations within institutions, published reports of CQI programs are valuable on many levels. Information from published CQI programs can broaden awareness of available options, provide guidance and insight, and offer possible applications to the ANE's institution.

Program Improvement Models

In addition to models used to guide program design and evaluation, several models have been developed to improve program outcomes. In this section, two models designed to improve achievement of undergraduate nursing program outcomes are reviewed, the Knowledge, Anxiety control, and Test-Taking Skills (KATTS) Framework and the Academic Center for Evidence-Based Education (ACE) Star Model.

The KATTS Framework

The KATTS model was developed as a comprehensive framework for improving student performance and evaluation outcomes on the NCLEX-RN (McDowell, 2008) (Box 5-7). According to McDowell, each of the components must be in proper balance to enable the student to achieve the maximum test score (2008). McDowell provides specific strategies for strengthening students' knowledge base, controlling anxiety, and improving test taking skills. The strategies can be implemented by individual students or integrated into the curriculum.

BOX 8-5 · Model for Reflective Self-Study

K = Knowledge base

A = Anxiety control

TTS = Test-taking skills

Data from McDowell, B. (2008). KATTS: A framework for maximizing NCLEX-RN performance. *Journal of Nursing Education, 47*(4), 183–186.

The knowledge base component of the KATTS framework uses the NCLEX-RN test plan to identify areas needing further study. During the student's final year or final semester in the program, a standardized examination that addresses the content areas of the NCLEX-RN test blueprint is completed. From the analysis of the standardized examination, strengths and weaknesses are identified, and an individual study plan is created. Rather than focusing on reviewing notes and textbooks, the recommended way to study is using question drills, completing content-focused tests, and completing a comprehensive NCLEX-RN pre-examination (McDowell, 2008).

Anxiety control is also important for successful test taking. Strategies used in the KATTS framework involve reducing or eliminating fear of the unknown, familiarizing the student with conditions similar to those found in the NCLEX-RN examination, maintaining a positive attitude, and keeping a focus on the ultimate goal (McDowell, 2008). Self-care life style practices, such as adequate rest, exercise, balanced diet, and recreation are foundational. The use of stress management techniques in daily living activities, as well as before and during test taking, is recommended. To reduce the fear of the unknown, students are encouraged to become familiar NCLEX-RN testing by completing computerized practice questions and visiting the test site before the exam, if possible.

The test-taking skills component of KATTS focuses on completing practice tests. Emphasis is placed on keeping the amount of time spent on question drill activities at least twice as high as time spent on content review. According to McDowell (2008), this is a departure from typical study strategies, which emphasize high content review and fewer practice questions. Students should plan to complete a minimum of 2000 test items. If the student is at risk because of high anxiety, history of poor test-taking skills, learning disability, or other factors, many authors recommend completing up to twice that number of test items (McQueen, Shelton, & Zimmerman, 2004; Stark, Feikema, & Wyngarden, 2002; Williams & Bryant, 2001). To accomplish these study goals, McDowell recommends the student establish a regular weekly review time and schedule the sessions as he or she would a recurring appointment. The conclusion of the test-taking component of KATTS is marked by competing targeted and comprehensive NCLEX preparation examinations at a level that is predictive of successful NCLEX testing.

The KATTS framework has been used to develop remediation programs for individual students and as a program for first-time testers. McDowell (2008) reports that after implementing KATTS program-wide at her university, the NCLEX pass rate increased from 85% to 97%, without implementing any other major curriculum changes. Because KATTS can be used by individual students or implemented as a program-wide initiative, the improvements in test scores and pass rates can benefit the individual student as well as improve program outcomes.

The ACE Star Model

The ACE Star Model of Knowledge Transformation has also been used to improve nursing program outcomes such as NCLEX pass rates (Box 5-8). The model describes a process used to discover and use evidence-based knowledge and enhance achievement of program outcomes. The first step is the discovery of evidence-based knowledge from the literature. The second step involves evaluating individual studies and synthesizing the key findings into a summary statement. The summary statement is then translated into specific practice recommendations. The fourth step calls for taking action to integrate the practice recommendation into the curriculum. The final step involves evaluation to determine the effect of the strategies on student learning and goal achievement (Bonis, Taft, & Wendler, 2007). After applying the ACE Star Model to a baccalaureate nursing program, Bonis and colleagues (2007) noted that stu-

---

BOX 5-8   Steps in the ACE Star Model

Step 1: Review evidence-based literature.

Step 2: Evaluate studies; write a summary statement.

Step 3: Translate summary statement into practice recommendations.

Step 4: Take action to integrate practice recommendation into curriculum.

Step 5: Evaluate effect of implementing practice recommendation.

Data from Bonis, S., Taft, L., & Wendler, C. (2007). Strategies to promote success on the NCLEX-RN: An evidence-based approach using the ACE star model of knowledge transformation. *Nursing Education Perspectives, 28*(2), 84–85.

dents' pass rates on the NCLEX-RN exam increased over previous years and were higher than the national norm. Program improvement models such as the KATTS and ACE Star Model provide a generic format for program improvement that can be easily adapted by a variety of programs to increase pass rates on the NCLEX-RN.

CONCLUSION

The ANE plays an essential role in curriculum design and program evaluation activities. These range from developing or implementing a new course, or revising existing courses, to designing or revamping the curricular structure for an entire nursing program. Knowledge of the curriculum components, such as program outcomes and curricular philosophy; and knowledge of program evaluation processes are essential for effective curriculum design and program evaluation. In addition, the ANE who is equipped with knowledge and skills related to the change process will be able to anticipate and respond to curricular change in a timely and effective manner and ultimately improve the achievement of program outcomes.

SUMMARY

- The scope of Competency 4 involves all components of curriculum development, from assessment of program needs, to the evaluation of program outcomes.
- A curriculum is a sequence of courses or set of lessons in a related field of study designed to achieve specific learning outcomes or objectives.
- The process of curriculum development begins with the identification of a learning or service need, and then gaining the necesssary support from faculty, administration, and community stakeholders.
- Change theories, either prescriptive or analytical, can be used to guide faculty in the curriculum development process.
- A curricular philosophy is an extension of the overall philosophy of the program, which identifies the perspective, values, and beliefs of the institution and the program.
- The institutional mission statement identifies the services and programs that the institution provides for the community.
- The institutional mission and philosophy should reflect values and beliefs of society, higher education organizations, the community, and the institution.
- The program's mission and philosophy statements represent the focused values, beliefs, and standards of the faculty and the nursing profession.

- Institutional outcomes are broad in scope, whereas program outcomes are discipline specific.
- Course objectives represent the learning outcomes for specific courses and are content specific.
- Taxonomies are used for developing cognitive, affective, and psychomotor outcomes and learning objectives that enable evaluation of course and program outcomes.
- The cognitive domain concerns mental or thinking processes used to acquire and use knowledge.
- Cognitive taxonomies describe hierarchical thinking processes used when acquiring or using knowledge
- Affective domain is concerned with acquiring values, beliefs, and attitudes.
- Affective taxonomies describe the hierarchical processes used to develop and integrate values, beliefs, and attitudes into one's daily life.
- The psychomotor domain is concerned with the development of physical skills or performance of technical tasks.
- Psychomotor taxonomies describe the hierarchical processes used to learn and refine one's performance of new motor skills.
- Effective performance of nursing skills requires a combination of cognitive, affective, and psychomotor domain knowledge.
- Two formats are commonly used to develop objectives include the three-part general format, and Mager's five-part format.
- The general format for objectives includes identifying who the objective is for, what will be done, and how it will be done.
- Mager's format for writing objectives builds on the general format, adding conditions of the performance and the level of expected performance.
- The Interactive Model of Program Planning described by Caffarella (2002) is distinguished from other models by its comprehensive design, recognition of the importance of people and the environment in the planning process, consideration of cultural differences in the planning process, and its practicality and usefulness.
- The Nursing Residency and Clinical Home Community Models are design models for undergraduate nursing programs that are concerned with structure and content emphasis, respectively.
- Program evaluation is an ongoing process of data collection to determine compliance with professional and educational standards.
- Purposes of program evaluation are summarized in Box 5-4.

- A systematic evaluation plan consists of an evaluation framework, identification of existing program resources, data collection, and a timeline for evaluation.
- Successful planning and implementation of curriculum change involves open communication with community stakeholders to determine the needs of the community, the resources needed and available, and the type of student learning experiences possible.
- Iwasiw's Components of Curriculum Evaluation include: (1) congruence of philosophical approaches, (2) curriculum outcomes, (3) curriculum design, (4) courses, (5) teaching and evaluation strategies, (6) resources, (7) policies, and (8) learning climate.
- Chen's Program Evaluation Model provides a comprehensive mechanism for determining the relationship between program elements and outcomes.
- The Learning Evaluation and Program Effectiveness Model and the Educational System Analysis Model are evaluation models that consider the external and internal elements that affect the operation of the nursing program.
- External environmental factors that can affect the operation of a nursing program include: (a) legal, regulatory, political, and ethical issues, (b) societal values, (c) technology, (d) reputation of the institution and nursing program, (e) demand for educational services, and (f) competition with other institutions and nursing programs.
- The internal elements that affect the performance of a nursing program include the mission, goals, values, and culture of the program and institution, expectations of employers and students, the services and resources offered, and program outcomes.
- The CIPP Model describes the context, inputs, process, and products that can be used to develop a comprehensive program evaluation framework.
- A Visual Analog Scale is a reliable and easy tool for program outcome evaluation.
- Continuous Quality Improvement is a process of problem solving used to ensure the maintenance of high-quality outcomes.
- KATTS Framework and the ACE Star Model are used to improve undergraduate nursing program outcomes.
- The KATTS Framework involves providing students with strategies to address three common sources of failure when taking objective examinations: (1) the need for Knowledge, (2) the need for Anxiety control, and (3) Test-Taking Skills.
- ACE Star Model describes a process used to discover and use evidence-based knowledge and enhance achievement of program outcomes (see Box 5-8).

RECOMMENDED RESOURCES

- The American Association of Colleges of Nursing has published a toolkit for implementing the baccalaureate essentials into the nursing programs. The toolkit is available for downloading at http://www.aacn.nche.edu/Education/pdf/BacEssToolkit.pdf.
- The American Association for Advancement of Curriculum Studies is an organization for faculty interested in the advancement of curriculum studies as an academic discipline. Access to the Journal of the American Association for the Advancement of Curriculum Studies is available through their Web site at http://calvin.ednet.lsu.edu/~aaacs/index.html.
- The American Educational Research Association—Division B—Curriculum Studies, offers a listserv focusing on curriculum issues and an informative newsletter. Select the Division menu option at http://www.aera.net.
- The goal of the American Association for Teaching and Curriculum is to promote the scholarly study and discussion of teaching and curriculum. The Web site at http://www.aatchome.org houses a discussion and a refereed journal published annually.
- Febey and Coyne (2007) developed an innovative board game to teach and assess player's knowledge of the program evaluation process. The players move through a series of 44 squares by rolling dice and correctly answering questions related to the program evaluation process. For more information see Febey, K., & Coyne, M. (2007). Program evaluation: The board game: An interactive learning tool for evaluators. *American Journal of Evaluation, 28,* 91–101.

REFERENCES

1. American Association of Colleges of Nursing. (2008). *The essentials of baccalaureate education for professional nursing practice.* Washington, DC: Author.
2. American Association of Colleges of Nursing. (2009, February). *Nurse faculty tool kit for the implementation of the baccalaureate essentials.* Retrieved April 10, 2009 at http://www.aacn.nche.edu/Education/pdf/BacEssToolkit.pdf.
3. Benefield, L. D., Walker, W. P., Halpin, G., Halpin, G., & Trentham, L. (1996). *Assessment and quality in higher education: A model with best practices.* Paper presented at the Conference on Assessment and Quality of the American Association of Higher Education. Retrieved May 4, 2009, from http://www.eric.ed.gov/ERICDocs/data/ericdocs2sql/content_storage_01/0000019b/80/14/a0/61.pdf.
4. Bevis, E.O. (1989). *Curriculum building in nursing: A process.* (3rd ed.), New York, National League for Nursing.

5. Bevis, E. O. (2000). Illuminating the issues. In E. O. Bevis, & J. Watson (Eds.), *Toward a caring curriculum: A new pedagogy for nursing* (pp. 13–35). Sudbury, MA: Jones and Bartlett.

6. Billings, D., & Halstead, J. (2009). *Teaching in nursing: A guide for faculty*. St. Louis: Saunders Elsevier.

7. Bloom, B. (Ed.). (1956). *Taxonomy of educational objectives: The classification of educational goals. Handbook I: Cognitive domain*. New York: David McKay.

8. Boland, D. L. (2009). Developing curriculum: Frameworks, outcomes and competencies. In D. Billings, & J. Halstead (Eds.), *Teaching in nursing: A guide for faculty* (pp. 137–153). St. Louis: Saunders Elsevier.

9. Bondy, K. (1983). Criterion-referenced definitions for rating scales in clinical evaluation. *Journal of Nursing Education, 22*(9), 376–382.

10. Bonis, S., Taft, L., & Wendler, C. (2007). Strategies to promote success on the NCLEX-RN: An evidence-based approach using the ACE star model of knowledge transformation. *Nursing Education Perspectives, 28*(2), 82–87.

11. Brown, J. F., & Marshall, B. (2008). Continuous quality improvement: An effective strategy for improvement of program outcomes in a higher education setting. *Nursing Education Perspectives, 29*(4), 205–211.

12. Buchanan, D., & Badham, R. (1999*). Power, politics, and organizational change: Winning the turf game*. London: Sage.

13. Caffarella, R. (2002). *Planning programs for adult learners: A practical guide for educators, trainers, & staff developers*. San Francisco: Jossey-Bass.

14. Cervero, R., & Wilson, A. (1994). *Planning responsibly for adult education: A guide to negotiating power and interest*. San Francisco: Jossey-Bass.

15. Cervero, R., & Wilson, A. (1996). What really matters in adult education program planning: Lessons in negotiating power and interests. *New directions for adult and continuing education*. San Francisco: Jossey-Bass.

16. Chen, H. (1990). *Theory-driven evaluations*. Newbury Park, CA: Sage Publishing.

17. Clark, M. J. (2004). Finding the way: A model for educational system analysis. *International Journal of Nursing Education Scholarship, 1*(1), Art. 11.

18. Collins, D. (1998). *Organizational change: Sociological perspectives*. London: Routledge.

19. Csokasy, J. (2009). Philosophical foundations of the curriculum. In D. Billings, & J. Halstead (Eds.), *Teaching in nursing: A guide for faculty* (pp. 105–118). St. Louis: Saunders Elsevier.

20. Dawson, P. (1994). *Organizational change: A processual approach*. Adelaide, Australia: Paul Chapman Publishing.

21. Deming, W. E. (1986). *Out of the crisis*. Cambridge, MA: Massachusetts Institute of Technology, Center for Advanced Engineering Study.

22. Diefenbeck, C. A., Plowfield, L. A., & Herrman, J. W. (2006). Clinical immersion: A residency model for nursing education. *Nursing Education Perspectives, 27*, 72–79.

23. Febey, K., & Coyne, M. (2007). Program evaluation: The board game: An interactive learning tool for evaluators. *American Journal of Evaluation, 28*, 91–101.

24. Foley, D. (2008). Development of a visual analog scale to measure curriculum outcomes. *Journal of Nursing Education, 47*(5), 209–213.

25. Frost, P., & Robinson, S. (1999 July/August). The toxic handler: Organizational hero- and causality. *Harvard Business Review*, 96–106.

26. Gard, C., Flannigan, P., & Cluskey, M. (2004). Program evaluation: An ongoing systematic process. *Nursing Education Perspectives, 25*, 176–179.

27. Glennon, C. (2006). Reconceptualizing program outcomes. *Journal of Nursing Education, 45*(2), 55–58.

28. Halstead, J. (2007). *Nurse educator competencies: Creating an evidence-based practice for nurse educators.* New York: National League for Nursing.

29. Hamner, J. B., & Bentley, R. W. (2003). A systematic evaluation plan that works. *Nurse Educator, 28*(4), 179–184.

30. Hardy, C. (1996). Understanding power: Bringing about strategic change. *British Journal of Management, 7* (Special Issue), S3–S16.

31. Holaday, S. D., & Buckley, K. M. (2007). A standardized clinical evaluation tool-kit: Improving nursing education and practice. In M. H. Oermann, (Ed.), *Annual review of nursing education* (Vol. 6, 2008). *Clinical nursing education* (pp. 123–149). New York: Springer.

32. Iacovini, J. (1993). The human side of organization change. *Training and Development, 47*(1), 65–68.

33. Iwasiw, C., Goldenberg, D., & Andrusyszyn, M. (2009). *Curriculum development in nursing education.* Sudbury, MA: Jones and Bartlett.

34. Knowles, M. (1980). Malcolm Knowles on "Lifelong" learning—Buzz word or new way of thinking about education. *Training & Development Journal, 34*(7), 40, 3p.

35. Lewin, K. (1947). Frontiers in group dynamics: Concept, method, and reality in social science; social equilibria and social change. *Human Relations, 1*(1), 5–41.

36. Lewin, K. (1951). *Field theory in social science: Selected theoretical papers.* New York: Harper & Row.

37. Lewin, K. (1958). Group decisions and social change. In E. E. Maccoby, & E. L. Hartley, (Eds.), *Readings in social psychology* (pp. 197–211). New York: Holt, Rinehart, & Winston.

38. Mager, R. F. (1984). *Preparing instructional objectives.* Belmont, CA: David S. Lake.

39. McDowell, B. (2008). KATTS: A framework for maximizing NCLEX-RN performance. *Journal of Nursing Education, 47*(4), 183–186.

40. McQueen, L., Shelton, P., & Zimmerman, L. (2004, May/June). A collective community approach to preparing nursing students for the NCLEX RN examination. *The ABNF Journal, 15*(3), 55–58.

41. Menix, K. D. (2007). Evaluation of learning and program effectiveness. *Journal of Continuing Education in Nursing, 38*(5), 201–208.

42. Montano, C. B., Hunt, M. D., & Boudreaux, L. (2005). Improving the quality of student advising in higher education—A case study. *Total Quality Management, 16*(10), 1103–1125.

43. National League for Nursing Board of Governors (2003, August). *Innovation in nursing education: A call to reform,* National League for Nursing, pp. 1–5. Retrieved February, 27, 2009 from http://www.nln.org/aboutnln/PositionStatements/innovation082203.pdf.

44. National League for Nursing Certification Governance Committee. (2005). *The scope of practice for academic nurse educators.* New York: National League for Nursing.

45. Pettigrew, A. M. (1990). Longitudinal field research on change: Theory and practice. *Organizational Science, 3*(1), 267–292.

46. Porter-O'Grady, T. (2001). Profound change: Twenty-first century nursing. *Nursing Outlook, 49*(4), 182–186.

47. Sauter, M., Johnson, D., & Gillespie, N. (2009). Educational program evaluation. In D. Billings, & J. Halstead, (Eds.), *Teaching in nursing: a guide for faculty* (pp. 467–509). St. Louis: Saunders Elsevier.

48. Shanley, C. (2007). Management of change for nurses: Lessons from the discipline of organizational studies. *Journal of Nursing Management, 15*, 538–546.

49. Singh, M. D. (2004). Evaluation framework for nursing education programs: Application of the CIPP Model. *International Journal of Nursing Education Scholarship, 1*(1), 1–16.

50. Sork, T. J. (1997). Program priorities, purposes, and objectives. In P. S. Cookson, (Ed.), *Program planning for the training and education of adults: North American perspectives.* Malabar, FL: Krieger.

51. Sork, T. J. (2000). Planning educational programs. In A. Wilson, & E. Hayes, (Eds.), *Handbook of adult and continuing education* (pp. 171–190). San Francisco: Jossey-Bass.

52. Stark. M., Feikema, B., & Wyngarden, K. (2002). Empowering students for NCLEX success: Self-assessment and planning. *Nurse Educator, 27*, 103–105.

53. Stuart, R. (1996). The trauma of organizational change. *Journal of European Industrial Training, 20*(2), 11–16.

54. Stuffelbeam, D. L. (2000). The CIPP model for program evaluation. In G. F. Madaus, M. Scriven, & D. L. Stuffelbeam (Eds.), *Evaluation models: Viewpoints on educational and human service evaluation.* Norwell, MA: Kluwer Academic Publishers.

55. Warner, J., & Misener, T. (2009). Forces and issues influencing curriculum development. In D. Billings, & J. Halstead (Eds.), *Teaching in nursing: A guide for faculty* (pp. 92–104). St Louis: Saunders Elsevier.

56. Williams-Barnard, C., Sweatt, A., Harkness, G., & DiNapoli, P. (2004). The clinical home community: A model for community-based education. *International Nursing Reviews, 51*, 104–112.

57. Williams, D., & Bryant, S. (2001). Preparing at-risk baccalaureate students for NCLEX success. *Kentucky Nurse, 49*(1), 17.

58. Yearwood, E., Singleton, J., Feldman, H., & Colombraro, G. (2001). A case study in implementing CQI in a nursing education program. *Journal of Professional Nursing, 17*, 297–304.

CHAPTER 6

Function as a Change Agent and Leader—Competency 5

1. Compare theoretical perspectives and models of change, leadership, and advocacy.
2. Identify strategies for developing leadership and advocacy skills and implementing organizational change.
3. Explore strategies for evaluating organizational effectiveness in nursing education.
4. Identify innovative practices and changes within academic institutions and nursing programs.
5. Explore programs and initiatives effective in meeting nursing and educational needs of the local and regional communities and beyond.

KEY TERMS

Action centered leadership model
Advocacy
Change agent model
Creative leadership
Rogers' diffusion of innovation theory
Empowerment theory

LEAD project
New Science Leadership Theory
Open systems theory
Organizational change
Servant leadership

DEFINITION AND DESCRIPTION OF COMPETENCY

Functioning as a change agent and leader is integral to the teaching, scholarship, and service role functions of the ANE. Change and leadership processes work interdependently, hand-in-hand. A leader's functioning is enhanced by understanding the complexities of the leadership role and the change process within the organization. Theoretical knowledge and skills in change, advocacy, empowerment, diffusion of innovations, and leadership theory provide a foundation for functioning as a change agent and leader.

THEORY AND RESEARCH RELATED TO COMPETENCY _____

Virtually every profession is interested in the concept of leadership and change. Leadership is central to building and maintaining the structure and function of professional disciplines, facilitating the advancement of knowledge, and the achievement of goals and outcomes. Change is inevitable and influenced by multiple factors. Therefore, research and theory development concerned with leadership and change have been progressive and extensive.

In this chapter, several aspects of leadership are explored including leadership theories, tasks, styles, and competencies for nurse leaders. Change theories including Lewin's Change Process Model, Rogers' Diffusion of Innovation Theory, and factors that enhance sustainability of change are reviewed. Research related to change and leadership; and suggestions for application to practice are integrated throughout.

Evolution of Leadership Concepts and Theories

For the academic nurse educator (ANE), leadership is inherent in the daily functions of teaching in the classroom and clinical settings. The ANE also functions as a leader and change agent when establishing clinical partnerships, participating in academic governance, or serving as an officer in professional organizations. Awareness of a variety of leadership theories and perspectives can be empowering because it allows the ANE to draw from and utilize a range of concepts to achieve goals, and to change and manage the teaching/learning environment.

Leadership theories can be classified into categories representing an overlapping evolution of leadership perspectives (Table 6-1). Leadership theories such as the great man theory fall within the category of trait-based leadership theory. An assumption of the trait-based theories is that the leader has unique or especially strong leadership abilities that others in the organization do not manifest. Behavioral and situational leadership theories represent a shift from focusing on the leader to focusing on the leader's behaviors. In behavioral leadership theories the leader's relationships and performance behaviors are paramount. In situational leadership theories there is a movement from focusing solely on the leader, to focusing on the leadership environment and the leader's ability to adapt to different environments. Situational theories appreciate the differences and changes in an organization and the leader's ability to adapt to the situation.

Servant Leadership, Path-Goal Theory, and Belbin's Team Roles Theory can be classified as transactional theories that share an emphasis on valuing the nature of the relationship between the leader and followers. Transformational Theory is also linked

TABLE 6-1   Comparison of Leadership Theories

Leadership Perspective	Examples	Characteristics
Trait Theories: Emphasis on abilities of leader	Great Man Theory	• Persons are born with innate leadership qualities
	Trait Approach Theories	• Leadership associated with traits such as charisma, intelligence, task motivation, social skill, administrative skills, and emotional control (Gosling, Marturano, & Dennison, 2003, p. 7)
	Keirsey's Temperament Theory and Leadership	• Identified four types of roles assumed by leaders (diplomat, strategic, tactical, and logistical). The type of leadership role assumed depends on temperament. • Leadership is enhanced by matching talents to the leadership task (Keirsey, 1998, p. 289).
Behavioral Theories: Focus on the types of relationships and the performance of leaders	Theory X and Theory Y Managers	• Theory X managers believe people lack motivation and need direction. • Theory Y managers believe people actively seek responsibility, and can be self-directed to achieve goals (McGregor, 1960).
	Managerial Grid	• Leaders are categorized based on concern for people and production (Blake & McCanse, 1991; Blake & Moulton, 1985).
Situational Theories: The leader's adaptability to the environment is important	Fiedler's Contingency Model	• Relationships, type of task, and leader power influence leader effectiveness (Fiedler, 1996).
	Hersey-Blanchard Model of Leadership	• Leadership types include participating, delegating, telling, and selling.

(continues)

TABLE 6-1 Comparison of Leadership Theories *(continued)*		
Leadership Perspective	**Examples**	**Characteristics**
		• Leader effectiveness is influenced by task behavior, matching of leadership style with situation, and the readiness of the followers (Hersey & Blanchard, 1993).
	Tannenbaum & Schmidt's Leadership Continuum	• A continuum of leadership based on the levels of freedom that a manager chooses to give to a team, and the level of authority used by the manager (Tannenbaum & Schmidt, 1973)
	Action-Centered Leadership Model	• Responsibilities include achieving the task, managing the group, and managing individuals (Adair, 1973).
	Normative Decision Model of Leadership	• Focus is on conditions in which decisions should be made either autocratically, democratically, or in consultation with the group members (Blau, 1964).
	Reframing Organizations	• Different situations require different cognitive approaches depending on political, structural, human resources, or symbolic aspects (Bolman & Deal, 2003).
Transactional Theory: Values the nature of the relationship between the leader and followers	Servant Leadership	• A philosophy that emphasizes being of service as the precursor for aspiring to the role of leader (Greenleaf, 1977)
	Path-Goal Theory	• Emphasis on motivation of followers to achieve goals (House, 1971)
	Team Role Theory	• Defines nine team roles; the specialist, finisher, implementer, evaluator, team worker, shaper, coordinator, plant (idea person), and resource locator (Belbin, 1993, 2009)

(continues)

TABLE 6-1   Comparison of Leadership Theories *(continued)*

Leadership Perspective	Examples	Characteristics
Transformational Theory: Leadership outcomes are guided by moral vs. functional outcomes.	Transformational Leadership	• Appeals to the values and beliefs of followers to stimulate creative vision and change in the organization's performance. • Leader is seen as proactive (Burns, 1978). • Follower's awareness of the importance of the task, focus on goals, and higher order needs are important (Bass, 1985 & 1990).
Dispersed Leadership Theories: Emphasis on shared responsibility	Distributed Leadership	• Responsibility for leadership is shared throughout the organization. • Focus is on interdependence of relationships (Gronn, 2000).
	Multidimensional Leadership	• Effective leader varies leader behaviors based on situational demands and members' preferences (Chelladurai & Saleh, 1978). • Results are achieved through joint efforts at multiple levels (Peterson, 1997).
	Chaos Theory	• Characterized by collaborative, decentralized process, yielding unpredictable outcomes (Heifetz, 1994; Wheatley, 1992; 2006)
Social-Cultural Leadership Theories: Emphasis on understanding history, context, values, meaning, and interpretation	Women's Leadership Theory	• Emphasis on responsibility and empowerment • De-emphasis of hierarchical relationships (Kezar *et al.,* 2006, p. 53)
	Organizational Culture Theory	• The type of leader behavior considered desirable and workable varies with the organizational culture. • The leader creates and changes organizational culture based on his or her values and beliefs (Schein, 1992).

Some data from Eddy, P. L., & Vanderlinden, K. E. (2006). Emerging definitions of leadership in higher education. *Community College Review, 34*(1), 20; and Kezar, A., Carducci, R., & Contreras-McGavin, M. (2006). Rethinking the "L" word in higher education: The revolution of research on leadership. *ASHE Higher Education Report, 31*(6), 31–70.

to values. Transformational theory is outcome focused and sees the leader as guided by moral versus functional outcomes.

Dispersed leadership theories such as Distributed Leadership, Multidimensional Leadership, and Chaos Theory represent a new emphasis away from leader-focused theories to a focus on the members within the organization. These theories envision a shared responsibility or mutual effort in the leadership and change processes. Leadership is characterized as interdependent, decentralized, and collaborative.

The final classification, social-cultural leadership theories, place an emphasis on understanding the context, the organization's history, its values, and the meaning and interpretation of change. Unlike previous theories that focused on the leader, or leader behaviors and values, the social-cultural leadership theories are concerned with understanding the change and the context in which it is occurring. Although these leadership theories share some similarities, each also provides a unique perspective that contributes to our understanding of leadership.

Application of leadership theory to the ANE's work setting first requires familiarity with a range of leadership perspectives and processes. The ANE needs to adapt approaches to unique and changing situations and often needs to combine aspects of one or more theories. Therefore, familiarity with diverse theoretical perspectives will provide a foundation for integrating selected leadership concepts into practice. Selected leadership theories are reviewed in this section to provide a basic foundation. The reader who desires more information about selected theories is directed to the resources and reference sections at the end of this chapter.

Overview of Selected Leadership Theories

Hartley and Allison's Leadership Framework

Hartley and Allison (2002) offer a concise framework to describe leadership that does not fall neatly into one category. They view leadership as related to the three Ps, person, position, and process. The person aspect describes personal attributes, behaviors, and skills important in leadership. The person's position within an organization is the second aspect of leadership. The position or title a person holds is seen as an indication of power and authority within an organization but not necessarily a condition for leadership. Often people without an administrative title demonstrate leadership and are considered leaders within an organization. The ANE is an example. Nursing faculty who do not hold an administrative title may provide leadership for the classes they teach, or may be involved in developing community partnerships, implementing changes in curriculum, clinical, or educational practice, all of which require skills and attributes commonly associated with leadership.

The final aspect of leadership described by Hartley and Allison (2002) *is* "process." This involves working with others to achieve movement toward a goal. The leader uses influence, appreciation, and people skills to motivate and help those within the organization move closer to the goal. The ANE utilizes selected leadership processes when implementing changes in curriculum, engaging in student and faculty recruitment efforts, developing and implementing program infrastructure, strategic planning, developing research projects, and establishing community partnerships.

Servant Leadership

Servant leadership was proposed by Greenleaf (1977) as a type of leadership philosophy characterized by a leader who values being of service to followers more than his or her own personal interests (Rennaker, 2005, p. 2). Servant leadership is also distinguished from other leadership types by the personal value system of the leader. Spears (1998) identified servant leadership characteristics as empathy and the ability to listen, persuade, and build community. Personal values identified from the literature that are apparent in servant leaders include trust, caring, authenticity, altruism, and appreciation of others (Rennaker, 2005, p. 2).

Application of servant leadership to the role of the ANE involves aligning with values that focus on and facilitate service to others and modeling behaviors consistent with those values when interacting in the workplace. Chonko (2007) took the application of servant leadership a step further and identified principles of servant leadership that defined his teaching practice and gave it purpose (Box 6-1). By using the servant leadership philosophy, Chonko found a rekindled focus and passion for teaching and active learning.

The desired outcome of effective servant leadership can be as straightforward as enhancing the performance of others or increasing the positive orientation of others toward service. To learn more about servant leadership and how to apply it to your setting, see the Greenleaf Center for Servant Leadership Web site listed in the resource section.

Creative Leadership

Clark (2009) presents a new perspective on leadership referred to as creative leadership. The emphasis in creative leadership is on "producing or inventing new solutions to challenging situations and using imagination and skills to apply relevant theory and concepts" (p. 5). Creative leadership calls for the leader to have knowledge of a broad range of theories that enhance the understanding of individuals as well as the social and environmental influences that affect the institution. Thus, creative leadership is

---

BOX 6-1   Principles of Servant Leadership as Applied to Teaching

Principle 1: Teaching must be a subversive activity (i.e., emphasizing the inquiry method).

Principle 2: Inquiring minds must drive education (teachers are open to learning from students).

Principle 3: Servant teachers are stewards (students are entrusted to the teachers to be stimulated toward growth).

Principle 4: Servant teachers engage students in a lifetime of learning paradigm.

Principle 5: The servant teacher teaches to the learner's needs, not wants.

Principle 6: Students are people of worth.

Principle 7: Servant teachers practice patience, tolerance, and professionalism.

Principle 8: Servant teachers translate knowledge into active learning.

Principle 9: Servant teachers act as a servant first (ensuring the needs of the student are meet first).

Data from Chonko, L. B. (2007). A philosophy of teaching . . . and more. *Journal of Marketing Education, 29,* 111–118.

---

founded in an awareness and assessment of the institutional setting and the trends that influence practice. Clark suggests the leader can readily apply selected aspects of various theories by determining which theoretical concepts are relevant to the situation. This can be achieved by asking questions such as, Which theoretical ideas can help explain the behaviors and responses of those within my institution? What actions, if any, does the theory suggest that could be useful in the current situation? Does the theory provide a rationale for understanding the outcomes of specific leadership actions?

Although Clark's text is written for clinical nursing leaders, the key components of creative leadership are applicable to other leadership settings including nursing education. Clark (2009) also identifies six competency areas as essential for creative leaders. These include: technology master, problem solver, change maker, ambassador, great communicator, and team player (p. 5). These creative leadership competencies easily translate to the activities of the ANE such as managing educational and clinical based technology, and modeling and assisting students in problem solving. The ambassador, change maker, communicator, and team player competencies are demonstrated through a variety of clinical and classroom interactions.

Situational Leadership

As change occurs in society, the demands, stressors, relationships, and resources also change and necessitate organizational adaptation. Meeting changing needs requires a flexible leadership style to adjust to new goals of the institution. Situational leadership has been identified as a leadership style that addresses the variability in the situation. Taylor (2007) refers to situational leadership style as one in which "the preferred leadership styles [are] adapted to meet the demands of different situations" (p. 32).

To determine the leadership style that will be most well received and most effective, the ANE determines the degree of competency, commitment, and motivation needed to accomplish the goal. Taylor adapted four approaches from Northouse (1997) that combine varying degrees of support and directive behaviors, depending upon the competency, motivation, and commitment of the individuals involved. The four approaches vary from high to low in terms of directiveness and support (Table 6-2).

Taylor (2007) acknowledges that the situational leadership approach is widely utilized in leadership training despite a lack of research support. An inherent difficulty with the situational leadership approach is that the use of different degrees of support and directiveness could be perceived by some individuals as biased or preferential

TABLE 6-2 Situational Leadership Approaches Using Directive and Supportive Behaviors

Level of Support	Low Directive	High Directive
Low Support	• For dealing with individuals who do not need high degree of guidance, who are motivated and competent • Leader facilitates individuals to take action.	• Useful for dealing with individuals who lack knowledge and skills needed to achieve goals but are highly motivated • Leader is highly directive and commanding.
High Support	• For dealing with individuals who are competent but lack motivation to engage in change • Leader offers praise and encouragement.	• Useful when individuals are lower in terms of competence and are not motivated to engage in the change process • Leader gives verbal encouragement, praise, direct guidance, and feedback.

Data from Taylor, V. (2007). Leadership for service improvement. *Nursing Management-UK, 13*(9), 30–34.

treatment. It may also be difficult to apply varying levels of support and directiveness to groups who are highly mixed in terms of knowledge, skills, competence, and motivation.

Belbin's Team Role Theory

Belbin defines a team role as "a tendency to behave, contribute, and interrelate with others in a particular way" (Belbin, 2009, para. 1). Belbin, a management consultant and author of several books on leadership and management, identified nine behaviors or team roles relevant to leadership (Box 6-2). "Each team role has its particular strengths and allowable weaknesses, and each has an important contribution to make to a team" (para. 2). Most of the roles are clearly reflected by the titles; however, the characteristics of those assuming the *plant* and *shaper* roles may not be as transparent. The "plant" team role is symbolized by a light bulb and represents someone who uses creativity and imagination to solve difficult problems. The shaper is symbolized by a whip and represents someone who is driven to overcome obstacles and thrives on challenge and pressure.

Because leadership occurs within groups, understanding the roles inherent in a team or work group is beneficial. Awareness of team role preferences of each group member can facilitate group work by providing members with knowledge of what

---

BOX 6-2   Beldin's Team Role Behaviors

- Plant

- Resource Locator

- Co-coordinator

- Shaper

- Monitor/Evaluator

- Teamworker

- Implementer

- Completer/Finisher

- Specialist

Data from Belbin, M. R. (2009). *Belbin team role theory*. Retrieved April 20, 2009 from http://www.belbin.com/rte.asp?id=8.

types of behavioral tendencies to expect. According to Belbin (1993; 2009), individuals have 3–4 team role preferences that are not fixed and may change over time or with certain circumstances. Factors such as newness to the work setting, a promotion, or changes in circumstances at home or in key relationships can influence the individual's team role preferences (Belbin, 2009). Those interested in more information can visit the Belbin Web site listed in the reference section.

Action Centered Leadership Theory

As implied by the theory name, action centered leadership describes the actions leaders need to take to be most effective. The theory was developed by Adair (1973), while teaching at a British military academy. Since then, the theory has become widely adapted for use in industry, business, and education settings. The theory describes three categories of actions that a leader must attend to, including: (1) action related to achieving the task, (2) building and managing the team, and (3) developing individuals within the team. Each of these action categories is interdependent and all must be addressed for the group to be effective in meeting the goals of the organization.

To become an effective leader, Adair (1973) identified eight leadership functions that need to be developed and practiced (see Box 6-3). The first function is to define the task by developing clear objectives that are specific, measurable, achievable, realistic, and time constrained. The second task involves planning and looking for alternatives and contingencies. Third is briefing individuals on the goals, task, and status. The fourth function—controlling—refers to using delegation and monitoring skills and ensuring that good control systems are in place. Leaders also need to be good at evaluating all aspects of the situation. They should possess organizational skills, be able to provide motivation for group members during the change process, and be able to role model or set an example for group members.

Chaos Theory

One approach to studying the complexity of leadership has been to explore the application of chaos theory to the organizational environment and leadership processes. Chaos theory was originally developed as a branch of mathematical physics to deal with events and processes that could not be predicted using conventional laws and theorems. Since its inception in the 1960s, chaos theory has been applied to many other fields such as natural sciences, social sciences, and business. Although the term chaos is typically thought to refer to a state of disorder and randomness, when used in science it is more accurate to think of chaos as "apparent randomness" that actually follows laws or rules that may not be immediately obvious. This apparent chaos or

BOX 6-3   Functions of Action Centered Leaders
• Define the task
• Plan
• Debrief
• Control
• Evaluate
• Motivate
• Organize
• Set an example
Data from Adair, J. (1973). *Action centered leadership*. London: McGraw-Hill.

randomness, results from interactions among complex systems. A key postulate of chaos theory is that complex natural systems, such as organizations, obey specific rules and are sensitive to small initial changes. It is the sensitivity of complex systems to minute changes, that can cause unexpected results, thus giving the impression of random events (Society for Chaos Theory in Psychology and Life Sciences, 2009).

Several authors including Heifetz (1994) and Wheatley (1992; 2006) have applied the ideas underlying chaos theory to organizational systems and the leadership process. Heifetz emphasizes that complex organizational systems require adaptive and novel responses. Thus, according to Kezar *et al.* (2006), "Leadership is no longer a predictable process that requires the application of a set of characteristics, skills, or behaviors" (p. 40). Chaos theory has led to a reexamination of the common assumptions of leadership such as task differentiation, authority, and hierarchy; and instead looks at flexibility, adaptability, decentralized processes, and collaboration within the organization (Wheatley, 2006).

A review of chaos research by Kezar *et al.* (2006) found that leaders who considered organizational complexity showed improved effectiveness. In the area of leadership, chaos theory has encouraged researchers to look at the leadership processes from a much broader perspective that considers social and technical aspects. Chaos theory has also changed the way leadership contexts and processes are perceived. According to Kezar *et al.* (2006), chaos theory recognizes the changing nature of the organizational environment and incorporates new and emerging structures and processes including: networks, systems thinking, partnering, and collaboration. Grossman and Valiga (2009) summarize the influence of chaos theory as "assisting us in understanding how disorder and confusion . . . in our work settings" reflect the same process that occur in nature (p. 31).

New Science Leadership Theory

New Science Leadership Theory is derived from chaos and quantum theories (Wheatley & Kellner-Rogers, 1996; Wheatley, 2006). Chaos theory provides a broad perspective for examining the functioning of an organization as opposed to examining a small part of the organization. According to proponents of new science theory, proj-ects that initially seem disordered tend to show increased organization with time because of the tendency for self-organization (Doyle, 2004). Another differentiating feature of New Science Leadership Theory involves the roles of those engaging in the process. Instead of focusing on tasks, or on the hierarchy involved with power, control, and communication, the focus is on relationships and the capacity to form flexible relationships. In fact, in New Science Leadership Theory, participants may share and take turns in assuming the role of the leader (Doyle, 2004).

Another unique characteristic of New Science Leadership Theory is the recognition of the influence of quantum theory on organizational systems. According to quantum theory, observation of a phenomenon affects or changes the phenomenon. Thus, ideas of predictability and control of a situation are not absolutes. Instead, less prediction, prejudgment, and compartmentalization occur (Grossman & Valiga, 2009). Thus, New Science Leadership Theory takes an approach that shifts from rule based leadership to one that emphasizes relationships and progression that is non-linear (Doyle, 2004).

Several authors have reported on the application of New Science Leadership Theory to nursing education (Doyle, 2004; Grossman & Valiga, 2009). The theory was used by Doyle in the planning stages of the development of an international practice experience for nursing students. The flexibility and emphasis on shared and alternating leadership roles and relationships, allowed students and faculty involved in the planning to work independently and in small groups. Grossman and Valiga (2009) discuss how growth and change in nursing is stimulated by chaos and disequilibrium. They note that "changes in worldview, similar to any type of growth, occur as a result of disequilibrium" (p. 29). Both people and organizations go through developmental changes that are often stimulated by challenging experiences. Thus, the experience of disequilibrium is not a negative thing but a necessary experience that enhances growth within individuals and within the organization.

Leadership Styles and Practices

A style is defined as "a particular form of behavior directly associated with an individual . . . the way in which something is said or done" (Moiden, 2002, p. 23). Therefore, leadership style reflects the ways in which leaders interact with others to accomplish goals. There are many classification systems used to describe leadership styles. Moiden (2002) reviews three styles classified as authoritarian, democratic, and laissez-faire. The authoritarian style represents as a range of behaviors. At one end of the continuum, the authoritarian style is rigid, controlling, and coercive; at the other end, the authoritarian leader may be less controlling but firm and self-assured. The democratic leadership style is more person-focused and concerned with human interactions and collaboration. The person engaging in democratic leadership style seeks input from others and fosters the groups' sense of responsibility and decision-making. In contrast, the laissez-faire style of leadership is characterized as valuing the individual over the group and over the task to be completed. Laissez-faire leaders typically relinquish control and responsibility to members of the group and limit their influence to providing resources and responding to questions. Ideally, the use of the authoritarian, democratic, and laissez-faire styles will vary depending on the type of situation and the skill and motivation of the members. However, the democratic style is often viewed as an effective balance between the two approaches and is amendable to a variety of situations.

Another classification of leadership styles was developed by the Hay Group based upon a survey of healthcare organizations (Kenmore, 2008). Six leadership styles were delineated including: affiliative, coaching, directive, pace-setting, participative, and visionary. The affiliative style is a good fit for situations that are progressing without incident and in which the group members are motivated to continue working toward the established goals. The coaching style is a good fit for situations where there is minimal conflict and there is a sense of teamwork. When dealing with urgent matters or crisis situations, the directive style facilitates prompt completion of tasks. The pace-setting style is characterized by setting and achieving high standards and works best with well-motivated and competent group members. When the group needs to reach a consensus in terms of goals and processes used, the participative style is useful. The participative style stimulates involvement of all members through discussion. The final category, the visionary leadership style, is appropriate when new, untried approaches and solutions need to be considered and when there is a need for long-term planning.

In a survey of clinical managers and staff, 50% of the managers rated as high performers regularly used more than three of the six leadership styles, whereas only 20%

of the low performing managers used three or more styles (Kenmore, 2008). Although these styles have not been studied in nursing faculty, the categories describe generic leadership characteristics and behaviors that can be seen in teaching, in the development of community partnerships, and in academic governance activities. Additional research in educational settings is needed to determine which styles are used most frequently, under what circumstances the styles are used, and the perceived effectiveness of the styles.

Kezar and colleagues (2006) draw some insightful observations about past and present leadership theories. They note that earlier theories and research have tended to be leader-centered; whereas emerging research is more concerned with understanding the processes and contextual variables that influence leadership. As a result, earlier theories and research have tended to focus on the study of individual leaders and their characteristics, while emerging theory and research are more concerned with understanding the collaborative processes that occur between the leader and others.

Choosing a Leadership Style

According to Kezar *et al.* (2006), a major shift in the study of leadership is in the emphasis on the relationships between followers and leaders. Thus, research that in the past had emphasized the leader's power and hierarchical relationships has shifted to focus on understanding mutual power and influence between leaders and followers. Research and theory development have also shifted from a reductionist perspective, which looked at separate traits, to understanding the complexity and changing nature of leadership within the context of the organization and its members.

Awareness of a range of leadership styles and perspectives is a precursor to taking deliberate action and choosing an appropriate leadership style for the setting and circumstance. In a classic article by Tannenbaum and Schmidt (1973), the authors explore how to select a leadership pattern. First, they identified a continuum of leadership behavior that depicts how much influence and control the leader and his or her subordinates should assume for decision making. Leadership behaviors ranging from "boss-centered" to "subordinate-centered" are outlined in Box 6-4. Each behavior depicts varying degrees of involvement and control by either the leader or the group members (p. 164).

To decide which leadership approach should be used, Tannenbaum and Schmidt (1973) suggest identifying the forces that affect the leader, subordinates, and the situation. Forces that affect the leader include personal values related to responsibility, shared decision-making, and his or her perspective on the importance of organizational efficiency and cost effectiveness. The leader also brings to the situation, a level

> **BOX 6-4   Continuum of Leadership Behaviors**
>
> The leader:
>
> 1. Makes a decision and informs the group
>
> 2. Makes a decision and persuades the group about the decision
>
> 3. Presents the decision and invites questions
>
> 4. Presents a tentative decision and seeks input from group
>
> 5. Presents the problem, solicits ideas, and makes the final decision
>
> 6. Asks the group to make the decision within specific parameters
>
> 7. Allows group to identify problem and generate solutions within specific parameters
>
> Data from Tannenbaum, R., & Schmidt, W. H. (1973, May/June). How to choose a leadership pattern. *Harvard Business Review, 51*(3), p. 163–165.

of confidence in the group's ability to handle the situation, personal leadership preferences, and the ability to tolerate uncertainty. Considering these forces enables the leader to answer a key question, "who is best qualified to deal with this situation?" (p. 175). Another set of factors to consider are the forces operating within the group such as the groups' knowledge, experience, and interest in dealing with the problem. Questions to consider include, Does the group expect shared decision-making? Does the group have strong need for independence in problem-solving? How ready is the group to assume responsibility for decision-making? And finally, how does the group's ability to tolerate uncertainty and ambiguity compare to the degree of ambiguity and uncertainly that is inherent in the situation?

Tannebaum and Schmidt (1973) also recognize the importance of situational forces in the choice of leadership behavior. The organization's characteristics, the groups' effectiveness, the nature of the problem, and time constraints need to be considered. The organization's characteristics, such as values and traditions, can influence expectations of the leaders and subordinates within the organization. When considering the group's effectiveness, factors such as how long the group members have worked together and similarities in background will also play a role in the group's effectiveness.

The nature of the problem may have an impact on the amount of authority and responsibility the leader chooses to control or delegate to the group. According to Tannenbaum and Schmidt (1973), the degree of complexity of the problem does not always indicate that the leader should engage others in the decision-making process.

There may be times when the leader has all of the factual data relevant to the problem and it would be easier and more efficient for the leader to work through the problem-solving process alone. However, when one person does not have the knowledge or expertise, it may be wise to obtain ideas from experts or from the group as a whole. The question that should guide the decision is, "Have I heard the ideas of everyone who has the necessary knowledge to make significant contributions to the solution of this problem?" (p. 179).

The final aspect to consider is the urgency of the problem and the amount to time that can be devoted to decision making. The more urgent the need for a decision, the less likely the leader will be able to involve others in the process. A less urgent problem will afford more opportunity to involve the group and explore a variety of ideas. In any given situation, the urgency of the problem, and the amount of time for decision making will have a direct influence on leader behaviors and on determining the actions that will be most effective.

Gardner's Leadership Tasks

Gardner (1989) described nine tasks common to leadership (Box 6-5). The first task is "envisioning goals" to guide group activities. Second is to affirm shared values that underscore the short and long-term goals and purpose of the organization. The task of motivating involves discovering the underlying motives of the group members and encouraging, acknowledging, and appreciating the efforts of individuals and the group as a whole. The task of managing involves using systematic processes to plan and make decisions that will move the group closer to the established goals. Clarifying goals and values, and motivating group members will help in the next task which is "achieving a workable unity" (Gardner, 1989, p. 386). Group unity relies on respect, trust, and loyalty of the group members to the group's mission and goals. Facilitating discussion and sharing will enhance the understanding and respect between individual members and foster valuing of the group mission.

Another leadership task identified by Gardner (1989) involves explaining. Providing explanations and the rationale for certain procedures and policies, and helping group members see the big picture can help avert conflicts and help maintain a cohesive work group. Through many of the previous leadership tasks, the leader also engages in symbolic behaviors such as becoming a central source of group unity and providing continuity. The leader also assumes the task of being the identified group representative who is able to advocate for the group and speak to others about the group's mission and goals. The final task Gardner describes is "renewing," which involves sharing information and power, building the confidence of followers in their

BOX 6-5   Leadership Tasks
1. Envisioning goals
2. Affirming values
3. Motivating
4. Managing
5. Achieving a workable unity
6. Explaining
7. Serving as a symbol
8. Representing the group
9. Renewing
Data from Gardner, J. W. (1989). *On leadership*. New York: Free Press.

own ability to achieve goals through their own efforts, resolving conflicts, and removing barriers that are inhibiting the individual's expression of energy and talent. Gardner's leadership tasks provide general guidelines which are not discipline specific, and can be applied to leadership functions within the ANE's teaching, scholarship, and service activities.

Practices of Exemplary Leadership

Kouzes and Posner developed a leadership model that outlines five practices of exemplary leadership (2002). The model describes processes faculty can use to facilitate change in the organization or in the classroom (Box 6-6). The first stage is called "model the way," which involves establishing relationships where students can observe and interact with faculty, preceptors, and nurse leaders who are excellent role models (p. 156). Leaders who "model the way" need to invest time in sharing information, reviewing the student's goals, and providing opportunities for the student to gain experiences that will facilitate goal achievement. During this process, the leader also guides students to appreciate theory and correlate theory to the situation by using questioning.

The second practice of exemplary leadership involves "inspiring a shared vision" (Kouzes & Posner, 2002, p. 157). This is characterized by a desire to do something significant and set far-reaching but attainable goals. The third practice is called "chal-

> **BOX 6-6   Practices of Exemplary Leadership**
>
> 1. Model the way
>
> 2. Inspire a shared vision
>
> 3. Challenge the process
>
> 4. Enable others to act
>
> 5. Encourage the heart
>
> Data from Kouzes, J. M., & Posner, B. Z. (2002). *The leadership challenge.* San Francisco: Jossey-Bass, (p. 14).

lenge the process" which involves fostering an attitude of fun, excitement, and determination. Kouzes and Posner describe the fourth process as "enabling others to act," which involves collaboration, sharing information, listening, and trusting others to carry out their responsibilities. Cardin and McNeese-Smith (2005) support the process of enabling others to act. They note that "effective leaders invoke a strong sense of sharing, creation, and responsibility and are skillful at building a climate of trust, facilitating positive interdependence, and supporting face-to-face interactions" (p. 159). These characteristics demonstrate the exemplary practice of "enabling others to act."

The final exemplary practice of Kouzes' and Posner's leadership model is called "encourage the heart," which involves recognition of participants and their contributions (2002, p. 21–22). Integral to this practice is the establishment of clear and high standards and expectations, and providing formal acknowledgement and recognition of each individual's contributions. Cardin and McNeese-Smith (2005) describe the application of Kouzes and Posner's five exemplary practices of leadership in a graduate nursing administration program. They used the five practices to guide development of course content, assignments, and most importantly to guide the interactions between faculty, preceptor, and student as they engaged in leadership activities. In addition to using the five practices to guide curriculum and teaching approaches, Cardin and McNeese-Smith note that the framework may be useful when the ANE serves in leadership roles with students, colleagues, and community members.

AONE Competencies for Nurse Leaders

The American Organization of Nurse Executives (AONE) recently revised the competencies deemed relevant to the leadership practice of nurse executives. These competencies are easily applicable to leadership practices inherent in the ANE's role as leader. The AONE competencies include: (1) communication and relationship build-ing, (2) knowledge of the healthcare environment, (3) leadership, (4) professionalism, and (5) business skills (AONE, 2005). The communication and relationship-building competency involves the ability to work with diverse groups, to communicate and in-teract effectively, to influence others, manage relationships, and carry out shared decision-making. The ANE demonstrates these behaviors through interactions with students and colleagues, and preceptors from diverse clinical settings. Knowledge of the healthcare environment is also an essential competency for nursing leaders. For the ANE, knowledge of clinical practice and the healthcare environment is needed for addressing teaching, research, and/or service responsibilities.

Leadership is the third competency, which is viewed as central and related to all other competencies. The AONE has delineated five attributes of leadership, includ-ing: (1) foundational thinking skills, (2) systems thinking, (3) succession planning, (4) change management, and (5) personal journey disciplines (AONE, 2005). Foun-dational thinking skills include consideration of diverse perspectives, visionary and reflective thinking, decision making skills, and intellectual curiosity. Systems thinking requires the ability to "synthesize and integrate diverse viewpoints for the good of the organization" (p. 54), and view the impact of change on not only on the institution but on the healthcare and educational systems. Succession planning is concerned with promoting and developing leadership of others through mentoring, identifying issues within the institution related to succession planning, and establishing a plan to deal with issues related to succession. The change management component involves using change theory to recognize reactions to change and adapt one's change management style to the needs of the situation. The term personal journey disciplines is concerned with the change agent's inward dialog and journey through the change process. En-gaging in self-assessment, learning from experiences and feedback, identifying per-sonal learning needs, and engaging in life-long learning are some of the ways the ANE can develop in the area of personal journey disciplines.

The competency of professionalism is delineated by six attributes: (1) personal and professional accountability, (2) career planning, (3) ethics, (4) evidence-based clinical and management practices, (5) advocacy, and (6) membership in professional organizations (AONE, 2005). Leaders demonstrating personal and professional ac-countability create an environment that allows team members to set expectations and produce results. The leader takes responsibility for his or her actions, and fosters an environment where team members also assume responsibility for their own actions. The career planning component involves encouraging and coaching others in devel-oping a career plan and evaluating one's progress. The ethics component involves set-ting high standards and creating an environment where upholding high standards is an expectation. Advocacy involves role modeling and ensuring that team members are actively involved in decisions affecting their work and that the goals of the group are being supported. The final component of professionalism involves maintaining active membership in professional organizations and encouraging similar expectations of team members.

The fifth competency of a nurse leader involves acquiring and using business skills such as: (1) financial management, (2) human resources, (3) strategic management, (4) marketing, and (5) information management and technology. Financial management involves using accounting principles, analyzing budgets, and financial statements. Human resource management involves supporting and managing personnel and the environmental conditions that facilitate safe and effective work by employees. The ability to develop goals and strategies to meet the mission of the institution and evaluate achievement are essential components of strategic management.

The first four competencies can be easily translated to the daily functions of the ANE. For example, the nurse educator needs to be able to communicate effectively and establish relationships in the classroom, clinical setting, and within academic governance committees (AONE competency # 1). The ANE also needs knowledge of the healthcare environment (AONE competency # 2), as this is where students will apply the knowledge and skills they acquire in their nursing program. Knowledge of the healthcare environment enables the ANE to provide effective, relevant, and timely educational experiences for nursing students. The ANE also demonstrates leadership skills in day-to-day classroom management, clinical interactions, and in faculty governance responsibilities. The fourth competency—professionalism—is modeled by the ANE who uses evidence-based knowledge and demonstrates an interest in the profession through active membership and involvement in organizations. The fifth competency of business skills is primarily applicable to the ANE who assumes an administrative position, such as dean or program director. However, at various points in time, faculty in nonadministrative positions may need business skills when administering a grant, marketing a project or program, or serving on an institutional or professional committee that oversees budgetary issues. The AONE concurs and notes that, "While all nursing leaders share these competency domains, the emphasis on particular competencies will be different depending on the leader's specific position in the organization" (AONE, 2005, para. 6).

Leadership Development

Leadership is an essential characteristic of the professional nurse and of the ANE who prepares students for nursing practice. Despite the importance of leadership to the progress and development of the nursing profession, there has been little documented research on what contributes to the development of the leadership role in nursing (Whitehead, Fletcher, & Davis, 2008). In reviewing the research on teacher leadership in middle and high schools, Whitehead *et al.* found that the school culture, climate, and opportunities for professional development enhanced teacher leadership. However, they found a lack of research on leadership development in teachers and were unable to find a leadership development theory specific to nursing faculty.

Attributes of Nurse Leaders

Regardless of the type of leadership style, philosophy, or theoretical approach adhered to, there appears be a core of attributes that are common to nursing leaders. Houser & Player (2004) interviewed twelve nationally known nurse leaders to determine a set of positive common traits (Box 6-7).

A grounded theory study of 10 informal leaders in nursing education revealed five themes (Whitehead *et al.*, 2008). Passion was the primary attribute found in all nursing education leaders. Passion was demonstrated by enthusiasm, drive, and commitment, and served to motivate and stimulate others. As important as passion is to leadership development, Whitehead *et al.* noted that passion was not deliberately developed in these nurse leaders, it simply existed.

BOX 6-7   Common Attributes of Nurse Leaders

1. Thoughtful
2. Responsive
3. Committed
4. Creative
5. Resilient
6. Visionary
7. Scholarly
8. Courageous
9. Innovative

Data from Houser, B. P., & Player, K. N. (2004). *Pivotal moments in nursing: Leaders who changed the path of a profession.* Indianapolis, IN: Sigma Theta Tau International.

Four additional attributes of informal nursing education leaders included factors that could be developed or enhanced such as self, foundation, atmosphere, and background (Whitehead *et al.*, 2008). Self includes the person's abilities as well as confidence in those abilities, such as interpersonal skills, listening, compromising when necessary, and being innovative. Another theme important in faculty leadership is the concept of "foundation." The informal leaders in nursing education reported that acquiring education to prepare for leadership was important; others commented that a lack of education had been a limitation for developing the leadership role (p. 283). Not only was formal educational preparation beneficial for many of the leaders, the individual's background and experiences also contributed to leadership development. Previous managerial and leadership experiences in clinical nursing practice were sited as beneficial. The final theme reflects the importance of "atmosphere" or the context in which one works. The encouragement provided through mentors, the support and confidence displayed by others, and the provision of resources, were important in developing leadership.

The study by Whitehead *et al.* (2008) represents the initial formation of a theory of faculty leadership development. Of the five themes identified by the researchers, four are factors that are developmental in nature and can be enhanced through education and experience. For example, "elements of self, such as critical reflection, leadership style, communication skills, and networking ability can be developed. Foundational knowledge can be enhanced through lifelong learning" (p. 284). The ANE can apply these concepts by seeking formal education in leadership development, seeking leadership experiences that provide gradual exposure to increasingly demanding leadership opportunities, and by seeking mentors, resources, and colleagues to create a supportive atmosphere for leadership development (Whitehead *et al.*, 2008).

Leadership Development Initiatives

Several programs for development of nursing faculty leadership have been implemented, including the Leadership Enhancement and Development (LEAD) Program, Maternal Child Health Leadership competencies, practice/academic partnerships, and the American Council on Education (ACE) Fellowship Program. Highlights of these initiatives are reviewed in this section.

Leadership Enhancement and Development Program

The LEAD project is a literature-based model developed and piloted by Bessent and Fleming (2003) to enhance and develop the leadership of minority nurses in educational settings. The model is based on six key elements: (1) knowledge of self,

(2) integrity, (3) vision, (4) communication, (5) collaboration, and (6) commitment to excellence (Box 6-8). The model served as a framework for Fellows in the LEAD program. LEAD Fellows attended quarterly seminars and were paired with and mentored by established nurse leaders. The mentors guided participants in exploring and developing knowledge and skills in key elements described in Box 6-8. LEAD Fellows were encouraged and supported in the process of applying the LEAD elements to the implementation of a change project in their home institution.

Abdur-Rahman (2007), a former LEAD Fellow, chronicled the application of knowledge and skills acquired during the LEAD program to the redesign of the undergraduate nursing curriculum at her home institution. Although the LEAD program was initially designed for minority nursing leadership development, the six elements represent a framework that could be useful for any ANE who wishes to develop a more solid leadership foundation through informal study and reflection on the LEAD elements.

Maternal Child Health Leadership Model

Maternal child health (MCH) professionals have articulated a set of core and applied competencies that serve as a model for leaders in MCH (Mouradian & Huebner, 2007). The core competencies reflect personal attributes (communication skills, critical thinking, self-reflection, and ethics/professionalism), which are believed to be "in-

---

BOX 6-8   Elements of the Leadership Enhancement and Development Model

1. Knowledge of self: Refers to insight into and confidence in one's abilities

2. Integrity: Involves taking responsibility, following through, keeping one's word

3. Vision: "ability to inspire, empower, challenge, and provoke through confidence" (p. 258)

4. Communication: Giving and receiving of information and feedback; listening, speaking, clarifying, and resolving conflicts

5. Collaboration: Functioning from a shared power base with others to address the needs and outcomes of the program

6. Commitment to Excellence: Motivation to incorporate an innovation within an institution or program, influenced by the alignment of the innovation with the institution/program visions and goals

Data from Bessent, H., & Fleming, J. W. (2003). The leadership enhancement and development (LEAD) project for minority nurses (in the new millennium model). *Nursing Outlook, 41*(6), 258–259.

fluenced by early experiences and reinforced by later experiences and opportunities" (p. 213). Although the core competencies represent preexisting characteristics and skills, they may be enhanced with specific training. The MCH Leadership Model involves "the practical application of one or more core competencies to complex situations and tasks faced by MCH leaders" (p. 213). The competencies can be acquired through formal education programs in mentoring, cultural competency, negotiation, conflict resolution, constituency building, management, and through the use and translation of evidence-based knowledge.

To utilize the MCH model, Mouradian & Huebner (2007) encourage self-assessment of knowledge and skills in each of the core and applied competencies. The ANE can use reflective journaling and formal and informal feedback mechanisms to provide assessment data. The model may also be used in teaching by providing students with information about the core competencies and providing opportunities for further exploration and study. The development of the MCH competencies in nursing graduates could then be monitored through alumni surveys or other assessment mechanisms.

Practice-Academic Partnerships

Throughout this section the reader may have noticed a divide between leadership in clinical practice and academics. According to Donaldson and Fralic (2000), the ANE is no longer fully immersed in what is happening clinically, and clinical nurses are not closely involved with trends and issues in nursing education. Various mechanisms have been instituted to close the gap and provide each party with an accurate and current perspective. Joint appointments between hospitals and universities, which are common in the medical profession, have been instituted by many nursing programs that are affiliated with large universities and medical centers. A nursing faculty with a joint appointment fulfills both a teaching role in the academic institution and a clinical or administrative role in the clinical agency, thus providing a person who is informed of issues and practices relevant to both academia and health care.

Another approach to creating practice and academic partnerships is the development of a joint institution. Donaldson and Fralic (2000) describe the development of a joint institution used to link the educational and clinical components at Johns Hopkins University School of Nursing and Johns Hopkins Hospital Department of Nursing. The process involved exploring potential partnerships with a selected facility, discussing the possibility of developing cooperative activities, exploring mutual goals, identifying needs, and negotiating arrangements for each facility to help meet the needs of the partner facility. Visit the Web site for the Institute for Johns Hopkins Nursing to find out more about the joint initiative.

ACE Fellows Program

The American Council on Education provides a higher education leadership development program open to professionals of all academic disciplines, referred to as the ACE Fellowship. The fellowship provides on the job experience, mentoring, and formal education in leadership for senior faculty and administrators. Each fellow designs an individualized learning plan for the year, attends educational conferences, and works with a mentor at another institution to gain experience. Since its inception in 1965, more than 1500 higher education leaders have participated in the ACE Fellows Program (ACE Fellows Program, 2009). After completion of the formal fellowship program, the fellows remain active and connected through a variety of initiatives including mentoring, nominating applicants, and ongoing professional development. Further information is available from the ACE Web site listed in the resource section.

Organizational Change

Changes in teaching and learning seem to parallel the rapid changes occurring in health care and technology. This creates an educational system faced with numerous demands, expectations, and stimuli for change. Porter-O'Grady identify the dilemma stating, "the question is no longer when will the educational framework for nursing learning change, but how fast?" (2001, p. 184). Changes in educational values, how teaching is conducted, and changes in the goals and outcomes of higher education are primary factors influencing how fast change occurs.

Porter-O'Grady (2001) identified several shifts that have implications for nursing education. Today greater emphasis is being placed upon facilitation of learning rather than merely providing learning opportunities. As a result, more emphasis is being placed upon evidence of achievement of competency (p. 184). Life-long learning is recognized as essential for profession practice, thus nursing faculty play a larger role in teaching the learner to learn. Rather than learning being instructor-controlled, today the trend in education is to give the student tools for independent, life-long learning.

Another change is the increasing complexity of health care and the need to provide care to people where they live. These changes have lead to a wider array of clinical sites and experiences being utilized than in the past. This in turn, leads to emphasis on developing "mobile rather than fixed skill sets" (Porter-O'Grady, 2001, p. 184). There also is more emphasis on interdisciplinary learning and the recognition that healthcare disciplines share a common core of knowledge. These changes in education along with changes in the content and context of learning combine to make the delivery of nursing education a challenge.

To effectively deal with change can be difficult. As with most types of change, awareness or recognition of the need to change is an essential first step. Phases of organizational change have been described as the letting go phase, the impasse phase, and the new beginning phase in which individuals experience a sense of renewal and risk taking (Iacovini, 1993). Change is inherently difficult because the process starts with the need to let go of old, familiar, and comfortable ways. Iacovini (1993) sees the lack of openness to change as based in fear, confusion, uncertainty, doubt, and or threats to self-esteem.

Whether the ANE is responsible for implementing a change or is in the midst of experiencing the phases of change, certain strategies can be helpful. Iacovini (1993) notes that dealing with negative emotional responses to change during the letting go phase can be handled by increasing the opportunities for informal interaction. Rather than focusing on the instability that is inherent in the change, look for areas where change is not dominant. As a leader in the change process, it is important for the ANE to acknowledge the difficulties encountered and offer visible support for those at varying levels of acceptance. To help individuals deal with uncertainty and fear, it is helpful to communicate information frequently and provide updates on the status of the change. During the impasse phase, individuals may experience frustration and resistance. Iacovini (1993) suggests using reflective strategies such as thinking about the past and reframing the vision for the future, reflecting on the current situation, encouraging creativity, and exploring new ideas. These strategies can help prevent individuals from becoming stuck in the impasse phase and facilitate movement toward the renewal phase.

During the renewal phase of organizational change individuals may experience new roles and begin practicing new ideas (Iacovini, 1993). According to Iacovini, "if the letting go and impasse (phases) have created positive memories, then employees are probably willing to embrace a continuous quality improvement concept" (1993, p. 68). No matter what phase of change is currently being experienced, identification of the phases of change can allow the ANE to select appropriate actions to help ease the transition.

Change Theories

When changes in curricular structure, content, or processes are initiated, a variety of factors may influence the change process and the ability to sustain the change. Understanding diverse theoretical perspectives can provide the ANE with a choice of frameworks for making informed decisions, implementing changes, and generating contingency plans. Several theoretical perspectives are discussed in this section, including Lewin's Change Process Model and Rogers' Diffusion of Innovations model. Key features of selected change theories are identified and suggestions for choosing a change theory are offered.

Lewin's Change Process Model

Kurt Lewin (1947, 1951) developed the change process model, which identifies three phases of change: unfreezing, changing, and refreezing. Lewin proposed that the progression through these phases is determined by analysis of the force field, or factors inhibiting and facilitating the change. In each phase of change, both inhibiting and facilitating influences are likely to be active. Therefore, the net effect of these forces is seen as an influencing factor.

In the unfreezing phase, the leader introduces ideas which will allow the organization to be ready for change. To determine actions that may be beneficial for the unfreezing process, a force field analysis is conducted. The forces (and strength of the forces) that support, as well as impede, the implementation of the change are identified. Once impeding forces have been identified, the leader may use research findings to disconfirm existing beliefs about the efficacy of the status quo. To further unfreeze the situation, the leader may strive to motivate individuals to change by offering statements about the rationale for the change. For example, using statements that indicate that the change will ensure that best practices are followed, or that the change will ensure that the best outcomes are achieved, may be beneficial. A final component of the unfreezing phase involves ensuring that mechanisms to provide psychological safety are in place for those involved in implementing the change. For example, phasing-in the introduction of the change to allow users time to become familiar with the change may be helpful. In addition, providing sufficient information about the implementation so that uncertainly and stress related to the implementation can be reduced is often beneficial.

The second phase of Lewin's theory is the change or implementation phase. It is important during this phase to anticipate some confusion, frustration, or resistance to the change and provide the group with a supportive environment for addressing these concerns. The leader creates a supportive environment by encouraging individuals to discuss feelings and problems related to the change, providing verbal support, feedback, and opportunities to experiment with the change.

The refreezing phase refers to using processes to help ensure that the change remains integrated into the organization. Clark (2009) suggests using strategies that will keep the change in forefront or keep "the change visible" to help sustain the change (p. 295). The leader can report on observed changes or outcomes using e-mail, letters, newsletters, annual reports, as well as informal verbal conversations. In addition, some changes will require periodic retraining workshops to keep group members informed and up-to-date. Incorporating the change into existing policies and procedures and providing ongoing education to enable implementation of the change also assists in the refreezing phase. Using Lewin's change Process Model requires the ANE to analyze the forces affecting the change and use the analysis to move through the phases of unfreezing, change, and refreezing.

Rogers' Diffusion of Innovation Theory

Rogers (2003) defines innovation as an "idea, practice, or object that is perceived as new" (p. 12). Diffusion is the process by which an innovation is communicated to individuals or groups over time and possibly adopted. Of course not all innovations are desirable and not all innovations should be adopted. Individuals will perceive the desirability of an innovation differently depending on several factors (Box 6-9). According to Rogers "Innovations that are perceived by individuals as having greater relative advantage, compatibility, trialability, observability, and less complexity, will be adopted more rapidly than other innovations" (p. 16).

Another component of the diffusion of innovation theory is the categories of adopters, which describe how readily and at what point in time individuals will likely adopt an innovation. Rogers identifies five categories of adopters: (1) the innovators, (2) early adopters, (3) early majority, (4) late majority, and (5) laggards (2003). Innovators are the first to adopt an innovation and tend to be individuals who can deal with higher levels of uncertainty about an innovation. Laggards on the other hand are the last to change or adopt an innovation. For the ANE who is considering institut-

---

BOX 6-9 Characteristics of Innovations that Influence Rate of Adoption

1. Relative advantage: The degree to which an innovation is perceive as an improvement

2. Compatibility: Congruence of the innovation with the values and needs of potential adopters

3. Complexity: The ease of understanding and using the innovation

4. Trialability: The ability to gradually adopt the innovation

5. Observability: The visibility of the results of the innovation to others

Data from Rogers, E. M. (2003). *Diffusion of innovations*. New York: Free Press. p. 15–16.

ing a change or innovation within the organization, identifying the types of adopters and examining the innovation in terms of relative advantage, compatibility, trialability, observability, and complexity may increase the likelihood of successful integration of the innovation.

Factors Influencing Sustainability of Change

Buchanan *et al.* (2005) surveyed the literature on sustaining organizational change and uncovered 11 factors that enhance sustainability (Table 6-3). Each of these factors has been identified by several authors as important in influencing sustainability. Evaluating the institution and situation for the presence of these factors can be helpful in enhancing sustainability. However, Buchanan *et al.* note that the weight or importance of these factors will vary with the institution and with the type of change being considered.

Advocating for Change

Advocacy refers to a process of influence and action that is directed toward achieving a change that will meet the goal or need of a program or specific group. Advocacy is a function of professional nursing that is incorporated into many nursing programs. Halpern (2002) explains that advocacy at the political or policy level is a natural extension of the patient care advocacy role of nurses. ANEs not only teach students about advocacy, they role model the patient care advocacy process. In addition, ANEs engage in political advocacy to achieve changes within the educational arena, the clinical setting, and within professional organizations. The focus in this section is on the broader concept of political advocacy, which encompasses patient, healthcare, and educational advocacy.

Much of the information on policy advocacy relative to nursing has been written from the healthcare provider perspective. However, ideas and processes related to healthcare advocacy can be easily adapted to educational practice. Taking the definition provided by Spenceley, Reutter, and Allen (2006), policy advocacy is defined as "knowledge-based action intended to improve health by influencing system-level decisions" (p. 184). They view involvement in policy change as a moral and ethical obligation. For ANEs, the definition of policy advocacy can be expanded to include knowledge-based action that may improve health indirectly by influencing nursing education policy and education outcomes.

A study of public health leaders' ability to influence policy development provides a foundation for identifying competencies, policy making knowledge, support systems, and barriers to effective policy development (Deschaine & Schaffer, 2003). The

TABLE 6-3   Factors Influencing Sustainability of Change

Factor Category	Description	Sources
Substantial	Degree of fit with the organization, the centrality of the change to the organization	Dawson (1994); Jacobs (2002); Pettigrew (1985); Rimmer, Macneil, Chenhall, Langfield-Smith, & Watts (1996)
Individual	Involves personal attributes such as knowledge, values, beliefs, skills	Dale *et al.* (1999); Jacobs (2002); Senge *et al.* (1999); Senge & Kaueffer (2000)
Managerial	Concerned with "style approach, preferences, behaviors" (Buchanan *et al.*, 2005, p. 201)	Dale *et al.* (1999); Dawson (1994); Kotter (1995); Pettigrew (1985); Rimmer *et al.* (1996); Senge *et al.* (1999); Senge & Kaueffer (2000)
Financial	Considers the cost benefit ratio of making or not making the change as planned	Rimmer *et al.* (1996)
Leadership	Defining the institution or program values, mission, and vision statements	Dale *et al.* (1999); Dawson (1994); Kotter (1995); Pettigrew (1985); Reisner (2002)
Organizational	Concerns the structure and function of the institutional system	Dale *et al.* (1999); Reisner (2002)
Cultural	The norms, values, and beliefs held by members of the group	Dale *et al.* (1999); Kotter (1995); Rimmer *et al.* (1996); Senge *et al.* (1999); Senge & Kaueffer (2000)
Political	Power and influence of individuals and groups	Dawson (1994); Kotter (1995); Pettigrew (1985); Rimmer *et al.* (1996)
Processual	Concerned with procedures and methods	Dale *et al.* (1999); Dawson (1994); Pettigrew (1985); Senge *et al.* (1999); Senge & Kaueffer (2000)
Contextual	Concerned with factors in the external and internal environment	Dale *et al.* (1999); Dawson (1994); Pettigrew (1985); Reisner (2002); Rimmer *et al.* (1996)
Temporal	Timing, pacing of change, and flow of events (Buchanan *et al.*, 2005, p. 201)	Dawson (1994); Kotter (1995); Pettigrew (1985); Rimmer *et al.* (1996)

Data from Buchanan, D., Fitzgerald, L., Ketley, D., Gollop, R., Jones, J., Lamont, S., Neath, A., & Whitby, E. (2005). No going back: A review of the literature on sustaining organizational change. *International Journal of Management Reviews, 7*(3), 189–205.

researchers used a model by Longest (2002) to develop interview questions and analyze interview responses for themes. According to Longest's model, individuals can become involved in the policy-making process by: (1) identifying issues that need to be dealt with, (2) helping to develop possible solutions, and (3) helping to create circumstances that will result in an action plan.

Research by Deschaine & Schaffer (2003) uncovered several barriers to participation in policy decision making, such as lack of skill and training in public policy, the need for leadership competency and education, and the inability to use research findings to support policy change. Each of these barriers can be alleviated through a variety of self-initiated means. The ANE can engage in self-study; obtain formal education in leadership, research, or policy development; or connect with a mentor who has the needed knowledge and skills. The researchers emphasize that understanding the factors that affect an individual's ability to participate in the policy-making process is essential for enhancing and strengthening the individual's policy-making role.

Advocacy Strategies

A variety of advocacy strategies are discussed by Galer-Unti, Tappe, & Lachenmayer (2004) including electioneering, direct lobbying, grassroots lobbying, media advocacy, acting as a resource person, and voting behavior (Box 6-10). They identify three levels of activities for each advocacy strategy that reflect good, better, and best actions in terms of advocacy impact. For example, a basic activity in electioneering is to contribute to campaigns of politicians who support causes of interest. More involved forms of electioneering may involve campaigning for an individual with congruent interests, or running for an elected office. Of course not everyone can engage in all forms of electioneering. According to Galer-Unti et al. (2004), some employees of government and nonprofit organizations may be prohibited from certain forms of electioneering.

For direct lobbying, Galer-Unti et al. (2004) identify good, better, and best activities ranging from contacting a policy maker, to meeting with a policy maker, to developing ongoing relationships with policy makers. Another advocacy strategy involves integrating grassroots lobbying into direct lobbying activities. Good, better, and best strategies for grassroots lobbying might include starting a petition drive related to a specific issue or policy, giving testimony at a policy making meeting, or creating a community coalition to stimulate specific policy changes.

For media advocacy, Galer-Unti and colleagues (2004) suggests writing a letter to the editor, writing an opinion editorial article, or developing and maintaining ongoing relationships with media personnel. Another advocacy strategy that involves the

---

BOX 6-10 Definitions of Advocacy Terms

- Electioneering: Influencing the outcome of an election through one's individual vote, campaigning for candidates, or running for an office

- Direct Lobbying: An individual attempts to influence the passage of specific legislation though contact with a political appointee

- Grassroots Lobbying: An attempt to influence a group to take action on a specific piece of legislation

- Media Advocacy: Use of interactions with the media to express opinion and inform the public

- Media Resource: Serve as a resource to print, radio, and television reporters on issues related to nursing, health care, or education

- Voting Behavior: Taking action to exercise one's personal right to vote or facilitate the voting behavior of others

Data from Galer-Unti, R. A., Tappe, M. K., & Lachenmayer, S. (2004). Advocacy 101. Getting started in health education advocacy. *Health Promotion Practice, 5*(3), 280.

---

media is to serve as a resource person. Many educational institutions maintain a list of faculty members who have expressed an interest or have expertise in specific topics. News reporters who contact the institution are then directed to contact individual faculty to obtain expert commentary on specific issues. The ANE who is interested in serving as media resource person can contact the public relations office of their institution or contact local media directly.

Empowerment Theory

A sense of empowerment is considered a desirable attribute that can facilitate the achievement of organizational goals. Individuals who feel empowered are "inspired and motivated to make meaningful contributions" . . . and they "have confidence that their contributions will be valued and recognized" (Larkin, Cierpial, Stack, Morrison, & Griffith, 2008, p. 2).

Kanter's Theory of Structural Empowerment (Kanter, 1993) identifies conditions that exist in institutions where individuals feel empowered (Box 6-11). First, individuals will have access to information that describes the context and history of the situation. Second, individuals will have access to resources necessary to achieve goals

---

BOX 6-11   Characteristics of Empowering Institutions

1. Access to information

2. Access to resources

3. Support for achieving goals

4. Opportunity to learn

5. Opportunity to develop skills

Data from Kanter, R. M. (1993). *Men and women of the corporation.* (2nd ed.). New York: Basic Books.

---

such as services and equipment. In addition, individuals in empowering institutions tend to receive support for exploring, monitoring, and achieving goals. And finally, empowered individuals have the opportunity to learn and develop their knowledge and skills.

The ANE can use Kanter's characteristics of empowered institutions as a framework for developing a greater sense of personal empowerment. Applying the framework requires the ANE to reflect on a situation to determine the specific needs and capabilities that may need to be developed. By seeking to learn about the history and context of the institution the ANE can obtain a broader awareness of factors which have contributed to the current environment. This awareness will allow the ANE to plan and implement changes more effectively. Empowered individuals also need to know what types of resources are needed and how they can be obtained. Finally, the ANE can take actions which will draw supportive individuals to the cause and help identify areas for further knowledge and skill development.

CONCLUSION

Leadership and change are interrelated and codependent processes. A key function of a leader is to use interpersonal skills to facilitate needed changes, and likewise, a change agent assumes a leadership role in the process of implementing change. The ANE assumes the roles of leader and change agent through a variety of teaching, scholarship, and service activities. Awareness of the phases of change and familiarity with a variety of leadership and change theories allows the ANE to anticipate issues and take informed actions to meet the needs of the community of interest.

SUMMARY

- Leadership and change are central processes for building and maintaining the structure and function of nursing education, advancing knowledge, and achieving goals and outcomes.
- Functioning as a change agent and leader is integral to the role functions of teaching, scholarship, and service.
- In the teaching role function, the ANE demonstrates serving as a change agent and leader through role modeling the patient care advocacy and political advocacy processes to achieve changes within the educational arena and clinical setting.
- In the scholarship role function, the ANE applies leadership knowledge and skills to plan and implement research studies and disseminate innovations.
- In the service role function, the ANE engages in advocacy for change within professional organizations, providing leadership in academic governance, and in professional and community organizations.
- Leadership theories have evolved from an emphasis on individual characteristics to relationships, to a focus on situational factors and outcomes (see Table 6-1).
- Hartley and Allison's leadership framework focuses on the concepts of person, position, and process.
- Servant Leadership is distinguished from other leadership theories by its emphasis on the leader's personal value system and the importance of the leader being of service.
- Creative Leadership calls for the leader to have knowledge of a broad range of leadership theories and selectively apply these to the situation.
- Six competency areas essential for creative leaders include technology master, problem solver, ambassador, change maker, communicator, and team player.
- Situational Leadership is a leadership style that addresses adapting to the variability in the situation (see Table 6-2).
- Belbin's Team Role Theory describes nine categorizes of roles that team members commonly assume. Individuals have three to four team role preferences which are not fixed and may change over time or with certain circumstances.
- Action Centered Leadership developed by Adair (1973), describes the action leaders need to take to be most effective (see Box 6-3).
- Chaos theory has encouraged researchers to look at the leadership processes from a much broader perspective that considers social and technical aspects.
- New Science Leadership Theory recognizes the influence of chaos theory and quantum theory on organizational systems.

- Leadership styles describe how leaders interact with others to accomplish goals.
- Leadership styles have been classified as authoritarian, democratic, and laissez-faire (see Moiden, 2002); or as affiliative, coaching, directive, pace-setting, participative, and visionary (see Kenmore, 2008).
- Tasks common to leadership include: (1) envisioning goals, (2) affirming values, (3) motivating team members, (4) managing, (5) achieving a workable unity, (6) explaining, (7) serving as a symbol, (8) representing the group, and (9) renewing.
- Five practices of exemplary leadership include the ability to: (1) model the way, (2) inspire a shared vision, (3) challenge the process, (4) enable others to act, and (5) encourage the heart.
- The American Organization of Nurse Executives has identified five competencies for nurse leaders: (1) communication and relationship building, (2) knowledge of healthcare environment, (3) leadership, (4) professionalism, and (5) business skills.
- Core attributes of formal nurse leaders include being thoughtful, responsive, committed, creative, resilient, visionary, scholarly, courageous, and innovative (see Houser and Player, 2004).
- Whitehead *et al.* (2008) present a theory of faculty leadership development that integrates "elements of self, such as critical reflection, leadership style, communication skills, and networking ability" (p. 284)
- Models for faculty leadership development include the Leadership Enhancement and Development (LEAD) Program, the Maternal Child Health Leadership competencies, practice-academic partnerships, and the ACE Fellowship Program.
- Changes in health care, educational technology, economics, demographics, and societal values serve as a stimulus for organizational change.
- As changes occur in society, the demands, stressors, relationships, and resources change and require organizational adaptation.
- Organizational change includes the phases of letting go, impasse, and new beginnings.
- Lewin's Change Process Model identifies three phases of change: unfreezing, changing, and refreezing.
- Unfreezing is the preparatory phase in which individuals are prepared for the change.
- The changing phase is the implementation phase.
- The refreezing phase involves using processes to help ensure that the change remains integrated into the organization.

- Using Lewin's Change Process Model requires analysis of the forces affecting the change and using the analysis findings to move through the phases of unfreezing, change, and refreezing.
- Rogers' Diffusion of Innovation Theory describes factors important in adopting or failing to adopt an innovation.
- Factors that influence the rate of adoption of an innovation include the relative advantage, compatibility, complexity, trialability, and observability of the innovation.
- Factors that enhance sustainability of change are categorized as substantial, individual, managerial, financial, leadership, organizational, cultural, political, processual, contextual, and temporal (see Table 6-3).
- Advocacy refers to a process of influence and action that is directed toward achieving a change that will meet the goal or need of a program or group.
- The ANE may engage in advocacy within the educational arena, the clinical setting, or within professional and community organizations.
- Political advocacy strategies include electioneering, direct lobbying, grassroots lobbying, media advocacy, acting as a resource person, and voting behavior (see Box 6-10).
- A sense of empowerment can facilitate the change process and the achievement of organizational goals.
- Empowering institutions provide individuals with access to information and resources, opportunities to learn and develop needed skills, and support for achieving goals.
- Kanters's Theory of Structural Empowerment identifies characteristics of empowering institutions as having access to information and resources, providing support for achieving goals, and providing opportunities to learn and develop skills.

RECOMMENDED RESOURCES

- American Organization of Nurse Executives Web site at http://www.aone.org/ houses a resource section with information on advocacy, leadership, and position papers related to leadership and organizational issues.
- American Council on Education Web site houses information about the ACE Fellowship Program at http://www.acenet.edu/AM/Template.cfm?Section= Home.
- Helpful sources of information on Belbin's Team Roles theory including an introductory flash animation and text resources are available at http://www.belbin.com/.

- Learn more about Margaret Wheatley and her perspective on leadership and organizational change at http://www.margaretwheatley.com/index.html. Full text articles and podcasts on a variety of leadership, change, and organizational topics are available.
- To learn more about John Adair and Action Centered Leadership theory visit http://www.johnadair.co.uk/.
- Greenleaf Centers for Servant Leadership are located in eleven countries. Obtain a free information packet about servant leadership from http://www.greenleaf.org/.
- For information on Situational Leadership Theory visit The Center for Leadership Studies—Home of Situational Leadership, founded by Hersey at http://www.situational.com/.

REFERENCES

1. Abdur-Rahman, V. (2007). My journey through project LEAD. *ABNF Journal, 18*(3), 83–87.
2. Adair, J. (1973). *Action centred leadership*. London: McGraw-Hill.
3. American Council on Education. (2009). *ACE fellows program*. Retrieved January 16, 2009 from http://www.acenet.edu/Content/NavigationMenu/ProgramsServices/FellowsProgram/index.htm.
4. AONE 2004 Education Committee. (2005). American organization of nurse executives (AONE) competencies. Retrieved January 2, 2009 from http://www.aone.org/aone/pdf/February%20Nurse%20Leader—final%20draft—for%20web.pdf.
5. Bass, B. (1985). *Leadership and performance beyond expectations*. New York: Free Press.
6. Bass. B. (1990, Winter). From transitional to transformational leadership: Learning to share the vision. *Organizational Dynamics,*140–148.
7. Belbin, M. R., (1993). *Team roles at work*. Oxford: Butterworth-Heinemann, Ltd.
8. Belbin, M.R. (2009). *Belbin team role theory*. Retrieved April 20, 2009 from http://www.belbin.com/rte.asp?id=8.
9. Bessent, H., & Fleming, J. W. (2003). The leadership enhancement and development (LEAD) project for minority nurses (in the new millennium model). *Nursing Outlook, 41*(6), 255–260.
10. Blake, R. R., & McCanse, A. A. (1991). *Leadership dilemmas-grid solutions*. Houston, TX: Gulf Publishing.
11. Blake, R. R., & Mouton, J. S. (1985). *The managerial grid III*. Houston, TX: Gulf Publishing.
12. Blau, P. M. (1964). *Exchange and power in social life*. New York: Wiley.
13. Bolman, L. G., & Deal, T. E. (2003). *Reframing organizations: Artistry, choice, and leadership*. New York: Wiley.
14. Buchanan, D., Fitzgerald, L., Ketley, D., Gollop, R., Jones, J., Lamont, S., Neath, A., & Whitby, E. (2005). No going back: A review of the literature on sustaining organizational change. *International Journal of Management Reviews, 7*(3), 189–205.
15. Burns, J. M. (1978). *Leadership*. New York: Harper Row
16. Cardin, S., & McNeese-Smith, D. (2005). A model for bridging the gap: From theory to practice reality. *Nursing Administration Quarterly, 29*(2), 154–161.

17. Chelladurai, P., & Saleh, S. D. (1978). Preferred leadership in sports. *Canadian Journal of Applied Sciences, 3,* 85–92.

18. Chonko, L. B. (2007). A philosophy of teaching . . . and more. *Journal of Marketing Education, 29,* 111–121.

19. Clark, C. (2009*). Creative nursing leadership and management.* Sudbury, MA: Jones and Bartlett.

20. Dale, B., Boaden, R. J., Wilcox, M., & McQuater, R.E. (1999). Sustaining continuous improvement: What are the key issues? *Quality Engineering, 11,* 369–377.

21. Dawson, P. (1994). *Organizational change: A processual approach.* London: Paul Chapman.

22. Deschaine, J. E., & Schaffer, M. A. (2003). Strengthening the role of public health nursing leaders in policy development. *Policy, Politics, & Nursing Practice, 4,* 266–274.

23. Donaldson, S., & Fralic, M. (2000). Forging today's practice-academic link: A new era for nursing leadership. *Nursing Administration Quarterly, 25*(1), 95–101.

24. Doyle, R. M. (2004). Applying new science leadership theory in planning an international nursing student practice experience in Nepal. *Journal of Nursing Education, 43*(9), 426–429.

25. Eddy, P. L., & Vanderlinden, K, E. (2006). Emerging definitions of leadership in higher education. *Community College Review, 34*(1), 20.

26. Fiedler, F. E. (1996, June). Research on leadership and training: One view of the future. *Administrative Science Quarterly, 41(2),* 241–250.

27. Galer-Unti, R. A., Tappe, M. K., & Lachenmayer, S. (2004). Advocacy 101. Getting started in health education advocacy. *Health Promotion Practice, 5*(3), 280–288.

28. Gardner, J. W. (1989). *On leadership.* New York: Free Press.

29. Gosling, B., Marturano, J., & Dennison, P. (2003). *A review of leadership theory and competency frameworks.* United Kingdom: Centre for Leadership Studies University of Exeter.

30. Greenleaf, R. K. (1977). *Servant leadership: A journey into the nature of legitimate power and greatness.* New York: Paulist Press.

31. Gronn, P. (2000). Distributed properties: A new architecture for leadership. *Educational Management and Administration, 28*(3), 317–338.

32. Grossman, S., & Valiga, T. (2009). *The new leadership challenge: Creating the future of nursing.* (3rd Ed.). Philadelphia: F.A. Davis.

33. Halpern, I. M. (2002). Reflections of a health policy advocate: The natural extension of nursing activities. *Oncology Nursing Forum, 29*(9), 1261–1263.

34. Hartley, J., & Allison, M. (2002). The role of leadership in the modernisation and improvement of public services. In J. Reynolds, I. Henderson, J. Seden, J. Chariesworth, & A. Bullman (Eds.), *The managing care reader,* Buckingham: Open University Press.

35. Heifetz, R. A. (1994). *Leadership without easy answers.* Cambridge, Mass: The Belknap Press of Harvard Press.

36. Hersey, P., & Blanchard, K. H. (1993). *Management of organizational behavior.* Englewood Cliffs, NJ: Prentice-Hall.

37. House, R. J. (1971, September). A path-goal theory of leadership effectiveness. *Administrative Science Quarterly, 16,* 321–328.

38. Houser, B. P., & Player, K. N. (2004). *Pivotal moments in nursing: Leaders who changed the path of a profession.* Indianapolis, IN: Sigma Theta Tau International.

39. Iacovini, J. (1993). The human side of organization change. *Training and Development, 47*(1), 65–68.

40. Jacobs, R. L. (2002). Institutionalizing organizational change through cascade training. *Journal of European Industrial Training*, *26*(2/3/4), 177–172.

41. Kanter, R. M. (1993). *Men and women of the corporation*. (2nd ed.). New York: Basic Books.

42. Keirsey, D. (1998). *Please understand me II: Temperament, character, intelligence*. Delmar, CA: Prometheus Nemesis Book Company.

43. Kenmore, P. (2008). Exploring leadership styles. *Nursing Management-UK*, *15*(1), 24–26.

44. Kezar, A., Carducci, R., & Contreras-McGavin, M. (2006). Rethinking the "L" word in higher education: The revolution of research on leadership. *ASHE Higher Education Report*, *31*(6), 31–70.

45. Kotter, J. P. (1995). Leading change: Why transformation efforts fail. *Harvard Business Review*, *73*(2), 59–67.

46. Kouzes, J. M., & Posner, B.Z. (2002). *The leadership challenge*. San Francisco: Jossey-Bass.

47. Larkin, M. E., Cierpial, C. L. Stack, J. M., Morrison, V. J., & Griffith, C. A. (2008). Empowerment theory in action: The wisdom of collaborative governance. *Online Journal of Issues in Nursing*, *13*(2), 10.

48. Lewin, K. (1947). Group decision and social change. In T. M. Newcomb, & E. L. Hartley (Eds.), *Readings in Social Psychology* (pp. 340–44). New York: Henry Holt and Co.

49. Lewin, K. (1951). *Field theory in social science: Selected theoretical papers*. New York: Harper & Row.

50. Longest, B. B. (2002). *Health policymaking in the United States*. Chicago: Health Administration Press.

51. McGregor, D. (1960). *The human side of enterprise*. New York: McGraw-Hill.

52. Moiden, N. (2002). Evolution of leadership in nursing. *Nursing Management-UK*, *9*(7), 20–25.

53. Mouradian, W., & Huebner, C. (2007). Future directions in leadership training of MCH professionals: Cross-cutting MCH leadership competencies. *Maternal Child Health Journal*, *11*, 211–218.

54. Northouse, P. G. (1997). *Leadership: Theory and practice*. San Francisco: Sage.

55. Peterson, M. (1997). Using contextual planning to transform institutions. In M. Peterson, D. Dill, L. A. Mets, & Associates (Eds.), *Planning and management for a changing environment*, (pp. 127–157). San Francisco: Jossey Bass.

56. Pettigrew, A.M. (1985). *The awakening giant: Continuity and change in ICI*. Oxford: Basil Blackwell.

57. Porter-O'Grady, T. (2001). Profound change: Twenty-first century nursing. *Nursing Outlook*, *49*(4), 182–186.

58. Reisner, R. A. F. (2002). When a turnaround stalls. *Harvard Business Review*, *80*(2), 45–52.

59. Rennaker, M. (2005). *Servant leadership: A chaotic leadership theory*. Servant Leadership Research Roundtable. School of Leadership Studies, Regent University. Retrieved September 20, 2008 at http://www.regent.edu/acad/global/publications/sl_proceedings/2005/rennaker_servant.pdf.

60. Rimmer, M., Macneil, J., Chenhall, R., Langfield-Smith, K., & Watts, L. (1996). *Reinventing competitiveness: Achieving best practice in Australia*. South Melbourne, Australia: Pitman.

61. Rogers, E. M. (2003). *Diffusion of innovations*. New York: Free Press.

62. Schein, E. H. (1992). *Organizational culture and leadership*. New York: John Wiley and Sons.

63. Senge, P., & Kaeufer, K. H. (2000). Creating change. *Executive Focus*, *17*, 4–5.

64. Senge, P., Kleiner, A., Roberts, C., Ross, R., Roth, G. & Smith, B. (1999). *The dance of change: The challenges of sustaining momentum in learning organizations*. London: Nicholas Brealey.

65. Society for Chaos Theory in Psychology and Life Sciences. (2009). Chaos and complexity resources for students and teachers. Retrieved July 14, 2009 from http://www.societyforchaostheory.org/.

66. Spears, L. C. (Ed.). (1998). *Insights on leadership: Service, stewardship, spirit, and servant leadership.* New York: Wiley.

67. Spenceley, S. M., Reutter, L., & Allen, M. N. (2006). The road less traveled: Nursing advocacy at the policy level. *Policy, Politics, & Nursing Practice, 7*(3), 180–194.

68. Tannenbaum, R., & Schmidt, W. H. (1973, May/June). How to choose a leadership pattern. *Harvard Business Review, 51*(3), 162–180.

69. Taylor, V. (2007). Leadership for service improvement. *Nursing Management-UK, 13*(9), 30–34.

70. Wheatley, M. (1992). *Leadership and the new science: Learning about organization from an orderly universe.* San Francisco: Berrett-Koehler.

71. Wheatley, M. (2006). *Leadership and the new science: Discovering order in a chaotic world.* San Francisco: Barrett-Koehler.

72. Wheatley, M., & Kellner-Rogers, M. (1996). *A simpler way.* San Francisco: Berrett-Koehler.

73. Whitehead, D., Fletcher, M., & Davis, J. (2008). Determination of how nurse educators successfully transition to leadership in nursing education. In M. Oermann (Ed.), *Annual review of nursing education, Vol 6, 2008. Clinical nursing education.* (pp. 271–285). New York: Springer Publishing.

CHAPTER 7

Pursue Continuous Quality Improvement in the Nurse Educator Role—Competency 6

OBJECTIVES

1. Identify theoretical perspectives and evidence-based practices for mentoring faculty colleagues.
2. Explore effective strategies for promoting socialization to the faculty role and continuous quality improvement as an ANE.
3. Examine issues and processes affecting the design and implementation of policies and procedures relevant to the educational environment.
4. Explore factors that impact the ANE's functioning in the areas of teaching, scholarship, and service.
5. Discover strategies to develop effective teaching, scholarship, and service practices in education.
6. Identify theoretical and evidence-based practices to elicit and utilize feedback and self-evaluation findings to enhance educational practice.

KEY TERMS

Benchmark
Benchmarking
Competitive benchmarking
Continuous quality improvement
Criteria
Evidence-based education
Evidence-based practice
Faculty development
Faculty evaluation triad
Generic benchmarking

Internal benchmarking
Longitudinal benchmarking
Mentoring
Objective-based education
Peer evaluation
Policy
Standards
Self-evaluation
Self-reflection
Teaching portfolio

DEFINITION AND DESCRIPTION OF COMPETENCY

Rapid changes in healthcare delivery, teaching strategies, and learning systems demand that ANEs focus on attaining and maintaining knowledge and skills related to both subject matter and teaching. The overall process of attaining and maintaining needed knowledge and skills is referred to as continuous quality improvement or CQI.

The National League for Nursing (NLN) Task Group on Nurse Educator Competencies (2005) describes the attributes of competency six using eight task statements. The task statements relate to obtaining and using feedback about one's teaching and role performance from multiple sources. Feedback is then used to determine areas in which additional knowledge and skills are needed. CQI is achieved through professional development activities and life-long learning. Quality improvement is also enhanced by engaging in mentoring and policy development activities that enhance functioning in the ANE role.

THEORY AND RESEARCH RELATED TO COMPETENCY

CQI, benchmarking, and total quality management reflect processes and programs instituted to attain and monitor the achievement of outcomes. Ensuring outcomes are met is essential for promoting quality. In this section several topics are explored, including the Total Quality Management Model and the Hallmarks of Excellence in Nursing Education, which can be used to guide quality improvement efforts. In addition, specific processes the ANE can use on a regular, ongoing basis to enhance the CQI process, such as professional development activities and using feedback from peer, student, and self-evaluation, will be reviewed. Concepts such as benchmarking, evidence-based education, and mentoring are also important vehicles for enhancing quality and role performance as an ANE. Educational policies provide structures and mechanisms that support quality improvement. Therefore, the ANE's role in educational policy development is also explored.

Total Quality Management

Total quality management (TQM) is a model used in business and other organizations to explore key issues involved in sustaining change. A central principle of TQM is that individuals within an organization should "listen to those whom they serve, (and) continually evaluate how well they are responding to the needs of their constituencies" (de Jager & Nieuwenhuis, 2005, p. 253). For the ANE this means listening to the needs of students and community partners and gathering evaluation data from these sources. TQM includes five sustaining factors and nine key elements that are considered when implementing a quality improvement project (Box 7-1). The sustaining factors represent broad organizational factors that can influence quality improvement efforts within the institution. These sustaining factors may also have a direct influence on the ANE's personal efforts in CQI. The key elements represent action oriented concepts that can be explored on a smaller scale by individuals within the institution. The TQM model provides a comprehensive framework that can be used to guide quality improvement efforts on an individual or institutional level.

BOX 7-1   Attributes of total Quality Management

Sustaining Factors:

- Environment (internal and external)

- Management style

- Policies

- Organizational structure

- Process of change

Key Elements:

- Commitment

- Leadership

- Planning/organization

- Applying tools /techniques

- Education

- Involvement

- Teamwork

- Measurement and feedback

- Cultural change

Data From Dale, B. G., Boaden, R. J., Wilcox, M., & McQuater, R. E. (1999). Sustaining continuous improvement: What are the key issues? *Quality Engineering, 11*(3), 369–377.

Authors de Jager & Nieuwenhuis state, "Although TQM was developed within the manufacturing environment, the benefits are equally applicable to service entities such as higher education institutions" (2005, p. 254). They correlated key concepts of TQM (i.e., leadership, scientific methods and tools, and problem solving through team work) to the concepts of objectives-based education (OBE). Both TQM and OBE emphasize the importance of meeting the needs of the consumer. In OBE, the emphasis is on active involvement of learners (who are the consumers) and on the achievement of learning outcomes.

According to de Jager & Nieuwenhuis (2005), leadership, scientific methods, and problem solving through team work interact to create the organizational climate and the education and training needed to provide meaningful data. Data can then be used to achieve the desired outcome of customer service. When these concepts are translated to academic education, the interaction between the TQM concepts produces standards, outcomes, and education and training that meets the learner's needs. Another similarity between TQM and OBE is the concern for moving the focus of control from outside the individual to within. The objective is to make those working within the institution "accountable for their own performance, and to get them to commit to attaining quality in a highly motivated fashion" (2005, p. 255).

Hallmarks of Excellence in Nursing Education

The NLN Task Group on Nursing Education Standards (2005) published a document outlining 30 hallmarks of excellence for nursing programs of all levels and types. These hallmarks of excellence refer to characteristics that indicate exceptional performance of an institution and of individuals within the institution. The hallmarks are categorized into 10 areas including: students, faculty, CQI, curriculum, teaching/learning and evaluation strategies, resources, innovation, educational research, environment, and leadership. The hallmarks provide guidance for faculty and administrators who seek to establish and maintain programs that perform at a high level. The CQI hallmark involves achieving accreditation from national nursing accrediting agencies and engaging in ongoing mechanisms that review program design, implementation, and evaluation. The NLN Hallmarks also recognize individual professional development as one of the hallmarks for faculty, noting specifically that "faculty model a commitment to lifelong learning, involvement in professional nursing associations, and nursing as a career" (para. 8). For more information and to access the Hallmarks of Excellence document please see the link in the resource section.

Benchmarking for Quality Improvement

Originating from a quality improvement approach used in industry, benchmarking involves identifying a point for comparison (i.e., benchmark) that reflects a best practice (Ellis, 2006, p. 378). "Benchmarks are the measure of a best practice; benchmarking is the process of identifying benchmarks and applying them for performance improvement" (Billings, 2007, p. 174). The process of benchmarking involves sharing successful program initiatives and learning from other's successes.

Billings (2007) defined four types of benchmarking as internal, competitive, generic, and longitudinal (p. 174). The process of internal benchmarking can be used to compare nursing with other academic departments in the same institution. Often internal benchmarking is used for promotion and tenure decisions, salary and equity, teaching evaluations, workload, and productivity. Competitive benchmarking is used when the goal is to improve outcomes by determining benchmarks of successful competitors and learning from the process they used. Generic benchmarking is concerned with processes and practices used by similar institutions. Typically the focus is on practices of comparable institutions that directly impact learning outcomes such as NCLEX preparation, remediation practices, and subject-specific learning outcomes. The longitudinal benchmarking simply refers to monitoring benchmarks over time so that that long-term trends can be determined.

BOX 7-2   Steps in the Benchmarking Process

1. Identify the area of interest

2. Define the benchmarks

3. Determine the type of benchmarking process to use

4. Identify attributes of benchmarking peers

5. Gather benchmark data

6. Analyze the data

7. Use data for improvement

8. Evaluate the results

Data from Billings, D. (2007). Using benchmarking for continuous quality improvement in nursing education. In M. Oermann & K. Heinrich (Eds.), *Annual review of nursing education, volume 5, 2007*, (pp.173–180). NY: Springer Publishing.

Benchmarking uses a structured process that generally involves eight steps (Box 7-2). Billings (2007) points out that the steps outlined in the benchmarking process can be use for institutional, program, course, or faculty level quality improvement efforts. Individual faculty can use aggregate data collected by their home institution as benchmarks for aspects of teaching, scholarship, and service. For example, aggregated student evaluation data can be used as a benchmark for teaching, or data concerning the number of grants and publications received by faculty of similar rank may serve as a benchmark for research productivity. To determine achievement in the service role, information on the number, type, and level of involvement in professional and academic service activities can be documented. Using benchmarks to assess processes, practices, and outcomes can provide comparative feedback that can guide the quality improvement process.

Professional Development Activities

Professional commitment to life-long learning is a common component of an institution's mission statement. Because of the changing nature of health care and education, life-long learning is especially valued in nursing education. It is important that the ANE seeks knowledge and skills to improve teaching practice and is able to model continuing professional development to their students. The American Nurse's Association (ANA, 1994) recognized the need for life-long learning as a necessary activity to maintain and increase the individual nurse's competence in nursing practice.

Researchers have explored a variety of aspects related to continuing education including nurses' attitudes and motivation toward continuing education (Thurston, 1992) and preferred methods of acquiring continuing education (Gessner & Armstrong, 1992; Hayes, Morin, Sylvia, & Bashford, 1995). The findings of two meta-analyses support the ability of continuing education to influence practice (O'Brien et al., 2001; Waddell, 1992). In a review of 32 studies, which included nearly 3000 subjects, O'Brien et al. (2001) found that interactive workshops with and without a didactic component produced a moderately large change in professional practice. In another review of 34 studies, analysis of the impact of continuing education on practice revealed an overall effect size of 0.73, indicating that participating in continuing education did have a positive influence on nursing practice (Waddell, 1992).

Despite the consensus that life-long learning and professional development are valuable and desirable for nurses, continuing education for nurses and ANEs is not mandated in all states. Yoder-Wise (1997) reported that only 20 states required continuing education for renewal of license. By 2007, the number of states requiring continuing education for licensure renewal increased to only 28 (The Journal of Continuing Education in Nursing, 2008).

Evidence-Based Education

Evidence-based practice has been strongly emphasized in nursing and healthcare literature as a necessary approach to ensure quality of care. Major drawbacks to fully implementing evidence-based knowledge in practice include a lack of time to uncover and review research, and lack of skill in applying the evidence-based process. One strategy to facilitate the use of current, high quality research findings comes from evidence-based education (EBE).

DePalma (2007) differentiates EBE from traditional educational sessions. One distinction is that in traditional educational sessions, references are provided at the end of the presentation. However, in EBE, references are provided directly next to the information on the slide or handout. This small change allows the learner to directly link content with the evidence-based source. This type of documentation allows the learner to easily access EBE recommendations at a later time and justify changes in practice, based on the documented evidence.

In addition to offering detailed reference citations supporting each piece of information, EBE presentations offer a summary of the best evidence, which is clearly documented in the handouts and slides for future reference. In EBE sessions, the presenter also provides a statement of the degree or strength of the evidence. Thus, at the end of the presentation, participants will be able to evaluate the strength and potential usefulness of the research.

Research supporting EBE is growing. DePalma (2007) cites a comparison study by Gruppen, Rana, & Arndt (2005) that used EBE and non-EBE approaches to teach medical students skills in effectively searching the literature. Students who attended the EBE session were able to conduct literature searches with fewer errors and the search results were determined to be of higher quality than those who did not attend the EBE session. Another study reviewed by DePalma compared prescribing practices of healthcare providers who attended an EBE session, a traditional educational session, and no educational session (Bernal-Delgado, Galeote-Major, Pradas-Arnal, & Peiro-Moreno, 2002). The providers who attended the EBE session showed greater changes in prescribing patterns when compared with those who received traditional education and no education.

Recommendations developed by participants at a national conference on continuing education in the heath professions also support the importance of EBE (Fletcher, 2008). "Participants generated a set of principles they believe should underlie and guide continuing education in the health professions" (p. 114). One of those principles calls for continuing education to be based on the strongest available evidence for practice. As consumers of continuing education programs, the ANE needs to be aware of EBE and seek continuing education offerings that use an EBE format, whenever possible. In addition, the ANE can begin using the EBE format when developing presentations, which will help establish the importance of EBP for current nursing students.

Utilizing Feedback

Utilizing feedback is an essential part of the CQI process. In academia, feedback may be obtained from self-reflection or self-evaluation, and peer and student evaluation of teaching. These sources of feedback are discussed in this section along with guidelines for conducting peer review.

Self-Reflection and Self-Evaluation

The processes of self-reflection and self-evaluation are essential skills for faculty to cultivate. Self-reflection is the process of looking inward to collect information about one's teaching practices. Reflection is a term used to describe a process of thinking about and analyzing a situation and reaching new understandings or insights. Self-reflection can enhance self-understanding and can provide useful guidance for professional development and continuing education. Self-evaluation is the process of judging the effectiveness of one's actions based on the data collected through self-reflection and external evaluators. Therefore, self-reflection provides a foundation for self-evaluation.

Self-reflection and self-evaluation both hinge on what Robbins (2001) calls "knowing what to look for" (p. 20). Robbins recommends that faculty develop the skill of self-observation while teaching by focusing on recognizing the barriers and motivators to learning (Table 7-1). Three easy-to-remember categories of self-observation include physical movements, visual support, and intellectual factors. Physical movements can range from distracting to enhancing mannerisms that emphasize key points and help the student stay focused on the message. Likewise, visual support can either contribute to confusion or add clarity. When providing effective instruction using visuals and text, the key goals are to clarify the content and make the material memorable. Often this means keeping the visuals uncluttered. The category of intellectual factors actually addresses several subcategories such as: organization and summary of the information, communication issues such as questioning students, digressing off the topic, and responding to student's questions.

TABLE 7-1 Categories of Self-Observation

Self-Observation Category	Barrier and Motivator Behaviors
Physical movement	Barrier—Distracting movements or nonsupportive gestures (pacing or nervous gestures)
	Motivator—Using movement to support what is being said or emphasize points
Visual support	Barrier—Visuals that are too small, or unclear, or too many
	Motivator—Visuals to illustrate and clarify key points
Intellectual factors	Barriers—Poor organization of content, posing ambiguous questions, digression of discussions
	Motivators—Clear summaries of key points, positive reinforcement for student questioning

Data from Robbins, L. (2001). Self-observation in teaching: What to look for. *Business Communication Quarterly, 64,* 19–37.

The ANE can gain insight into teaching performance and skills by recording and reviewing a teaching session, or having a colleague review a teaching session to look specifically for aspects that strengthen and diminish teaching effectiveness.

Research on Self-Reflection

Although self-reflection on the part of the ANE is valued, there is little theoretical or research support to describe effective reflection practices or substantiate how reflection influences professional development (Lockyer, Gondocz, & Thivierge, 2004: Lowe, Rappolt, Jaglal, & Macdonald, 2007). Furthermore, there is little research to establish whether healthcare professionals use reflection to integrate learning experiences into practice. However, one recent study by Lowe *et al.* (2007) did explore the use of reflection on learning and its application to practice. The researchers drew from a sample of thirty-three occupational therapists who attended a 3-day continuing education course and completed initial and follow-up surveys (i.e., the Self-Reflection and Insight Scale and the Commitment to Change Tool). From this pool, 10 respondents who showed the most variance in initial and follow-up responses were interviewed to provide a greater understanding of the influence of the continuing education course on the attendee's clinical practice.

From the data, the researchers generated a model depicting factors that influence the use of reflection on learning in practice (Lowe *et al.*, 2007). They found that reflection on learning was likely to lead to a change in practice based on the individual, the course, and the practice context. Individual factors included the person's interest in the topic, previous background or experience with the topic, and use of reflection. Course factors influencing reflection included the novelty, pace, and the amount of content presented. Content that was abstract, new or novel, and complex or challenging was more likely to involve reflection. Aspects of the practice context that influenced reflection included time demands, workload, resources, expectations, and whether the learning environment was open and supportive of reflection and innovation. Perhaps most importantly, the authors noted that "when [participants] learned without reflection, their learning had less effect on their practices" (p. 147). Learning without reflection is similar to what Moon (2004) refers to as "surface learning," which is retained only until the end of the course. In contrast, those who used reflection processes to make sense of new information and build on what they already understood, reported processes consistent with Moon's concept of deeper learning. For the ANE, these preliminary findings suggest that there is value in incorporating reflective practices along with most learning experiences, and reflection may facilitate the integration of new knowledge into clinical and teaching practice.

Peer Evaluation of Teaching

The peer evaluation process can be used to provide faculty with formative and summative evaluation feedback about teaching as well as provide useful information for faculty performance reviews. Peer review is defined as "informed colleague judgment about faculty teaching for either fostering improvement or making personnel decisions" (Van Note Chism & Chism, 2007, p. 3). For peer review to yield valid and reliable information it is important that data be obtained from multiple sources, using multiple methods, from multiple points in time (Box 7-3). In peer review, the issue of internal validity is concerned with measuring teaching effectiveness. To accomplish this, all parties need to agree on attributes of effective teaching so that when it occurs it can be readily identified. Reviewers also need to be aware of bias, which can stem from their specialization, teaching style preferences, and other internalized and often unrecognized values. Having criteria or standards for peer evaluation helps to counteract the "invisible bias . . . that can contaminate the peer review process" (p. 24).

Another issue of concern in peer review relates to lack of training and lack of observational skills of peer reviewers. This lack of skill can adversely affect the validity as well as reliability of observations. Fortunately this can be dealt with by providing

> ### BOX 7-3 Practices to Enhance Validity and Reliability of Peer Review
>
> 1. Use multiple reviewers
>
> 2. Review multiple aspects of teaching
>
> 3. Review at different points in time
>
> 4. Educate faculty in the peer review process
>
> 5. Partner inexperienced reviewers with experienced reviewers
>
> Data from Van Note Chism, N., & Chism, G. (2007). *Peer review of teaching: A sourcebook.* Bolton, MA: Anker Publishing.

educational preparation in peer reviewing, partnering inexperienced reviewers with more experienced reviewers, and by providing checklists to aid in observation and documentation. In addition, using multiple reviewers will negate this effect and will provide a more balanced and comprehensive review.

Using observations from a single peer reviewer who observes one classroom presentation has numerous limitations. The use of one faculty as a peer reviewer is problematic, because the reviewer is only able to offer a single perspective and may not have expertise in both the theory and classroom setting. Depending on the composition of faculty in a nursing program, it may be difficult to find a peer reviewer who has both content expertise and teaching expertise in the specific teaching methods used. Because nursing faculty teach in variety of settings and use a variety of approaches, it is important for the faculty member to be reviewed by someone who is comfortable and familiar with the content and the specific approaches used. Evaluation of clinical teaching, classroom teaching, and psychomotor skill demonstration in a practice laboratory are inherently different processes. It is safe to say that not all instructors would feel qualified evaluating peers from divergent teaching or clinical specialization settings. It is also important that content be evaluated for accuracy, currency, and appropriateness. Therefore, using multiple reviewers with different types of expertise can provide feedback on a broader scope than using a single reviewer.

To obtain evaluation data that truly reflects the ANE's teaching effectiveness, those who teach in a variety of settings such as clinical, face-to-face classroom, practice laboratory, or online should be evaluated in each setting. Likewise, those who use a variety of teaching approaches such as lecture, discussion, collaborative activities, or problem-based learning, should be observed when engaged in those activities. In addition, sampling teaching at various points in time can help provide a well rounded view of teaching. The type and nature of interactions between students and teacher, how early or late in the semester it is, and the proximity to stressful events such as examinations, can bias the evaluation findings.

Guidelines and Criteria for Peer Evaluation

Recommended guidelines for peer reviewers before, during, and after the peer review session are summarized in Box 7-4. First, before the peer review is undertaken the peer reviewer needs to develop knowledge and skills in classroom observation. This may involve the use of checklists or rating forms, videotaping, or more specialized systems such as teacher behavior coding, and mapping techniques (NC State University, Peer Review of Teaching, 2003). Prior to the peer review, the reviewer also needs background about the course, the students, and the specific expectations and goals that the ANE has for the students. Having knowledge of the context of the session will enable the reviewer to accurately interpret observations, evaluate whether the goals were achieved, and whether the teaching methods used were appropriate and effective for the situation.

BOX 7-4   Guidelines for Peer Reviewers

Prior to the peer review:

1. Acquire skills in peer observation

2. Establish the context of the class session

3. Review the peer review criteria or checklist

During the peer review process:

1. Be unobtrusive

2. Assure adequate length and frequency of observations

3. Utilize an established checklist or framework to guide observations and documentation

Soon after the peer review process:

1. Complete observation notes and write a formal report

2. Share observations and constructive feedback with the faculty

Data from North Carolina State University. (2003). *Peer review of teaching.* http://www.ncsu.edu/provost/peer_review/intro.html.

Once the criteria and procedural guidelines for peer review have been identified, the standards for peer review need to be defined. Whenever evaluation occurs, judgments are being made based on spoken or unspoken standards, thus for consistency in evaluation, the standards as well as the criteria and guidelines should be specified. According to Van Note Chism & Chism (2007), development of standards is the most challenging aspect of implementing a peer review system. "Standards are the guide to the expected quality of specific aspects of teaching. They help the reviewer to determine whether a given performance [or documented evidence] is poor, fair, good, excellent, or something in between. They are saturated with the values of the context" (p. 62). In the *Peer Review of Teaching* Van Note Chism & Chism (2007) provide a sample set of standards for content knowledge, course design, assessment, leadership, and scholarship that can serve as useful frame of reference for identifying excellent, satisfactory, and unsatisfactory teaching practices.

During the review session there is often an initial period of uneasiness as the faculty member is aware of being evaluated and students note the presence of the observer. In as much as possible, the reviewer should observe the instructor's typical teaching and the student's typical interactions. Therefore, it is important to be unobtrusive during the review session and to observe for a sufficient period of time to allow the students and faculty to resume typical interactions. Development of guidelines for peer review and a peer review template can provide a uniform structure enabling the evaluator to focus on key aspects. A typical structure for a peer evaluation may include: (1) evaluating the faculty member's knowledge and effective use of teaching strategies, (2) evaluating the faculty's knowledge of the subject matter, (3) the organization of content or other activities, and (4) appraisal of the teacher's overall effectiveness in using specific teaching and evaluation activities (Appling, Naumann, & Berk, 2001).

Van Note Chism & Chism (2007) describe three sets of criteria that can be used to develop peer evaluation tools. The criteria are derived from the works of Cohen & McKeachie (1980), French-Lazovik (1981), and Seldin (1984) (see Table 7-2). Cohen and McKeachie (1980) present the most detailed and enumerated set of criteria, which reflect concern with the teacher's direct teaching ability and strategies, as well as the development and use of teaching materials, assignments, and examinations. Peer evaluators are encouraged to make judgments of the appropriateness or suitability of the teaching strategies, materials, assignments, and teacher expectations based on the characteristics of the students in the class and the course objectives.

In contrast, French-Lazovik (1981) outlines a more concise yet in some ways more comprehensive set of peer evaluation criteria. Several criteria used by French-Lazovik differentiate this approach from the others. In criterion number three, the

TABLE 7-2 Criteria for Peer Review of Teaching

Cohen & McKeachie Criteria	French-Lazovik Criteria	Seldin Criteria
1. "Appropriateness of course goals" (p. 54)	1. Quality of teaching materials	1. Selection and knowledge of course content
2. Currency and coverage of course content	2. Faculty knowledge of subject	2. Appropriate objectives and teaching materials
3. Instruction and student assignments meet course goals	3. "Types of intellectual tasks set by teacher and students" (p. 55)	3. Appropriate teaching methods
4. Appropriate learning aids used	4. Teacher's responsibilities in department or institution (p. 55)	4. Appropriate strategies to enhance and evaluate learning
5. Reasonable time and effort required of students	5. Teacher's insight and motivation to provide quality teaching	5. Organization of course and content
6. Appropriate cognitive level evaluated		6. Student achievement
7. Appropriate grading criteria		7. Quality of assignments and teacher-developed materials
8. Integration and interpretation of student evaluation feedback		8. Teacher's concern and interest in teaching
9. Determination and weighting of criteria used for evaluation		

Data from Van Note Chism, N., & Chism, G. (2007). *Peer review of teaching: A sourcebook*. Bolton, MA: Anker Publishing, (p. 54–55).

emphasis is placed on the relationship between the teacher's goals and expectations for a particular activity and the student's performance, thereby valuing the teacher's ability to decisively achieve certain student outcomes. Criterion four values other teaching related activities outside of the classroom such as curriculum development or serving on governance committees that address teaching and learning. The fifth criterion recognizes the importance of the teacher's insight and motivation to develop as a teacher. Factors to be considered include the teacher's self-reflection on her or his teaching, use of feedback to improve teaching, and engagement in life-long learning to enhance teaching.

Seldin's (1984) criteria represent a blend of the specificity of Cohen and McKeachie's criteria with some of the unique criteria outlined by French-Lazovik. In addition, Seldin specifies looking at how the information was organized and the teacher's concern and interest in teaching. Commonalities between these sets of criteria include the instructor's use of teaching materials, the teacher's knowledge of the subject matter, and the congruence of these with the learning objectives.

Academic institutions, nursing programs, and individual nursing faculty will find the criteria helpful for developing an evaluation framework that aligns values of the institutional, program, and individual faculty, respectively. When adopting criteria to be applied to all faculty within a program or institution, weighting specific criteria to reflect the values of the program is recommended. This can be a difficult area in which to reach equitable agreement because not all criteria are equally significant for all courses and all instructors (Van Note Chism & Chism, 2007). Determining how much emphasis should be placed on each criterion versus evaluation of overall performance, and determining if the weighting should be flexible for faculty who engage in different types of teaching experiences are important considerations. However, in the absence of institution- or program-wide adoption of specific criteria, the ANE can elect to use some or all of the criteria as framework for conducting self-reflection on teaching.

A second type of peer review involves the evaluation of documentation submitted in a dossier or portfolio. The portfolio may contain samples of teaching materials, syllabi, documentation of teaching effectiveness from students and peers, and samples of students work. Activities that reflect the scholarship of teaching such as committee assignments and involvement with professional organizations that deal with education and curriculum issues may also be documented. Scholarly activities related to teaching such as obtaining grants for curriculum and program development, or publishing and presenting on topics in the field of nursing education are also relevant. This type of evidence evaluation is typically summative and used to provide feedback for administrative decisions such as tenure, promotion, or reappointment of the faculty.

Student Evaluation of Teaching

Student evaluation of teaching is the most widely used source of evaluation feedback. Simonson (2007) describes five hierarchical levels of student evaluation. Level one evaluation is the most commonly used type of student evaluation, which focuses on student reaction and student satisfaction. Level one evaluation asks the students' questions about their satisfaction with the teacher, the course content, and course management. The second level of evaluation is concerned with the student's learning, and asks questions such as, "What and how much did the student learn?" The third evaluation level is also concerned with learning outcomes but from a different perspective. It is not restricted to the student's perception of whether or not the course objectives were met or not met, but instead on the student's ability to transfer learning from the classroom to the real world.

The final two levels of evaluation deal with aspects that may not be immediately measurable. Evaluation at level four is focused on determining the long-term results of the program on improving quality or lowering healthcare or educational costs. The fifth level explores the return on investment and builds on the results of the previous levels. Table 7-3 provides a description of each evaluation level along with examples of typical evaluation questions used at each level.

Palloff and Pratt (2003) provide another view on student evaluation of teaching. They recommend that summative instructor/course evaluations should cover key elements such as (1) the overall course experience, (2) the orientation to the course, and (3) the course content including quantity and quality of material. Online course eval-

TABLE 7-3 Levels of Student Evaluation of Teaching		
Level of Evaluation	**Description**	**Evaluation Questions**
1. Student reaction	• Ask students for their reaction, opinions, likes or dislikes concerning the course or instructor	• What did you like best about this course? • What are the instructor's strengths? • Was the course content presented in a well-organized manner?
2. Student learning	• Ask students what was learned, how much their knowledge increased, if they met the course objectives	• What was the most important thing you learned in this course? • How much did your knowledge or skills improve in this course? • Did the course provide opportunities to meet the course objectives?

(continues)

TABLE 7-3	Levels of Student Evaluation of Teaching *(continued)*	
Level of Evaluation	**Description**	**Evaluation Questions**
3. Transfer of learning	• Ask student about application of knowledge to other classroom or clinical situations	• How has the learning in this course helped you in other courses? • How has it helped you in your clinical practice? • Which skills have you found most useful in clinical practice?
4. Results or program outcomes	• Look at employer and alumni survey data in terms of quality, productivity, and costs	• How do employers perceive graduates and the quality of their work? • How do alumni perceive the quality of their education? • What do alumni perceive as long-term benefits of their education? • How have work roles and responsibilities of alumni changed since completing their studies?
5. Return on investment	• Examine the cost/benefit ratio in terms of financial costs, time, and user satisfaction • Useful when extensive curriculum changes or new teaching technologies have been introduced	• What were the total costs of implementing this change? • What are the advantages and disadvantages of this change?

Data from Simonson, M. (2007). Evaluation and distance education: Five steps. *The Quarterly Review of Distance Education, 8*(3), vii–ix.

uations should ask questions about the discussion, technical support, the ease of use of the courseware system, access to resources, and the student's self-assessment of their performance in the course.

Developing Evaluation Tools

To enhance the evaluation process and ensure that valid student-generated faculty evaluations are obtained, faculty need to make certain that valid and practical evaluation tools are being used. General processes for developing evaluation tools are outlined in Box 7-5. If existing tools do not meet the predetermined evaluation needs of

BOX 7-5	Processes Used in Developing Evaluation Tools

1. Determine attributes of the desired evaluation tool

2. Review existing evaluation tools available from home institution, other institutions, and commercially

3. Determine if any tools address the desired attributes

4. Adapt or adopt existing tools

or

5. Develop a unique tool to address evaluation needs:

- Identify research-based attributes of effective teaching

- Translate attributes into rating scale items

- Develop overall rating scale format

- Identify subscales (i.e., content organization, teaching method, learning atmosphere)

- Select response anchors (i.e., agree/disagree)

- Review, edit, and approve items

- Field test the tool and revise as needed

Adapted from Appling, S. E., Naumann, P. L., & Berk, R. A. (2001). Using a faculty evaluation triad to achieve evidence-based teaching. *Nursing and Health Care Perspectives, 22,* 247–251.

the faculty, then development of a tailored evaluation tool can be initiated as described in step five.

After determining that existing tools did not meet the specific needs and constraints of their program, Appling *et al.* (2001) detailed the processes used to develop their own evidence-based, student-generated, faculty evaluation form. The end product was a 36-item evaluation tool that addressed five subscales: (1) course content and organization, (2) evaluation methods, (3) learning outcomes, (4) instructional methods, and (5) learning atmosphere (Appling *et al.*, 2001). A four-point rating scale of strongly disagree to strongly agree was used for each subscale item and a section for student's qualitative comments was provided at the end of the subscale. The tool was administered in 51 courses yielding over 1500 evaluations. Item-to-subscale correlations ranged from 0.70s to 0.80s, with the five subscales also demonstrating high alpha coefficients of 0.89 to 0.94. By using a systematic process to develop and analyze the evaluation tool, Appling and colleagues produced a valid and reliable tool for providing faculty feedback that will contribute to the CQI process for individual faculty.

Faculty Evaluation Triad

Traditionally, students' evaluations of faculty have played a dominant role in the evaluation process and serve as a major source of guidance for CQI efforts. However, it is widely recognized that the use of multiple sources of evaluation data will achieve a more comprehensive picture of a teacher's teaching skills and strengths. Faculty evaluation triad refers to combining data from self, peer, and student evaluation, in essence triangulating the information from all sources to arrive at a more complete picture of teaching effectiveness. Borrowing from the research concept of triangulation in which multiple sources of data are compared, the faculty evaluation triad provides a more holistic and comprehensive perspective than the use of a single evaluation method.

The faculty evaluation triad described by Appling *et al.* (2001) incorporates student evaluation of faculty, along with peer and self-evaluation, all of which are documented in a teaching portfolio. In addition to the self-evaluation narrative, the teaching portfolio contains concrete evidence or documentation of teaching activities such as the course syllabi, teaching materials developed, and student assignments. Other sources of portfolio content will depend on the institution's definition of teaching. For example, if teaching is defined as including academic advising, then the faculty may document the number of student advisees and any feedback received from advisees. If the institution defines the scope of teaching as including the scholarship of teaching, then activities such as curriculum development grants, action research projects related to teaching, and conference presentations on educational topics would be included.

Using a teaching portfolio to document data from the faculty evaluation triad provides additional benefits. Portfolios typically include a contextual narrative in which the teacher provides background information about teaching such as a description of courses taught, teaching responsibilities and activities, class size, and other student characteristics. In addition, the teacher can describe his or her teaching philosophy and any teaching activities outside of assigned courses such as student mentoring and guest lecturing. Providing teaching-related artifacts such as teaching materials and assignments and a contextual narrative about the nature of the teaching experience can help to substantiate the ratings and commentary provided by student, peer, and self-evaluations.

Promoting Socialization to the Role

Another aspect of competency six involves engaging in activities that promote socialization to the ANE role. In addition to the role functions of teacher, scholar, and collaborator discussed in Chapter 1, the ANE needs to integrate subject matter knowledge with clinical, and professional skills.

Educational Preparation

Graduate preparation as a nurse educator provides nurses who are transitioning from clinical to teaching practice with basic teaching knowledge and skills and often begins the socialization process. In many respects graduate preparation as a nurse educator is similar to teacher preparation for grades K–12. Both ANE students and K–12 student teachers acquire knowledge of teaching pedagogy, theory, and subject matter. In addition, they practice applying this knowledge to teaching students in a real learning setting. However, even with graduate preparation as a nurse educator, a new ANE will likely need additional mentoring, experience, and education to perform effectively in academia. A thorough orientation to the institution and program is needed to provide a foundation for socialization to the teaching, scholarship, and service expectations of the institution.

Learning From Experience

A framework developed by Hiebert, Morris, Berk, and Jansen (2007) outlines the skills needed to learn from experience. The authors recognize that academic preparation in teaching does not guarantee that students will be expert teachers upon graduation. New teachers need to be armed with skills that enable them to learn from their teaching experiences. According to Hiebert *et al.* (2007) "Assessing whether students achieve clear learning goals and specifying how and why instruction did or did not affect this achievement lies at the heart of learning to teach" (p. 48).

Four skills utilized daily by classroom teachers provide a framework teachers can use to learn from their teaching experiences (Box 7-6). The first and most essential skill involves specifying learning goals for a segment of instruction and assessing the effect of the instruction on goal achievement. "Formulating clear and explicit learning goals sets the stage for everything else . . . Until learning goals are expressed clearly, further analyses are impossible" (Hiebert *et al.*, 2007, p. 51). Unlike course objectives, which are typically broad, the more specific, detailed, and narrow the learning objectives are, the easier it will be to analyze the effect of the segment of instruction and collect observational data.

BOX 7-6 Framework for Self-Analysis of Teaching

1. Specify the learning goals for each learning task or activity

2. Compile observations to determine if learning goals were met

3. Develop hypothesis about the effect of teaching on student learning

4. Determine any revisions to teaching warranted

Data from Hiebert, J., Morris, A. K., Berk, D., & Jansen, A. (2007). Preparing teachers to learn from teaching. *Journal of Teacher Education, 58,* 47–61.

The second skill proposed by Hiebert *et al.* (2007) recognizes that evidence of student learning is essential to determining whether the teaching was effective. This differs from the typical emphasis in evaluation, which is on what the teacher does and how well the teacher does it. For example, when a teacher analyzes teaching in terms of how smoothly something was presented or how well a group activity was implemented, the focus is on the teacher versus on student learning outcomes. A shift to collecting evidence of student achievement of learning objectives demonstrates the development of this skill. Another component of this skill involves knowing what types of observations or evidence are best for determining how well students are learning the specific objective. Hiebert *et al.* suggests that one way to identify what would count as evidence is to review a lesson plan and speculate how students would indicate what they had learned. For example, the teacher can ask the students questions during the class session; observe their nonverbal behavior, such as affirmative nods or confused expressions; present case studies to analyze; or engage in a number of classroom assessment techniques (see Angelo & Cross, 1993; Silberman, 1998) to gather information about how well the students are learning.

Third, after the learning objectives are specified and evidence supporting or refuting student learning is collected, the teacher constructs a hypothesis that explains how a particular teaching segment facilitated or inhibited the students' learning (Hiebert *et al.*, 2007). A hypothesis in this case is a statement of the cause and effect relationship, or the link between a specific teaching approach and learning. As with developing learning objectives, the hypothesis should be as specific as possible to enable the teacher to develop and test the effectiveness of new teaching approaches. Hiebert *et al.* recommend reviewing principles of teaching and learning (see Chapter 2) and identifying principles that may have been operating in the specific teaching segment. When using the principles of teaching and learning, the educator is able to "offer explanations for why the learning did not occur and point to other instructional tasks, explanations, questions, and so on, that might have promoted such learning" (p. 54). This skill focuses on recognizing what the teacher did or didn't do that may have influenced the student's learning and identifying teaching learning principles to be tested in the future.

The three previous skills provide the foundation for making decisions about one's teaching practices and what needs to be revised. The fourth skill involves being able to act upon whatever recommendations stemmed from the hypothesis of step three. Hiebert *et al.* (2007) see the process of "making revisions to improve the instructional episode . . . a matter of following the implicit recommendations contained in the hypotheses" (p. 55). The ANE who engages in these skills will be using a systematic, disciplined process to identify areas for teaching improvement. The process enables the teacher to blend teaching learning theory with empirical observation and helps to bridge the gap between theory, research, and practice.

Mentoring

Mentoring is a valuable mechanism for ensuring quality education of students, and for facilitating the transition of new nursing faculty into academia. Researchers have found that both the mentor and mentee experience positive outcomes from the mentoring experience (Boice, 2000; Grossman & Valiga, 2005; Stewart & Krueger, 1996). The NLN position statement on mentoring of nursing faculty acknowledges that mentoring is not just for new faculty. Mentoring can be utilized throughout one's career continuum to enhance professional development and increase job satisfaction (NLN Board of Governors, 2006).

It is recommended that new faculty receive an orientation to the institution including key personnel, resources, institutional policies, and governance structures. A key component of the orientation should include assignment of a senior faculty mentor who will be available to the mentee for day-to-day questions and concerns (NLN Board of Governors, 2006). Faculty serving as a mentor for an inexperienced instructor may need to take a more direct, proactive role in the mentoring process rather than waiting for the new faculty to have an issue or concern needing to be addressed. New instructors will likely benefit from proactive guidance in teaching, classroom management, assessment, and evaluation practices.

In contrast to the mentoring of inexperienced faculty, mid-career faculty may seek mentors who can meet specific, well-defined needs. For example, mid-career faculty may seek mentors to facilitate a research agenda, or for transitioning to a specific leadership role, or to provide guidance in a specific teaching approach or technology. In this stage of career development, the mentoring process can be described as "eclectic, varied in content and process, and directed more by the faculty member (i.e., mentee) than the mentor" (NLN Board of Governors, 2006, p.3). Therefore, the mid-career mentoring relationship has a uniquely individual focus depending on the specific needs identified by the mentee.

Late career faculty mentors are experienced teachers who have typically served in leadership roles within the department or institution. The late career mentor plays an important role in sustaining the mentoring experience at the institution. The institution relies on seasoned faculty to establish relationships with new or mid-career faculty who show promise in developing into a leadership role (NLN Board of Governors, 2006).

If the institution does not have a formal mentoring program established, there are many ways the ANE can implement informal mentoring (See Box 7-7). First, spend time interacting together as a nursing community. For example, faculty lunches may provide a mechanism for mentoring. During faculty lunches, new faculty can talk with other nursing faculty and learn from personal stories and interactions shared informally. New faculty may also learn by observing others' teaching or through contacts with retired faculty. Assigning new faculty to co-teach courses with seasoned faculty before assuming full responsibility for course management will ease the transition process and provide the new faculty with opportunities to interact with and

---

BOX 7-7   Ideas for Informal Mentoring

1. Provide regular opportunities to talk and share such as faculty lunches

2. Encourage new faculty to observe experienced colleagues while teaching

3. Introduce new faculty to retired nursing faculty

4. Engage in brief, frequent interactions (i.e., one-minute mentor) (Oermann, 2001)

5. Assign new faculty to co-teach courses with experienced faculty

6. Develop a cadre of faculty interested in serving as resource persons

7. Circulate information to faculty about informal mentoring

8. Talk about informal mentoring during faculty orientation

9. Develop a resource packet for new faculty and for informal mentors

Some data from National League for Nursing, Board of Governors. (2006, January). *Mentoring of nurse faculty*. http://www.nln.org/aboutnln/PositionStatements/mentoring_3_21_06.pdf.

observe senior faculty on a regular basis. Oermann (2001) suggests that mentoring can also occur through brief, unplanned interactions referred to a being a one-minute mentor. Whether formal or informal mentoring processes are used, role performance and CQI of the ANE is enhanced through mentoring behaviors.

Designing and Implementing Educational Policies

In academia, policies play a central role in the CQI process. Implementation of formal CQI practices in evaluation of teaching, mentoring, and faculty performance reviews are guided by policies and procedures. Therefore, knowledge of policy development and implementation processes is helpful in the CQI process. This section reviews the structure of policies and outlines processes that the ANE can use for developing effective educational policies.

Policy Development Processes

A policy can be described as a plan of action that is to be used by individuals or groups to guide events and activities that promote the institution's values and beliefs. Policies typically stem from the need to deal with a real or anticipated problem. Processes that can be used to develop policies have been outlined by Rowe (2006) and Themba-Nixon (2002) and are summarized in Box 7-8. The first step is to identify the area of concern and define the problem. Various approaches can be used including looking at existing policies and identifying gaps, surveying stakeholders, gathering information related to legal requirements, and obtaining recommendations from professional organizations. At this stage of development, obtaining diverse viewpoints is helpful (Rowe, 2006).

Once the policy area and problem have been identified, broad goals for the policy are developed. The policy goals need to be congruent with the institution and program mission and goals. It is important, according to Themba-Nixon (2002), to determine how the policy will address the issue, and how it will impact individuals within the institution. The next step is to identify short-term objectives and the steps needed to meet each objective. Identifying steps needed to meet short-term objectives serves several purposes. It clarifies the potential impact of the policy on the institution and individual stakeholders, and is a precursor to determining capabilities and resources needed to implement the policy. In steps three and four, the capabilities and resources that will be needed to implement and enforce the policy are determined. Questions to consider include, Is the institution and or program able to implement the goals of the policy? How will implementing the policy impact the institution, the program, or the

---

BOX 7-8 Steps in Developing Educational Policy

1. Define the problem

2. Identify policy goals

3. Assess ability to implement policy goals

4. Determine resources needed to implement policy goals

5. Determine who will enact and enforce the policy

6. Determine ways to monitor the effectiveness of the policy

7. Submit a draft of the policy for faculty to review and approve

Data from Rowe, K. (2006). Developing a policy: Factsheet #4. *National Childcare Accreditation Council.* http://www.ncac.gov.au/factsheets/qias_factsheet_4.pdf; and Themba-Nixon, M. (2002). Developing a policy initiative. *The Praxis Project.* http://www.ThePraxisProject.org.

---

individual? The fifth and sixth steps involve determining who will have the power to enact and enforce the policy and determining how the effectiveness of the policy will be monitored. An underlying purpose of most policies is to provide guidance and ensure that certain actions are taken. Therefore, establishing markers to indicate that the policy is doing what was intended is recommended. The final step involves drafting the policy into document form for approval by faculty.

Components of Educational Policy

The actual components of written policies may vary from institution to institution. Recommendations for policy components and structure are outlined in Box 7-9. Because it is important that a policy is aligned with the program's values and beliefs, Rowe recommends a statement of the program's philosophy be included. Following the statement of the program's philosophy, a brief overview of what is covered in the policy and a rationale for the policy are provided. The rationale may be supported by research, recommendations of professional organizations, or other data. Next, a statement of purpose, and long- and short-term goals can be listed. The body of the policy should describe what needs to be done and what strategies need to be implemented. After the body of the policy is completed, a list of any references used to develop the policy, identification of related policies, appendices, and the date the policy was approved and implemented are included.

Institutions are likely to have many policies related to aspects of quality improvement such as faculty annual reappointment review, promotion, merit, mentoring, and

BOX 7-9   Components of a Policy

1. Philosophy statement

2. Policy overview or introduction including purpose and scope

3. Rationale for policy

4. Purpose and goals of the policy

5. Body of the policy (strategies and practices)

6. References used for policy

7. List of related policies, procedures, or forms

8. Appendices

9. Date policy approved and implemented

10. Who approved policy

11. Date of review or modification of policy

Data from Rowe, K. (2006). *Developing a policy: Factsheet #4*. National Childcare Accreditation Council. http://www.ncac.gov.au/factsheets/qias_factsheet_4.pdf; and University of Canterbury Policy Library. (2008, February). *Policies and procedures development and review policy*. http://www.canterbury.ac.nz/ucpolicy/documents/policyproc.pdf.

BOX 7-10   Policy Review Guidelines

Evaluate policies regularly for:

1. Effectiveness

2. Congruence with current trends

3. Congruence with new research

4. Congruence with new professional guidelines

5. Impact of organizational changes in structure, staffing, technology, and physical environment on the policy

Data from Rowe, K. (2006). Developing a policy: Factsheet #4. *National Childcare Accreditation Council*. http://www.ncac.gov.au/factsheets/qias_factsheet_4.pdf.

teaching evaluation policies. Although such policies may remain stable for many years, it is still important to conduct regular systematic reviews of existing policies. Rowe (2006) recommends that when reviewing policies the reviewers should explore the effectiveness of the policy, congruence with current trends, new research, and new professional guidelines. In addition, changes within the institution's organizational structure, staffing, and the physical environment may necessitate revision of the policy (Box 7-10). Rowe summarized policy review stating that, "Policies are 'living' documents that should be reviewed regularly to respond to the individual needs of those working with them to reflect new knowledge and to meet changing trends . . ." (para. 1).

CONCLUSION

Engaging in the process of continuous quality improvement is essential to achieving and maintaining competence in the roles of teacher, scholar, and collaborator. Using feedback from peers and students, engaging in self-reflection, and benchmarking performance outcomes can provide direction for professional development and mentoring activities. Engaging in policy development will also support quality improvement efforts on an individual and institutional level.

SUMMARY

- Competency six is concerned with activities that can be instituted on an individual or institutional level to help the ANE attain and maintain the knowledge and skills needed to fulfill teaching, scholarship, and service role functions.
- The CQI process involves professional development activities such as participation in continuing education programs, seeking and using feedback from peer, student, and self-evaluation.
- Total Quality Management is a model that identifies factors that influence the implementation and sustainability of quality improvement projects (see Box 7-1).
- The NLN has identified 10 Hallmarks of Excellence in Nursing Education related to students, faculty, continuous quality improvement, curriculum, teaching/learning and evaluation strategies, resources, innovation, educational research, environment, and leadership.
- A benchmark is an indicator of a best practice. Benchmarking is the process of using a benchmark as a goal or criterion for individual or institutional achievement.
- Four types of benchmarking include internal, competitive, generic, and longitudinal.

- Eight steps in the benchmarking process are presented in Box 7-2.
- Professional development in the form of life-long learning and continuing education is necessary to maintain competence in nursing and teaching practice.
- A Cochrane review of the effects of continuing education on professional practice supports the use of continuing education to change professional practice.
- Evidence-based education sessions facilitate the incorporation of evidence-based knowledge into practice by directly linking the content with research references, indicating the strength of the research evidence, and providing a summary of the research evidence.
- Feedback useful for continuous quality improvement may be obtained from self-reflection, self-evaluation, and peer and student evaluation of teaching.
- Self-reflection is the process of looking inward to collect information about one's teaching practices.
- Categories of self-observation may be classified as focused on physical movement, visual aspects of presentation, and intellectual factors.
- The ANE can gain insight into teaching performance through recording and reviewing a teaching session, or having a colleague review a teaching session, looking specifically for aspects that strengthen or diminish teaching effectiveness.
- Peer review is defined as "informed colleague judgment about faculty teaching for either fostering improvement or making personnel decisions" (Van Note Chism & Chism, 2007, p. 3).
- The peer evaluation process can be used to provide faculty with formative and summative feedback about teaching as well as provide useful information for faculty performance reviews.
- Criteria for peer review of teaching may include teacher attributes, content and teaching materials developed, teaching methods and assignments, and teaching related service and scholarship activities.
- Five levels of evaluation include student reaction, student learning, student transfer of learning, results or program outcomes, and return on investment.
- Processes for developing valid and practical evaluation tools include determining attributes of the desired tool, reviewing existing tools, determining if existing tools address the desired attributes, adapting or adopting an existing tool or creating a new tool (see Box 7-5).
- The faculty evaluation triad refers to the process of triangulating data from self-, peer, and student evaluations.
- The teaching portfolio may be used to describe the teaching context, document self, peer, and student evaluation data, and provide supporting documentation such as teaching materials and course syllabi.

- Four factors used by classroom teachers for self-analysis of teaching include, specifying the learning goals, collecting data to determine if goals were meet, developing a hypothesis about the effect of teaching on student learning, and determining the revisions needed.
- Adequate socialization to the ANE role is foundational for ensuring quality performance. Socialization is facilitated by formal educational preparation in the ANE role, thorough orientation to the institution, and formal or informal mentoring.
- Educational policies generally concern faculty and student roles and responsibilities throughout the educational process and reflect best practices for the specific institution.
- Institutions are likely to enforce many policies related to aspects of quality improvement such as faculty annual reappointment review, promotion, merit, mentoring, and teaching evaluation policies.

RECOMMENDED RESOURCES

Quality Indicators

- The AACN position paper on indicators of quality in research-focused doctoral programs in nursing is available online at http://www.aacn.nche.edu/Publications/positions/qualityindicators.htm.
- The NLN Hallmarks document "Hallmarks, Indicators, Glossary & References" lists 30 hallmarks for excellence in nursing programs and suggests indicators for all types of nursing programs. The Hallmarks document is available online at http://www.nln.org/excellence/hallmarks_indicators.htm.

Benchmarking

- Consortium for Higher Education Benchmarking Analysis (CHEBA) provides the opportunity for all levels of higher education around the world to exchange performance measurements and benchmarking data. Membership in the consortium is currently free, with fees assessed only when members want to join specific benchmarking efforts. Sign up for a free newsletter at http://www.cheba.com.
- The Institute for Higher Education has published benchmarks for Internet-based education available online at http://www.ihep.org/Publications/publications-detail.cfm?id=69.

Peer Review of Teaching

- North Carolina State University Peer Review of Teaching Web site offers information on types of peer reviews, guidelines, procedures, and best practices available at http://www.ncsu.edu/provost/peer_review/intro.html.

Educational Policy

- The American Council on Education is a membership organization for institutions of higher learning. The site features information on government and public policy including access to the latest news about public policy, legislation, and other government efforts that affect higher education. Visit at http://www.acenet.edu for more information.
- The Educational Policy Institute is focused on improving educational policy and practice through research and dissemination of information. The institute publishes scholarly reports as well as four newsletters (*Week in Review, Commentary, Student Success,* and *Policy Perspectives*), each dealing with policy-related issues. These reports and newsletters may be downloaded from the home page at http://www.educationalpolicy.org.
- The National Center for Public Policy and Higher Education provides analyses of policy issues facing the states and the nation. Policy analysis reports may be accessed online at http://www.highereducation.org.

REFERENCES

1. American Nurses Association. (1994). *Standards for nursing professional development: Continuing education and staff development.* Washington, DC: American Nurses Publishing.
2. Angelo, T. A., & Cross, K. P. (1993). *Classroom assessment techniques: A handbook for college teachers.* San Francisco, CA: Jossey-Bass.
3. Appling, S. E., Naumann, P. L., & Berk, R. A. (2001). Using a faculty evaluation triad to achieve evidence-based teaching. *Nursing and Health Care Perspectives, 22,* 247–251.
4. Bernal-Delgado, E., Galeote-Major, M., Pradas-Arnal, F., & Peiro-Moreno, S. (2002). Evidence-based educational outreach visits: Effects on prescriptions of non-steroidal anti-inflammatory drugs. *Journal of Epidemiology and Community Health, 56,* 653–658.
5. Billings, D. (2007). Using benchmarking for continuous quality improvement in nursing education. In M. Oermann, & K. Heinrich (Eds.), *Annual review of nursing education, volume 5, 2007,* (pp. 173–180). NY: Springer Publishing.
6. Boice, R. (2000). *Advice for new faculty members: Nibil nimus.* Needham Heights, MA: Allyn & Bacon.
7. Cohen, P. A., & McKeachie, W. J. (1980). The role of colleagues in the evaluation of college teaching. *Improving College and University Teaching, 28,* 147–154.

8. Dale, B. G., Boaden, R. J., Wilcox, M., & McQuater, R. E. (1999). Sustaining continuous improvement: What are the key issues? *Quality Engineering, 11*(3), 369–377.

9. de Jager, H. J., & Nieuwenhuis, F. J. (2005). Linkages between total quality management and the outcomes based approach in an education environment. *Quality in Higher Education, 11*(3), 251–260.

10. DePalma, J. A. (2007). The value of evidence-based continuing education. *The Journal of Continuing Education in Nursing, 38*(2), 52–53.

11. Ellis, J. (2006). All inclusive benchmarking. *Journal of Nursing Management, 14*, 377–383.

12. Fletcher, S. W. (2008). Chairman's summary of the conference: Continuing education in the health professions: Improving healthcare through lifelong learning. *The Journal of Continuing Education in Nursing, 39*(3), 112–117.

13. French-Lazovik, G. (1981). Peer review: Documentary evidence in the evaluation of teaching. In J. Millman (Ed.), *Handbook for college teachers*. Boston: Little, Brown & Company.

14. Gessner, B. A., & Armstrong, M. A. (1992). Reading activities of staff nurses from states with mandatory or voluntary continuing education. *The Journal of Continuing Education in Nursing, 23*(2), 76–80.

15. Grossman, S., & Valiga, T. (2005). *The new leadership challenge: Creating the future of nursing*. Philadelphia: F.A. Davis.

16. Gruppen, L. D., Rana, G. K., & Arndt, T. S. (2005). A controlled comparison study of the efficacy of training medical students in evidence-based medicine literature searching skills. *Academic Medicine, 80*, 940–944.

17. Hayes, E. R., Morin, K. H., Sylvia, B., & Bashford, M. R. (1995). Meeting the challenge of mandatory continuing education. *Journal of Nursing Staff Development, 11*(2), 89–94.

18. Hiebert, J., Morris, A. K., Berk, D., & Jansen, A. (2007). Preparing teachers to learn from teaching. *Journal of Teacher Education, 58*(1), 47–61.

19. The Journal of Continuing Education in Nursing. (2008).19th annual survey of state boards of nursing and selected national professional certifying boards/associations. *The Journal of Continuing Education in Nursing, 39*(1), 4–11.

20. Lockyer, J. M., Gondocz, S. T., & Thivierge, R. L. (2004). Knowledge translation: The role and place of practice reflection. *Journal of Continuing Education for Health Professionals, 24*(1), 50–57.

21. Lowe, M., Rappolt, S., Jaglal, S., & Macdonald, G. (2007). The role of reflection in implementing learning from continuing education into practice. *Journal of Continuing Education in the Health Professions, 27*(3), 143–148.

22. Moon, J. A. (2004). Using reflective learning to improve the impact of short courses and workshops. *Journal of Continuing Education in the Health Professions, 24*(19), 4–11.

23. National League for Nursing, Board of Governors. (2006, January). *Mentoring of nurse faculty*. Retrieved December 6th 2008 from http://www.nln.org/aboutnln/PositionStatements/mentoring_3_21_06.pdf.

24. National League for Nursing, Task Group on Nurse Educator Competencies. (2005). *Core competencies of nurse educators with task statements*. Retrieved September 10, 2008 from http://www.nln.org/facultydevelopment/pdf/corecompetencies.pdf.

25. National League for Nursing, Task Group on Nursing Education Standards. (2005). *Hallmarks, indicators, glossary & references*. Retrieved March 20, 2009 from http://www.nln.org/excellence/hallmarks_indicators.htm.

26. North Carolina State University. (2003). *Peer review of teaching*. Retrieved December 10, 2008 from http://www.ncsu.edu/provost/peer_review/intro.html.
27. O'Brien, M. A., Freemantle. N., Oxman, A. D., Wolf, F., Davis, D. A., & Herrin, J. (2001). Continuing education meetings and workshops: Effects on professional practice and health care outcomes. *Cochrane Database of Systematic Reviews*, Issue 1. Art. No.: CD003030. DOI:10.1002/14651858.CD003030.
28. Oermann, M. H. (2001). One minute mentor. *Nursing Management, 32*(4), 12–13.
29. Palloff, R., & Pratt, K. (2003). *The virtual student: A profile and guide to working with online learners*. San Francisco: Jossey Bass.
30. Robbins, L. (2001). Self-observation in teaching: What to look for. *Business Communication Quarterly, 64*, 19–37.
31. Rowe, K. (2006). Developing a policy: Factsheet #4. *National Childcare Accreditation Council*. Retrieved March 25, 2009 from http://www.ncac.gov.au/factsheets/qias_factsheet_4.pdf.
32. Seldin, P. (1984). *Changing practices in faculty evaluation*. San Francisco: Jossey-Bass.
33. Silberman, M. (1998). *Active learning: 101 strategies to teach any subject*. Boston: Allyn & Bacon.
34. Simonson, M. (2007). Evaluation and distance education: Five steps. *The Quarterly Review of Distance Education, 8*(3), vii–ix.
35. Stewart, B. M., & Krueger, L. E. (1996). An evolutionary concept analysis of mentoring in nursing. *Journal of Professional Nursing, 12* (5), 311–321.
36. Themba-Nixon, M. (2002). Developing a policy initiative. The praxis project. Retrieved March 25, 2009 from http://www.ThePraxisProject.org.
37. Thurston, H. (1992). Mandatory continuing education: What the research tells us. *The Journal of Continuing Education in Nursing, 23*(l), 6–14.
38. Van Note Chism, N., & Chism, G. (2007). *Peer review of teaching: A sourcebook*. Bolton, MA: Anker Publishing.
39. Waddell, D. (1992). The effects on continuing education on nursing practice: A meta-analysis. *The Journal of Continuing Education in Nursing, 23*(4), 164–168.
40. Yoder-Wise, P. (1997). Annual CE survey. *The Journal of Continuing Education in Nursing, 28*(l), 5–9.

CHAPTER 8

Engage in Scholarship—Competency 7

OBJECTIVES

1. Explore theories, research, and strategies relevant to faculty scholarship.
2. Identify knowledge and skills needed to design and implement scholarly activities.
3. Differentiate the scholarship of teaching, discovery, application, and integration in the ANE role.
4. Describe processes used to successfully develop and integrate scholarship activities into the faculty role.
5. Identify guidelines and resources for grant writing and dissemination of scholarly materials.

KEY TERMS

Action research	Nonrefereed journals
Boyer's Model of Scholarship	Refereed journals
Critical inquiry process	Scholarly teaching
Dissemination	Scholarship of application
Diffusion of innovation	Scholarship of discovery
Grantsmanship	Scholarship of integration
External funding	Scholarship of teaching
Evidence-based teaching process	Self-study of teacher education practices (S-STEP)
Internal funding	SMART objectives

DEFINITION AND DESCRIPTION OF COMPETENCY

In academia, the concept of scholarship is as broad and diverse as the disciplines within the institution. Engaging in scholarship involves activities that enhance teaching and nursing practice, and activities that develop the theory and knowledge base needed for teaching and nursing practice. Specific personal attributes and skills needed to engage in scholarship are identified in six competency task statements (NLN Task Group on Nurse Educator Competencies, 2005). The task statements reflect personal qualities such as a spirit of inquiry about teaching and the role of the academic nurse educator (ANE), and the qualities of "integrity, courage, perseverance, vitality, and creativity" (NLN Task Group on Nurse Educator Competencies,

2005, p. 7). The skills needed include the ability to use literature to guide practice, grant writing skills, and the ability to design and implement research and disseminate scholarly material.

Clarification of Terms

The literature contains various terms and meanings related to scholarship (Allen & Field, 2005; Boyer, 1990; Hutchings, 2001-2002; Kreber, 2003; Nicholls, 2004; Spath, 2007; Zeichner, 1999). The terms scholarship, scholarly teaching, scholarship of teaching, and scholarship of clinical teaching may seem similar on the surface; however, each has a distinct meaning that is discussed in this section.

Scholarship

Boyer's (1990) classic text, *Scholarship Reconsidered* has served as a major influence on the perspective of scholarship in academia. Boyer reconceptualized scholarship as including not only traditional research, referred to as the scholarship of discovery, but also scholarship of integration, application, and teaching. The scholarship of integration involves synthesizing existing knowledge in a new way to create new meanings. In nursing this may mean publishing literature reviews or participating in interdisciplinary endeavors in which existing information is synthesized from multiple perspectives and thus placed into broader contexts. The scholarship of application involves scholarly activities that facilitate utilization of the knowledge in one's field. For the ANE this could involve research utilization in clinical and teaching practice; taking actions to incorporate new knowledge into clinical practice through revision of policies, procedures, and clinical protocols. Similarly, in teaching practice, the scholarship of application could involve using new knowledge to revise teaching practices, curriculum, educational policies, and procedures. The scholarship of teaching involves conducting research about the teaching-learning process, and evaluating and transmitting information about the teaching process. For the ANE this may involve conducting action research, and presenting and publishing in the areas of teaching, learning, and evaluation. The scholarship of teaching is also demonstrated in the self-study of teacher education practices (S-STEP). S-STEP, which denotes the scholarly self-study of one's own teaching practices, is discussed later in this chapter, and resources for further exploration of this scholarly practice are provided in the resource section.

Although Boyer's work has broadened the perspective of scholarship, it has also generated more scholarly discussion, more writings about scholarship, and more diversity in scholarship terminology. Perhaps the most confusion relates to the terms scholarship and scholarly teaching. To help clarify the terms, Nicholls (2004) explored the use of various scholarship terms by academic educators. Interview responses revealed several themes. First, *scholarship* was delineated as the broadest term and was characterized as involving critical thinking and problem solving. Second, the terms *scholarly teaching* and *scholarship of teaching* were subsumed as aspects within scholarship.

Scholarly Teaching

Emerson and Records (2007) conducted a review of the literature to define the terms scholarly teaching and scholarship of teaching. The terms are differentiated based on scope of influence and focus. Scholarly teaching is a term that describes the faculty's reflection on teaching practices and the incorporation of ideas from the literature into his or her personal teaching practice. The scholarly teacher utilizes both knowledge of teaching and knowledge of the subject matter in her or his educational practices. Scholarly teaching only advances education at the individual student level; however, the scholarship of teaching and learning describes a type of research in which the process of teaching and learning is explored, tested, and results disseminated. It is important to note that this definition leaves out many teaching activities such as academic advisement, curriculum development and design, formation of positive learning environments, serving on teaching and curriculum related committees, and program coordination.

Richlin and Cox (2004) offer further clarification of the term *scholarly teaching*. They define it as what is done by the teacher to influence the teaching and learning process. Similarly, Allen and Field (2005) distinguish scholarly teaching as focused on teacher behaviors and the application of specific teaching strategies.

A broader terminology than scholarly teaching is the term evidence-based teaching (EBT, also called evidence-based education). EBT involves "the incorporation of the *doing* of teaching with the *study* of teaching, encompassing all of the roles and capacities from administrator to advisor" (Emerson & Records, 2007, p. 361). The processes used in EBT are parallel to those used in evidence-based practice (EBP), only specific to the teaching process (Box 8-1). For example, in EBP the process begins with identifying a clinical question of concern using the PICO format (patient, intervention, comparison, and outcome) to specify attributes of the question to explore. The EBT process uses a similar format, substituting student/problem for patient, and substituting teaching strategy for intervention.

Scholarly teaching has become an expectation of many institutions of higher education. As a result, many authors have delineated characteristics of scholarly teachers

---

BOX 8-1   Evidence-Based Teaching Process

1. Formulate a question to study using STCO format:

   (S = Student/problem, T = Teaching strategy, C = Comparison, O = Outcome)

2. Search for best evidence

3. Integrate personal teaching expertise

4. Consider student characteristics, knowledge, values, and preferences

5. Implement educational change appropriate for the situation and institution

6. Evaluate outcomes in terms of student, faculty, or employer feedback, or measurable performance

Data from Emerson, R. J., & Records, K. (2007). Design and testing of classroom and clinical teaching evalua-tion tools for nursing education. *International Journal of Nursing Education Scholarship, 4*(1), p. 362.

(Box 8-2). These characteristics include knowledge, values, and skills that will enable the instructor to engage in scholarly teaching.

Scholarship of Teaching

Boyer (1990) defined scholarship of teaching as one of the four types of scholarship (i.e., teaching, application, integration, and discovery) as discussed in Chapter 1. Since that time there has been much discussion among educators about what consti-tutes scholarship of teaching and what make it distinct from scholarship and scholarly teaching. One distinction noted by Allen and Field (2005) is that the scholarship of teaching goes beyond scholarly teaching. Whereas scholarly teaching is concerned with implementing effective teaching practices and is therefore teacher-focused, the scholarship of teaching is learning-focused and seeks to understand the learning process and factors influencing learning. Allen and Field describe two components of the scholarship of teaching; one involves the development of creative learning mate-rials that are disseminated to a broader audience than the teacher's own classroom. The second aspect involves study and exploration of teaching, learning, curriculum, and/or evaluation practices that are disseminated widely through publication and pro-fessional presentations. Richlin and Cox (2004) add to the definition, noting that scholarship of teaching is an aspect of scholarship that involves contributing to the discipline's knowledge base.

BOX 8-2 Characteristics of Scholarly Teachers

1. Demonstrates knowledge of the discipline and knowledge of teaching and learning

2. Sets clear teaching and learner goals

3. Tends to be learner- and learning outcome-focused

4. Consults the literature on the design, implementation, and evaluation of teaching strategies

5. Selects and effectively applies appropriate information from the literature to the teaching setting

6. Values peer consultation on instructional matters

7. Modifies teaching approaches to meet changing needs and circumstances

8. Systematically evaluates of the effects of their teaching

9. Shares insights on effectiveness of teaching strategies with colleagues

10. Contributes to the program's overall curriculum effectiveness (i.e., design, development, on-going maintenance, and evaluation)

Data from Allen, M. N., & Field, P. A. (2005). Scholarly teaching and scholarship of teaching: Noting the difference. *International Journal of Nursing Education Scholarship, 2*(1), 1–14; Glassick, C. E., Huber, M. T., & Maeroff, G. L. (1997). *Evaluation of the professoriate.* San Francisco: Jossey Bass; and Richlin, L., & Cox, M. D. (2004). Developing scholarly teaching and the scholarship of teaching and learning through faculty learning communities. *New Directions for Teaching and Learning, 97,* 127–135.

Scholarship of Clinical Teaching

Most academics will agree that scholarship has value in terms of developing the knowledge base of the profession, enhancing the instructor's teaching practice, and enhancing student learning and scholarship. Unfortunately, scholarship of teaching is primarily perceived as synonymous with traditional classroom teaching. Although lecture is the dominate mode of instruction across disciplines, practice professions such as nursing rely heavily on clinical and practice laboratory instruction, which demand different approaches for demonstration of scholarship. Clinical scholarship has been defined as "an approach that enables evidence-based nursing and development of best practices to meet the needs of clients efficiently and effectively" (STTI, Clinical Scholarship Task Force, 1999, p. 4). According to the task force report, clinical scholars possess skills in systematic observation, problem solving, quality improvement, use, dissemination of current research, leadership, and consultation. In nursing programs, clinical teaching is an essential vehicle for demonstrating the scholarship of teaching and the scholarship of application.

Although the research literature on classroom teaching and distance teaching has grown over the years, little research on clinical teaching and what makes a clinical teacher effective is available. Scanlan (2001) explored the concept of clinical teaching by conducting interviews and reviewing journals and concept maps of five novice and five expert clinical teachers. Participants were asked about factors that influenced their clinical teaching practices, how they learned to do clinical teaching, and changes they have made in their teaching over time. Novice teachers reported learning clinical teaching skills primarily on the job, by trial and error. "They use cognitive processes such as reflection, intuition, problem solving, and hypothesizing, as aids in understanding their clinical teaching experiences. They sometimes consulted the literature or attended conferences or workshops and used intangible processes that they believed contributed to the development of clinical teaching expertise" (p. 243). Although it is not clear from the report whether the clinical faculty had formal educational preparation in the nurse educator role, the findings provide a glimpse into the processes clinical teachers use to develop the scholarship of clinical teaching.

Spath (2007) sees the lack of agreement in terminology as crucial to the development of the profession. "Without conceptual clarity and subsequent operationalized application of these terms, tenure and promotion criteria may be misguided, the development of a quality professoriate may be impaired, research supporting educational science may be jeopardized or monopolized, and defining what constitutes teaching quality may be ambiguous" (p. 235). Therefore it is important that each academic institution clarify the meaning of terms so that scholarship within the institution can be fully realized and valued.

THEORY AND RESEARCH RELATED TO COMPETENCY

In this section, theoretical models and strategies to enhance the knowledge and skills needed for scholarship are explored. Strategies are identified that can be used by the program or institution as a whole or by individual faculty. Components of grant writing and dissemination of scholarly findings are reviewed.

Models For Fostering Scholarship

This section includes a review of two models for fostering scholarship that have been implemented at the program or institutional level: Boyer's Model of Scholarship and a modification of Boyer's model called the Pillars of Scholarship.

Boyer's Model of Scholarship

Boyer's (1990) Model of Scholarship has been adopted by many nursing programs across the United States and internationally to classify and guide scholarly activity. Boyer's four categories of scholarship (i.e., the scholarship of teaching, application, integration, and discovery) were addressed earlier in this chapter and introduced in Chapter 1. Boyer's model has had tremendous influence on the perspective of scholarship held by institutions and faculty alike. Along with a broader definition of scholarship have come greater expectations for scholarly activity.

Boyer's Model of Scholarship has expanded the view of scholarship as primarily conducting research and publishing to include other activities that generate and apply new knowledge. Using Boyer's terminology, the scholarship of discovery, which involves conducting research and disseminating findings, is recognized as only one of four categories of scholarship. The other three categories of scholarship (application, integration, and teaching) emphasize the educator's ability to interact with new knowledge and make it useful to a wider audience.

Pillars of Scholarship Model

Nursing programs vary in the types of resources, administrative support, and faculty expertise available and thereby vary in the emphasis given to each of the four types of scholarship outlined by Boyer (1990). Stull and Lants (2005), two faculty from a nonresearch-intensive institution, conceptualized scholarship as a Parthenon-like structure in which each type of scholarship (discovery, application, integration, and teaching) serves as a pillar for scholarship in general. They redefined Boyer's terms to create a more holistic perspective of scholarship that is more inclusive of the activities and processes of faculty at a nonresearch-intensive environment. They viewed the scholarship of discovery as a life-long process that involves inquiry into a topic to "validate and refine existing knowledge and/or generate new knowledge" (p. 495). Using this perspective, activities such as writing evidence-based manuscripts and giving evidence-based presentations are included. They redefined the scholarship of application as the "reflective interaction of current nursing knowledge, theory, and practice from which new understandings can occur" (p. 495). The scholarship of teaching was redefined as "a creative process that evolves constructing environments that support student and faculty engagement in learning" (p. 495). Elements of teaching such as course revision and coordination, role modeling, using evidence-based teaching strategies, self-reflection, and dissemination of teaching-learning methods were included within this definition. The final pillar, the scholarship of integration, was defined as a "holistic synthesis of knowledge that incorporates and promotes interdisciplinary and collaborative relationships" (p. 495). Activities such as consulting, performing integrative reviews of the literature, promoting interdisciplinary practices and projects, and reviewing and critiquing research, are examples of the scholarship of integration. Within these definitions, faculty were able to develop a workable perspective of scholarship that was congruent with the mission and resources of a nonresearch intensive institution.

Program and Institutional Strategies for Enhancing Scholarship

Boyer's Model of Scholarship has served to expand our concept of scholarship and bring expectations of scholarship to the forefront of academia. To address the growing expectations for scholarship, Cash and Tate (2008) and Lansang and Dennis (2004) identified several approaches for developing scholarship capacity and the strengths and weaknesses of each approach (Table 8-1). One approach is to provide advanced academic preparation for faculty. Disadvantages of this approach include the cost and time. Obtaining an advanced degree is expensive, especially when instituted for an entire department. In addition, it takes a significant amount of time for all faculty to get the desired training. Another approach is the use of research mentors. This can be more cost effective; however, there may not be a sufficient number of local mentors to accommodate the needs of all faculty members. A third approach is to create a center for research, which typically provides research leadership in specific areas. Cash and Tate (2008) note that research centers may not be flexible enough to accommodate large numbers of faculty or those with diverse research interests. A fourth approach is to develop partnerships that link together people who have diverse experiences and knowledge to create a scholarly project (Lansang & Dennis, 2004). The advantages of this approach are the inclusion of a large number of teachers and the use of the individual's strengths in the research project. Additional advantages are the limited costs involved and the relatively short time needed to establish partnerships. A fifth approach, referred to as the blended approach, combines several strategies to provide a comprehensive program for developing faculty scholarship. An example of the blended approach called the nurse educator scholarship project is described later in this next section.

Evidence-Based Nursing Committee

Strategies for promoting scholarship in clinical settings have been utilized that may be transferable to academic nursing programs. For example, Mohide and Coker (2005) describe the development of an evidence-based nursing committee to foster

TABLE 8-1   Approaches for Fostering Scholarship in Nursing Programs

Approach	Benefits	Drawbacks
1. Advanced academic preparation of faculty (i.e., grantsmanship or specific research preparation)	• Advanced knowledge base is established	• Expensive • Length of time to acquire preparation • Faculty may still need experience
2. Connect with research mentors	• One-to-one relationship is established • Minimal expense	• Limited number of mentors • Need to match mentors to interests and needs of individual faculty
3. Create a center for research	• Provides a formal structure • Provides visibility and marketability	• May lack flexibility in dealing with diverse research interests or large numbers of faculty • Requires in-house experts, development time, and administrative support
4. Research partnerships with institutions and agencies in the community	• Uses expertise of individual faculty from the community • Potential to involve large numbers of faculty	• Time commitment for initial development • Coordination with multiple agencies • Establishing a mutually agreeable infrastructure
5. Blended approach	• Approaches can be combined and tailored to meet the institution's needs	• Variable depending upon the approaches used

Data from Cash, P., & Tate, B. (2008). Creating a community of scholars: Using a community development approach to foster scholarship with nursing faculty. *International Journal of Nursing Education Scholarship, 5*(1), Art 6, 22 p; and Lansang, M. A., & Dennis, R. (2004). Building capacity in health research in the developing world. *Bulletin of the World Health Organisation, 82*, 764–770.

evidence-based changes in clinical practices. Initially, the committee focused on familiarizing the members with the processes used in evidence-based practice. They established a mission statement, identified responsibilities of the committee, and articulated an evidence-based nursing (EBN) model for implementing change. Once these tasks were completed, the committee began utilizing the EBN model to determine areas in need of change, and began identifying and evaluating the literature (Box 8-3). The committee used abstraction journals, such as *Evidence-Based Nursing*, that provided balanced reviews to help the members decide about the appropriateness of applying the findings to the current situation. In nursing education settings, a similar process could be utilized to explore scholarly solutions to educational issues.

Research Advisory Committee

The majority of nursing programs are not based in research-intensive institutions, and as a result, they need to develop organizational structures and processes that fit the unique scholarship abilities and needs of the faculty and institution. One approach discussed by Howland *et al.* (2008) is the formation of a departmental Research Advisory Committee (RAC). The RAC was structured as a standing committee composed of externally funded faculty, the PhD program director, and eventually an Associate Dean for Research and a staff member. Activities of the RAC included conducting a survey of faculty research interests, developing grant proposal guidelines and processes for engaging in mock grant reviews, developing a visiting scholar program, obtaining external consultants, and establishing mentors within the institution.

One of the key activities of the RAC was conducting mock grant reviews prior to submission for external funding. After instituting the mock review process, Howland *et al.* (2008), reported a 79% increase in the number of funded proposals. Witnessing the success of the RAC helped administrators justify the addition of an Associate Dean for Research and a grant coordinator, who were able to provide expertise, guid-

---

BOX 8-3   Evidence-based Nursing Process for Implementing Change

1. Assess need for change

2. Ask a research question

3. Synthesize the literature

4. Design a change in practice

5. Implement change

6. Evaluate effectiveness

7. Return to step 1

Data from Mohide, E. A., & Coker, E. (2005). Toward clinical scholarship: Promoting evidence-based practice in the clinical setting. *Journal of Professional Nursing, 21*(6), 375.

ance, and consultation. The RAC experiences described by Howland and colleagues may provide guidance and ideas for other faculty seeking to enhance scholarship within their nursing programs.

Nurse Educator Scholarship Project

Cash and Tate (2008) describe the establishment of a community development project that used a blended approach by combining mentoring, education, partnerships, and the establishment of formal structures for fostering scholarship. The Nurse Educator Scholarship Project (NESP) involved the collaboration of 400 nursing faculty from 12 colleges and universities and was designed to move faculty from an emphasis on teaching and service to one of teaching, service, and scholarship. Cash and Tate utilized a community development approach to create a community of scholars who worked together on scholarly projects to better the community. Central components in the community development approach included the creation of scholarship committees at each institution and the formation of an advisory committee consisting of one representative from each institution. Workshops were offered at each institution to foster the research development of the faculty. Interaction and relationships were facilitated by establishing mentoring opportunities, providing joint workshops, and teleconferences. An annual colloquium was conducted, which provided the opportunity to brainstorm about scholarly ideas and develop group research projects. By the end of the second year of the NESP, 58 faculty members were engaged in a total of six cross-site scholarly projects. As a result of the collaboration, the NESP faculty reported a growing appreciation for scholarship. The colloquia and participation on scholarly project teams that evolved from the colloquia, were crucial factors in the development of a community of scholars.

Individual Strategies for Fostering Scholarship

There are numerous options the ANE can utilize to foster the development of a program of scholarship. Several of the approaches mentioned in Table 8-1 can be instituted effectively on an individual level as well as an institutional level. These include seeking specialized training such as postdoctorate or specialized education in grant writing, or seeking career development grants. Another approach is for the ANE to find a mentor. Faculty who have little experience in research/scholarship will benefit from establishing mentoring relationships with successful researchers or building a cadre of research colleagues within the nursing program or university. In addition, Nolan *et al.* (2008) provide ideas that faculty may implement on an individual level

---

BOX 8-4 Individual Strategies for Enhancing Scholarship

Faculty Enrolled in Graduate School:

1. Obtain a research assistantship position

2. Consider the manuscript option in lieu of a dissertation, if available

3. Allot time to write and submit a manuscript while in school

Newly Degreed Faculty:

1. Present an aspect of your thesis/dissertation at professional conferences

2. Convert presentations into publications

3. Collaborate with others on scholarly projects

4. Obtain internal funding for small projects and pilot studies that build a foundation for a larger study

5. Schedule time for scholarship activities

6. Develop grant writing and publishing skills by serving as a reviewer

Data from Nolan, M. T., Wenzel, J., Han, H., Allen, J. K., Paez, K. A., & Mock, V. (2008). Advancing a program of research within a nursing faculty role. *Journal of Professional Nursing, 24*(6), 364–370.

(Box 8-4). They emphasize working smarter in achieving scholarship goals by turning presentations into manuscripts and using the latest technologies to search literature databases and manage reference citations. They note that productive scholars often collaborate with a small group of colleagues who have similar research interests, to develop a research and publication team. Together the team members share responsibilities in obtaining grants, conducting research, and disseminating findings through presentations and publications.

The unique nature of each nursing program and the individual faculty teaching within those programs means that one approach for developing faculty scholarship will not likely be effective for all programs. The scholarly productivity of faculty is influenced by multiple factors including the institution's mission, type of program (associate, bachelors, masters, or doctoral), and the types of resources and support provided for faculty scholarship. Research-intensive programs, which typically provide baccalaureate through doctoral level education, have developed organizational structures and processes that facilitate scholarship. These include adequate space and equipment for research, and support personnel for statistical and grant writing consultation.

Action Research

In education, the term *action research* is viewed as research conducted by teachers about a teaching/learning issue or concern. Action research may encompass qualitative research methods such as self-study and critical inquiry of teaching practices and quantitative research about aspects of one's teaching practices. Although action research is a legitimate type of research, it is viewed by many as less rigorous than controlled quantitative designs. Cochran-Smith & Lytle (1990) debunk some of the misconceptions about the foundation of action research methodology and discuss standards for establishing rigor of teacher research.

Cochran-Smith & Lytle (1990) acknowledge that although the goal of action research may not be to generalize the findings to other populations, the findings may still be useful for teachers in other contexts. Unfortunately the lack of "generalizability has been used to discount the value of . . . research conducted by individual teachers and conducted in single classrooms" (p. 6). However, they note an important inconsistency in this argument. By definition, the ability to generalize research findings requires the findings to be context free, but in qualitative research methodology contextual influence is always valued. Therefore, applying generalizability criteria from a quantitative paradigm to qualitative research methodology that is context dependent is inappropriate.

Another discrepancy explored by Cochran-Smith & Lytle (1990) is the documentation and analysis of data. Action research actually uses forms of data collection and analysis similar to other qualitative approaches such as interviews, field notes, teaching materials, student assignments, and test scores. Like other forms of qualitative research, in action research, data analysis is often strengthened by triangulation of data in which one or more sources serve to validate the other. An aspect that is often challenged in action research is the researcher's point of view and potential bias in data collection and analysis. However, Cochran-Smith & Lytle point out that teachers who explore their own teaching practices, such as in action research, do so from an emic point of view that may be more insightful than a researcher who has no personal knowledge of the research context. They conclude that "teacher research has the potential to play a significant role" (p. 9) in education, provided the nature, strengths, and underpinnings are understood and valued within the institution.

Action research is a vehicle for faculty scholarship that also facilitates optimal student learning and effective teaching practice. Therefore, "The ultimate imperative facing nursing today" according to Emerson and Records (2007) "is the creation of a culture that values the practice of nursing education and expands evidence-based education through the design, testing, and refinement of education strategies from nursing and other disciplines" (p. 359). Self-study of teaching, which is discussed in the next section, is another viable form of action research and scholarly practice.

Self-Study as Scholarship

"In self–study research, faculty members study both themselves and the act of teaching, resulting in a clearer understanding of who they are as teachers" (Drevdahl, Stackman, Purdy, & Louie, 2002, p. 414). Reflection, which is the underlying process in self-study, has been a topic in educational literature since *How We Think* was published by Dewey (1910/1997). Later, the importance of self-reflection was popularized in the book, *The Reflective Practitioner* by Schon (1983). In a literature review by Drevdahl *et al.* (2002), collaborative self-study involving colleagues was found to improve curriculum and instruction (Munby, 1996) and improve the teacher's teaching practice (Zeichner, 1999). However, Drevdahl *et al.* explain that awareness about one's teaching is not enough; deliberate self-reflection that stems from planned and systematic processes is essential.

A model developed by Drevdahl *et al.* (2002) provide a systematic process for reflective self-study that consists of three phases; assessment, implementation, and dissemination (Box 8-5). During the assessment phase, the literature on the topic of concern is explored. Topics may include clinical evaluation practices, providing student feedback, or fostering critical thinking in students. In addition, the readiness of the teacher to engage in self-reflection, the collaboration environment, and resources are assessed. The implementation phase focuses on determining data collection and analysis methods and conducting data collection and analysis to achieve valid and reliable interpretations. A narrative methodology can be used in the form of analysis of critical incidents, autobiography, and life history; or data from questionnaires, journals, interviews, focus groups, or class assignments can be analyzed. Drevdahl *et al.* emphasize that whatever method of data collection is used, the teacher's "practices, activities, beliefs, and feelings must be documented carefully" (p. 417) as these provide a means for validating the data analysis. The dissemination phase is concerned with answering the question, "How do the research findings (i.e., self-study findings), add to the body of teaching knowledge?" Drevdahl encourages publication of self-study research that provides documentation of the processes used, reasons for data collection, analysis, and interpretation of findings.

The emergence of self-study as a legitimate form of scholarly activity has been credited to Joseph Schwab, an educator and scholar in teaching and curriculum (Clark & Erickson, 2004; Craig, 2008). The processes used in self-study involve self-reflection, thinking, a spirit of scholarly inquiry, and self-dialog about one's teaching practices and the beliefs underlying practice (Bailey, 2007; Chapman, n.d.; Smith, 2006). Smith further described the self-study process as one in which the teacher notices, names, and reframes experiences and observations about his or her teaching to derive insights that enhance teaching practice.

> **BOX 8-5   Model for Reflective Self-Study**
>
> - Assessment phase—Is this the right time to assess? Is the context right? Is support available?
>
> - Implementation phase—Are the data collection and analysis methods appropriate? Have measures been taken to enhance validity?
>
> - Dissemination phase—How can the findings be used to improve teaching practice? What additional questions stem from the findings?
>
> Data from Drevdahl, D. J., Stackman, R. W., Purdy, J. M., & Louie, B. Y. (2002). Merging reflective inquiry and self-study as a framework for enhancing the scholarship of teaching. *Journal of Nursing Education, 41*(9), 413–419.

Chapman (n.d.) notes that self-study is a process that "paves the way for understanding, deepening, and/or restructuring . . . [of one's] . . . thinking and teaching practice" (para. 11). She emphasizes that beliefs play a central role in self-study of teaching and learning by influencing the personal knowledge, dispositions, and actions of the teacher; and by changing beliefs and influencing the learning processes in the teaching environment. For more information about teacher self-study and other forms of action research please explore the teacher self-study resources provided in the resource section.

Critical Inquiry Process

Very little has been written about the cognitive processes the ANE engages in when conducting evaluation, or on the values and beliefs that influence judgments. To explore the scholarly teaching processes used in nursing education, Mahara & Jones (2005) conducted a critical inquiry case study of a teacher's thinking processes during clinical evaluation of students. The process incorporates critical inquiry, which is a useful skill when engaging in self-study of teaching.

Over a 6-week clinical rotation, one of the authors engaged in critical inquiry using a hand-held recorder and a "talking out loud" approach to record her evaluative thinking process (Mahara & Jones, 2005). The authors found that the faculty member gained greater awareness of actual teaching practices and identified discrepancies between values, beliefs, and actual practices. Increased awareness on the part of the faculty led to the initiation of several positive changes in teaching practice. The authors concluded that a critical inquiry process, in which a faculty member explores her or his own evaluative practices and the factors that influence those practices, is beneficial.

Grantsmanship

Developing skill in grantsmanship is necessary when developing research studies that will require funding for implementation and dissemination in the form of equipment, personnel, supplies, or travel. Grantsmanship involves matching the goals and objectives of a research proposal to the goals and mission of a funding agency. The grant writer develops a well-designed research proposal that clearly describes how the proposed study meets a crucial need and fits with the granting organization's goals.

Types of funding may be referred to as a grant, contract, or award and may be sought from internal funding sources within the academic institution or from external funding sources such as foundations, professional organizations, and governmental agencies. Funding may be sought for research, project development, or teaching and curricular initiatives. Institutions with a strong research focus typically offer faculty a variety of internal funding sources. In addition, they provide a centralized department for reviewing and approving research proposals, awarding grant funding, and processing expenditures for grants and contracts. In this section, the processes involved in grant writing are briefly reviewed.

Geever (2007), author of *The Foundation Center's Guide to Proposal Writing*, outlines the following steps in preparing a grant or contract proposal:

- Commit your ideas to paper
- Clearly describe your program
- State the goals and objectives of your program
- Construct a timeline
- Estimate costs for staff, materials, and equipment
- Plan the program evaluation
- Write job descriptions for program staff

The actual components of a written proposal are outlined in the request for proposals published by the granting institution. The components commonly required in a proposal are presented in Box 8-6. These consist of a statement of need; data supporting the need; clearly identified objectives for the project; a description of the project including timeline for completion; an evaluation plan; and a budget including supplies, equipment, and personnel needs. The Foundation Center (2009) recommends developing program objectives using the SMART acronym, which will help to ensure that the objectives are clear and can be readily evaluated. SMART objectives are:

1. Specific
2. Measurable
3. Achievable

BOX 8-6   Components of a Grant Proposal

1. Executive Summary

2. Statement of Need

3. Project Description

4. Budget

5. Organizational Information

6. Conclusion

Data from Foundation Center. (2009). *Proposal writing short course.* (p. 4). Retrieved from http://foundation center.org/getstarted/tutorials/shortcourse/.

---

4. Realistic
5. Time bound.

External grant proposals submitted to agencies outside the institution will typically require background information about the organization, identification of the resources and partnerships needed to support the project, and background on the members of the project team. An executive summary is often included, as it provides a concise overview of the project designed to convince the reader of the need for the project and the ability of the organization to oversee the project. The executive summary typically consists of a brief statement of the problem, description of the project and how it will solve the problem or meet the need, a summary of the organization that emphasizes its capacity to support the proposal, and a summary of budget requirements.

Dissemination of Knowledge

A key aspect of all research and project development should include plans for dissemination of findings so that others may benefit from the researcher's efforts. Many methods currently exist for dissemination of research findings (Box 8-7). Publication in refereed journals indicates that the manuscript has been peer reviewed and approved for publication by experts. Book format is a common way to present a synthesis of knowledge on specific topics, theoretical models, and research studies, (see Benner (1984), *From Novice to Expert*). Other venues for dissemination include presenting scholarly projects at professional conferences. Most conferences include opportunities for peer reviewed podium or poster presenta-

BOX 8-7	Methods of Dissemination of Scholarly Materials

1. Refereed journals (print and electronic)

2. Nonrefereed journals, magazines, and newsletters (print and electronic)

3. Books (print and electronic)

4. Conference presentations (local, regional, national, international; podium or poster)

5. Educational media (Websites, CDs, PowerPoint presentations, streaming videos, or podcasts)

6. News media (newspaper, radio, or TV interviews)

7. Local presentations (within the department, institution, or community agency)

8. Scholarly teaching—integrate research findings into course content

tions. In addition to these venues, dissemination can occur through refereed and nonrefereed journals, newsletters, nonpeer-reviewed conferences, and institutional or community presentations.

Technological advances have afforded multiple venues for dissemination. Electronic journals (both refereed and nonrefereed), books, and newsletters provide additional opportunities for publishing, often with shorter submission to publication times than print formats. CDs, Web sites, video streaming, podcasts, and blogs can be used to disseminate scholarly information, although these venues are not typically peer reviewed. Interviews with local news media can also be used to disseminate information to the public about a completed study or other scholarly project. And finally, the incorporation of research findings into one's teaching practice, referred to as scholarship of teaching, is a vehicle for dissemination.

Deciding on a dissemination format depends on multiple factors. The intended audience, such as peers, students, or the public, and the relevance of the project to either local, regional, national, or international audiences, are key factors. Scholarly materials that are perceived to be well designed, significant, or groundbreaking will be validated through the peer review process that is incorporated into refereed journals, as well as conference presentations and books that are reviewed by peers. The desired timeline for dissemination and the skills and expertise of the scholar also influence the choice of venue. Peer-reviewed print formats generally take the longest time from submission to publication, whereas conference presentations and media can generally be developed and disseminated in a shorter time frame.

Diffusion of Innovation Theory

As an educator engaged in scholarship, the ANE is both a producer of scholarly material and a consumer of scholarly information disseminated by others. In the book *Diffusion of Innovations*, Rogers (2003) describes how a new idea comes to be adopted by individuals in society. Diffusion refers to the process of adopting or integrating an innovation. An innovation is anything that is perceived as new such as new knowledge, conclusions from a review of literature, a description of a project implementation, or research findings. As consumers and producers of innovations, it is helpful to be aware of the processes described by the diffusion of innovation theory.

According to Rogers (2003), individuals in society follow a bell curve distribution in terms of their likelihood of adopting innovations (Box 8-8). At the far left of the curve are the innovators who are the first to adopt, followed by early adopters, early majority, late majority, laggards, and on the far right of the curve the persistent skeptics who fail to adopt innovations.

Robinson (2009) offers suggestions for dealing effectively with different types of adopters, which may be helpful in planning, implementing, marketing, and/or promoting certain innovations. Innovators are the earliest to buy into a new idea or concept, therefore they often make good partners in planning, and designing projects. The early adopters are described as networkers who are well connected. These adopters can also be valuable in early stages of project testing and getting the word out about the innovation. The next group of adopters is the early majority who tend to be pragmatic and need proof of benefits. They are more likely to adopt innovations that involve a minimal disruption of time and energy, and innovations that are easy to learn and implement. The late majority adopters tend to be more conservative and

---

BOX 8-8   Categories of Innovation Adopters

1. Innovators

2. Early adopters

3. Early majority

4. Late majority

5. Laggards

6. Persistent skeptics

Data from Rogers, E. M. (2003). *Diffusion of innovations*. New York: Free Press.

are adverse to the perceived risks of changing or adopting an innovation. This group will eventually adopt the innovation as they become convinced that it is becoming the standard. The last adopters are laggards and skeptics who see the disadvantages and risks of adopting a new innovation. When seeking to diffuse an innovation to this group, Robinson says it is helpful to let them see other laggards successfully adopting the innovation, or provide statistics on the numbers and types of people who have already adopted the change.

CONCLUSION

Boyer's (1990) conceptualization of scholarship as the scholarship of teaching, application, integration, and discovery, has broadened the scope of scholarly activity in academia. The ANE engages in individual strategies for fostering scholarship such as self-study of teaching and critical inquiry, grant writing, and dissemination of findings. The ANE may also engage in program wide strategies for enhancing scholarship such as research, evidence-based practice committees, and partnerships. Engaging in scholarship is essential for building knowledge related to teaching and nursing practice; and utilizing that knowledge in teaching, clinical practice, and service activities.

SUMMARY

- Competency 7 involves engaging in scholarship, which includes the processes of (1) critical thinking, (2) problem solving, and (3) dissemination.
- Boyer's model of scholarship identifies four types of scholarship, the scholarships of teaching, application, integration, and discovery.
- Scholarly teaching is focused on the application of teaching strategies, the teacher's reflection on teaching practices, and the incorporation of ideas from the literature into teaching practice.
- Scholarly teaching advances education at the individual student level.
- Scholarly teaching is concerned with implementing effective teaching practices and is therefore teacher-focused.
- The scholarly teacher utilizes knowledge of teaching and knowledge of the subject matter in educational practice.
- The scholarship of teaching is learning-focused and seeks to understand the learning process and factors influencing learning.

- The scholarships of teaching and learning are distinct aspects of scholarship that describe a type of research in which the processes of teaching and learning are explored, tested, and disseminated.
- Clinical scholars possess skills in systematic observation, problem solving, quality improvement, utilization and dissemination of current research, leadership, and consultation.
- Action research is conducted by teachers about a teaching/learning issue or concern.
- Rogers' diffusion of innovation theory identifies factors that influence the adoption of an innovation and characteristics of adopters and non adopters.

RECOMMENDED RESOURCES

Research Support

- American Nurses Foundation (ANF) is an arm of the American Nurses Association (ANA) that provides research grants to promote the welfare of nurses, advance nursing, and enhance health. Information on grant funding offered by the ANF is available at funding http://www.anfonline.org.
- Membership in the Midwest Nursing Research Association (MNRA) is open to nurses and students within the 13-state Midwest region and beyond. The organization offers research grants for dissertations and small pilot studies and provides a venue for presentation of research findings through an annual conference. Membership includes unlimited participation in over 25 research interest groups. For more information visit http://www.mnrs.org.
- The Southern Nursing Research Society (SNRA) membership encompasses nurses and students in 14 southern states and the Caribbean, Latin America, and the Bahamas. Membership includes a free, online journal and newsletter, and participation in research interest groups. Information is available at http://www.snrs.org/index.html.
- In 2000, the Council for the Advancement of Nursing Science was established as an offshoot of the American Academy of Nursing (AAN), to facilitate research policy and research opportunities. Council membership is open to all nurses wishing to support nursing science. For more information visit the Web site at http://www.nursingscience.org.

- The Association for the Study of Higher Education (ASHE) promotes collaboration among its members and others engaged in the study of higher education through research. Membership is open to faculty and graduate students at http://www.ashe.ws/.

Teacher Self-Study

- Faculty interested in Self-Study of Teacher Education Practices (S-STEP) can explore the S-STEP Special Interest Group of the American Educational Research Association housed at the Kansas University Web site at http://sstep.soe.ku.edu/.
- Queens University in Kingston, Ontario houses a repository of conference papers related to teacher self-study and action research at http://educ.queensu.ca/ar.html.
- A free, downloadable manual titled *Action Research in Workplace Education* is available at http://www.nald.ca/Clr/action/action.pdf.

Publications Related to Scholarship

- The American Association of Colleges of Nursing has published a position statement on the definition of scholarship in nursing, which is available at http://www.aacn.nche.edu/Publications/positions/scholar.htm. In addition, a position statement on nursing research is available at http://www.aacn.nche.edu/Publications/pdf/NsgResearch.pdf.
- Full text peer reviewed articles on the scholarship of teaching can be accessed through the Journal of the Scholarship of Teaching and Learning (JoSoTL) at http://www.iupui.edu/~josotl/.
- Fashioned after the Cochrane Collaboration for healthcare and medical research, the Campbell Collaboration is involved in preparing, maintaining, and disseminating systematic reviews in education, crime and justice, and social welfare. For information on conducting systematic reviews and searching the Review Library go to http://www.campbellcollaboration.org/systematic_reviews/index.php.
- Sigma Theta Tau International Honor Society for Nursing Web site at http://www.nursingsociety.org/default.aspx includes resource papers on clinical scholarship.

Multidisciplinary Organizations

- American Association of Higher Education and Accreditation, founded in 1870, is the oldest organization focused on higher education. Information on accreditation and access to selected articles from the *AAHE Bulletin* are available through the Web site at http://www.aahea.org.
- Association of American Colleges and Universities is concerned with promoting the quality of undergraduate liberal education. The Web site contains links to an informative newsletter, publications, podcasts, and more at http://www.aacu.org/.
- The Association of Institutional Research Web site at http://airweb.org/ contains extensive links to resources and offers a grant program for faculty and doctoral students.
- The Center for the Study of Higher Education (CSHE) is an intellectual community center for those interested in improving higher education policy and practice. CSHE was one of the first research centers established specifically to study postsecondary education policy issues. Visit http://www.ed.psu.edu/educ/cshe to find out more.
- The American Educational Research Association (AERA) promotes dissemination of educational research from all disciplines. The AERA offers grants, numerous referred publications, conferences, and free webcasts available at http://www.aera.net. Faculty who are members of AERA may nominate graduate students at the masters and doctoral level for membership at reduced membership fees.
- The American Association of University Professors (AAUP) provides faculty support and resources on issues concerning faculty role performance, research, and research ethics. Free access to the publication *Academe Online* is available at http://www.aaup.org.

Grant Writing

- The Grantsmanship Center Provides education and grant consultation. Free podcasts may be accessed at http://www.tgci.com.
- A to Z Grant Writing offers basic through advanced grant writing courses and a free newsletter containing links to funding sources at http://www.atozgrantwriting.com.
- The Foundation Center features free online training programs and free funding-related newsletters focused on health, education, and more available at

http://foundationcenter.org. Plus, search the Foundation's list of Cooperating Collections for funding information centers located in your area. Cooperating Collections provide a core collection of Foundation Center publications and a variety of supplementary materials for grant seekers.

* An audiobook version of *The Foundation Center's Guide to Proposal Writing* by Geever is available for free download at http://foundationcenter.org/getstarted/learnabout/audiobook.html.

REFERENCES

1. Allen, M. N., & Field, P. A. (2005). Scholarly teaching and scholarship of teaching: Noting the difference. *International Journal of Nursing Education Scholarship, 2*(1), 1–14.
2. Bailey, J. (2007). Mathematical investigations: A primary teacher educator's narrative journey of professional awareness. In J. Watson, & K. Beswick (Eds.), *Mathematics: Essential research, essential practice—Volume 1 (Proceedings of the 30th annual conference of the mathematics education research group of Australasia, Tasmania, Australia* (pp. 103–112). Sydney: MERGA Inc.
3. Benner, P. (1984). *From novice to expert. Excellence and power in clinical nursing practice.* Menlo Park, CA: Addison-Wesley.
4. Boyer, E. (1990). *Scholarship reconsidered: Priorities of the professoriate.* Princeton, NJ: The Carnegie Foundation for the Advancement of Teaching.
5. Cash, P., & Tate, B. (2008). Creating a community of scholars: Using a community development approach to foster scholarship with nursing faculty. *International Journal of Nursing Education Scholarship, 5*(1), Art 6, p. 22.
6. Chapman, O. (n.d.). Self-study in mathematics teacher education. Retrieved June 30th, 2009 from http://www.unige.ch/math/EnsMath/Rome2008/ALL/Papers/CHAPMAN.pdf.
7. Clark, A., & Erickson, G. (2004). Self-study: The fifth commonplace. *Australian Journal of Education, 48*(2), 199–211.
8. Cochran-Smith, M., & Lytle, S. L. (1990). Research on teaching and teacher research: The issues that divide. *Educational Researcher, 19,* 2–11.
9. Craig, C. (2008). Joseph Schwab, Self-study of teaching and teacher education practices proponent? A personal perspective. *Teaching and Teacher Education: An International Journal of Research and Studies, 24*(8), 1993–2001.
10. Dewey, J. (1910/1997). *How we think.* Mineola, NY: Dover Publishers.
11. Drevdahl, D. J., Stackman, R. W., Purdy, J. M., & Louie, B. Y. (2002). Merging reflective inquiry and self-study as a framework for enhancing the scholarship of teaching. *Journal of Nursing Education, 41*(9), 413–419.
12. Emerson, R. J., & Records, K. (2007). Today's challenge, tomorrow's excellence: The practice of evidence based education. *Journal of Nursing Education, 47*(8), 359–370.
13. Foundation Center. (2009). *Proposal writing short course.* Retrieved May 10, 2009 from http://foundationcenter.org/getstarted/tutorials/shortcourse/.
14. Geever, J. C. (2007). *The foundation center's guide to proposal writing.* New York: The Foundation Center. Audiobook. Retrieved May 30, 2009 from http://foundationcenter.org/getstarted/learnabout/audiobook.html.

15. Glassick, C. E., Huber, M. T., & Maeroff, G. L. (1997). *Evaluation of the professoriate*. San Francisco, CA: Jossey Bass.

16. Howland, L., Sullivan-Bolyai, S., Bova, C., Klar, R., Harper, D., & Schilling, L. (2008). The research advisory committee: An effective forum for developing a research dynamic environment. *Journal of Professional Nursing, 24*(4), 241–245.

17. Hutchings, P. (2001–2002). Reflections on the scholarship of teaching and learning. *Teaching Excellence: Toward the Best in the Academy, 13*(5), 1–2.

18. Kreber, C. (2003). Teaching excellence, teaching expertise, and the scholarship of teaching, *Innovative Higher Education, 27*, 5–23.

19. Lansang, M. A., & Dennis, R. (2004). Building capacity in health research in the developing world. *Bulletin of the World Health Organisation, 82*, 764–770.

20. Mahara, M., & Jones, J. (2005). Participatory inquiry with a colleague: An innovative faculty development process. *Journal of Nursing Education, 44*(3), 124–130.

21. Mohide, E. A., & Coker, E. (2005). Toward clinical scholarship: Promoting evidence-based practice in the clinical setting. *Journal of Professional Nursing, 21*(6), 372–379.

22. Munby, H. (1996). Being taught by my teaching: Self-study in the realm of educational computing. In J. Richards, & T. Russell (Eds.), *Proceedings of the First International Conference on Self-study of Teacher Education Practices* (pp. 62–66). Kingston, Ontario, Canada: Self-study of Teacher Education Practices Special Interest Group of the American Educational Research Association.

23. National League for Nursing, Task Group on Nurse Educator Competencies. (2005). *Core competencies of nurse educators with task statements*. Retrieved September 10, 2008 from http://www.nln.org/facultydevelopment/pdf/corecompetencies.pdf.

24. Nicholls, G. (2004). Scholarship in teaching as a core professional value: What does this mean to the academic? *Teaching in Higher Education, 9*(1), 29–42.

25. Nolan, M. T., Wenzel, J., Han, H., Allen, J. K., Paez, K. A., & Mock, V. (2008). Advancing a program of research within a nursing faculty role. *Journal of Professional Nursing, 24*(6), 364–370.

26. Richlin, L., & Cox, M. D. (2004). Developing scholarly teaching and the scholarship of teaching and learning through faculty learning communities. *New Directions for Teaching and Learning, 97*, 127–135.

27. Robinson, L. (2009). *Summary of diffusion of innovations theory*. Retrieved on March 12, 2009 from http://www.enablingchange.com.au/Summary_Diffusion_Theory.pdf.

28. Rogers, E. M. (2003). *Diffusion of innovations*. New York: Free Press.

29. Scanlan, J. M. (2001). Learning clinical teaching: Is it magic? *Nursing and Health Care Perspectives, 22*(5), 240–246.

30. Schon, D. A. (1983). *The reflective practitioner*. New York: Basic Books.

31. Smith, T. (2006). Self-study through narrative inquiry: Fostering identity in mathematics teacher education. In P. Grootenboer, R. Zevenbergen, & M. Chinnappan (Eds.), *Identities, cultures and learning spaces. (Proceedings of the 29th annual conference of the mathematics research group of Australasia, Canberra)*. (pp. 471–478). Sydney: MERGA. Retrieved June 30, 2009 from http://www.merga.net.au/documents/RP542006.pdf.

32. Spath, M. L. (2007). A need for clarity: Scholarship, scholarly teaching, and the scholarship of teaching and learning. *Nursing Educational Perspectives, 28*, 235–236.

33. STTI, Clinical Scholarship Task Force. (1999). *Clinical scholarship resource paper.* Retrieved February 9, 2009 from http://www.nursingsociety.org/aboutus/PositionPapers/Documents/clinical_scholarship_paper.pdf.
34. Stull, A., & Lants, C. (2005). An innovative model for nursing scholarship. *Journal of Nursing Education, 44*(11), 493–497.
35. Zeichner, K. (1999). The new scholarship in teacher education. *Educational Researcher, 28*(9), 4–15.

CHAPTER 9

Function Within the Educational Environment—Competency 8

OBJECTIVES

1. Recognize current and historical factors that influence nursing education and higher education in general.
2. Explore strategies and collaborative initiatives that enhance the functioning of the nursing program.
3. Identify personal and organizational attributes that enhance development of faculty, students, and the academic community.
4. Identify processes and strategies used in political advocacy for nursing education.
5. Explore the development and implementation of leadership roles in the academic community.

KEY TERMS

Advocacy	Mentoring
Faculty review committee	Organizational climate
Global flattening	Political advocacy
Institutional governance	Tenure

DEFINITION AND DESCRIPTION OF COMPETENCY

Competency 8 calls for the academic nurse educator (ANE) to "function within the educational environment" (NLN Task Group on Nurse Educator Competencies, 2005, p. 8). The NLN has identified eight task statements that delineate the ANE's functioning within the educational environment. These tasks reflect skills and processes used to operationalize the goals, mission, and philosophy of the program and institution. A key factor is to understand the context in which the organization and program operate. This includes the social, economic, political and institutional history, and trends that impact nursing and education. The task statements also call for the ANE to set professional goals that are in alignment with the program and the academic community goals. These tasks require the ANE to understand the context in which the nursing program and the educational organization operate. The ANE uses leadership, change, and advocacy skills (see Chapter 6) to operationalize the goals, mission, and philosophy within the institution's organizational structure.

THEORY AND RESEARCH RELATED TO COMPETENCY

To function effectively within the educational environment requires the ANE to appreciate many factors and interrelationships that affect the individual faculty member, the program, and the institution as a whole. As depicted in Figure 9-1, factors influencing functioning within academia include past and current social, economic, political, and technological trends. These past and current trends influence the organizational climate, institutional governance practices, policy development, political advocacy, and faculty mentoring practices. Understanding the influences of these trends and factors can facilitate smooth transitioning of new faculty to the faculty role and enable seasoned faculty to effectively contribute to the ongoing development of students, and the achievement of institutional and program goals.

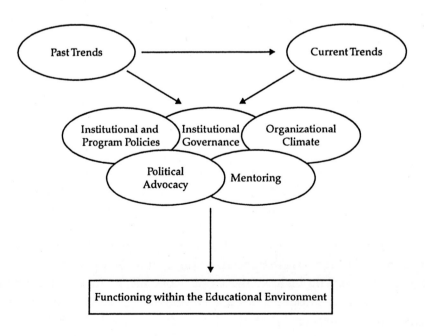

FIGURE 9-1   Factors Influencing Functioning Within the Educational Environment

Educational Trends

To a large extent educational trends that impact the role of the ANE reflect the changes we see in society in general. In 1994, Oermann predicted that healthcare reform, changing demographics, greater emphasis on health promotion, increasing healthcare costs, a focus on community-based care, and technology would be factors influencing health care and nursing education. Nursing education is now in the midst of these influences. The ability to anticipate and respond to these changes involves adjusting teaching, scholarship, and service activities to meet emerging needs.

Over the past several decades, rapid technological developments have affected how nurses practice clinically, how ANEs teach, and the geographical limits of education have been expanded. The growing number of older adults, combined with changes in healthcare reimbursement, and the increased cost of health care, have produced a hospital environment where patients are more acutely ill and experience shorter hospital stays. More people are returning to their communities to recuperate from surgery and illness, placing more emphasis on health care in the communities where people live. These changes affect the clinical learning environment and increase the complexity of patient care. As a result, there are higher expectations for critical thinking skills, ethical decision-making, competence, and accountability for health care than in the past. In addition to changes in population age distribution, exposure to individuals from diverse ethnic and racial backgrounds is increasing, demanding a culturally competent workforce.

As a result of these trends, what should be taught in nursing programs and where nursing students are receiving clinical education is changing. Expectations of what should be taught in nursing programs are being redefined by changes in society, technology, and shifting demographics. For example, national level curriculum initiatives are being developed and supported by professional nursing organizations, ANEs, and nurse researchers. Notable examples include recently published competencies in nursing informatics (Staggers, Gassert & Curran, 2001), genetics (National Coalition for Health Professional Education in Genetics, 2007), geriatrics (American Association of Colleges of Nursing & The John A. Hartford Foundation Institute for Geriatric Nursing, 2005), and culture in nursing education (American Association of Colleges of Nursing, 2008). These initiatives represent the growing expectation of competence in specific content areas deemed essential because of changing societal trends.

Increased patient acuity and rapid turnover of patients in the hospital setting make it more difficult to assure that all nursing students will acquire skills and experiences in caring for specific types of patients. As a result, nursing programs are incorporating more experiences in the practice laboratory and clinical simulation settings. Such experiences have an additional benefit in that they help ensure that students have minimal competence before entering the clinical setting. Nursing programs are also incorporating more learning experiences outside of acute care settings such as service-learning and community-based practicums to address the need to care for people where they live.

Accountability

More than ever before, ANEs and their students are being held accountable for meeting specific knowledge and performance standards. In today's increasingly fast-paced and complex healthcare system, it is vital that healthcare providers have certain knowledge and skill sets prior to assuming patient care responsibilities. In nursing education, this means that students and faculty are often required by clinical agencies to attend lengthy orientation programs and engage in performance checks to validate meeting established standards prior to entering the clinical setting. In many cases "on the job training" is no longer acceptable practice for learning to use common clinical technologies such as glucometers, intravenous infusion systems, and patient controlled analgesia pumps. Likewise, students and faculty are expected to have knowledge of how to utilize the institution's computerized documentation, medical records systems, and medication administration systems; implement HIPAA; infection control practices; and more.

Adherence to performance standards provides a reference point, or a basis for comparison, and facilitates achievement of a greater degree of excellence. One way to ensure adherence to minimal performance standards is to require faculty and students to complete agency-specific training sessions, tutorials, and orientation sessions. Meeting the specific training requirements of each clinical agency can be cumbersome, especially for nursing programs that use multiple clinical agencies. However, one benefit is that meeting established standards can help control costs and maintain the quality of health care in the long run (Seok, 2007). Adherence to standards also enhances efficiency by enabling smoother operations and allows "greater interoperability between systems" (p. 388).

One of the most far-reaching trends in education is the impact of educational technology. Technology has provided new opportunities for teaching strategies through the use of synchronous and asynchronous modalities, course management software, social networking, and more. Technology has expanded the ways learners receive information and feedback, interact with other learners, and communicate with faculty. In addition, technology has enabled courses to be offered outside the campus grounds to distant geographic locations. Additional information on the trends in educational technology is presented in Chapter 2.

Community and Educational Partnerships

Oermann (1994) also predicted that the healthcare system of the future would be more community oriented, with patients being discharged from hospitals much earlier than in the past, resulting in the need to continue receiving complex health care while at home. Thus, more acute and complex patient care opportunities now exist in homes, schools, shelters, outpatient clinics, long-term care facilities, day care centers, and other facilities. Many nursing education programs are partnering with these agencies to provide clinical experiences for students while meeting the needs of the agencies. Nurse-managed centers are another way that educational programs have established collaborative relationships with the community. Nurse-managed centers provide benefits to the community and to the nursing program by (1) addressing the healthcare needs of clients in the community, (2) providing learning opportunities for students, and (3) providing a clinical practice site for faculty.

Orientation of New Faculty

The growing complexity of academic institutions and healthcare settings has led to the development of formalized programs for faculty orientation. A review of over 20 years of research on faculty orientation programs by Morin & Ashton (2004) found that effective orientation programs shared common characteristics. From the research, they developed five evidence-based guidelines for faculty orientation programs (Box 9-1).

The first recommendation is that orientation programs should occur over an extended period of time ranging from 1 month up to a year (Morin & Ashton, 2004). Extending orientation over an entire semester allows the new faculty to work through all stages of teaching from initial preparation for the first day, through mid-term, and through final evaluation and grading. Second, orientation programs should provide a foundation for acculturation into academia and should be built into the faculty's development plan. The faculty member's professional development plan should involve setting annual goals for professional development. Specific strategies to fulfill the goals, such as meeting regularly with a mentor and completing continuing education workshops, can be included in the plan.

A third recommendation for faculty orientation programs is to foster a sense of collegiality, which can reduce the stress experienced by new faculty (Morin &

> **BOX 9-1   Guidelines for Faculty Orientation Programs**
>
> 1. Provide prolonged orientation (1month to 1year)
>
> 2. Integrate orientation into the personal development plan
>
> 3. Provide a welcoming environment
>
> 4. Provide information about role and behavioral norms
>
> 5. Provide a mentor or resource person
>
> Data from Morin, K. H., & Ashton, K. C. (2004). Research on faculty orientation programs: Guidelines and directions for nurse educators. *Journal of Professional Nursing, 20*(4), 239–250.

Ashton, 2004). Fourth, providing information about the issues and expectations related to teaching, scholarship, and service can facilitate the faculty's immersion in these role functions. The fifth guideline includes identifying a resource person or mentor for new faculty. The mentor can serve as a resource for new faculty and can facilitate the realization of other guidelines. For example, mentoring can provide a mechanism for ongoing interaction and "orientation" by answering questions about teaching, scholarship, and service roles; thus extending the formal orientation beyond the initial classroom session. The mentor can also tailor the learning process to help meet the individual's development plan and provide the personal contact that creates an inviting, welcoming environment.

The recommendations outlined by Morin & Ashton (2004) stem from a review of research. Each recommendation is supported by an average of three or more studies at the third level of quality of evidence. Although this does not represent the highest possible level of evidence, it does represent a moderate degree of evidence, which can be used as a foundation for program development to enhance the functioning of new faculty in the academic setting.

Mentoring

A valuable component of an orientation program for new faculty is an effective mentoring program. Recognizing the stages of mentoring relationships is helpful in developing and monitoring the mentor/mentee relationship. Using the mentoring continuum from Johnson (2007), the mentoring dyad moves through the initiation, cultivation, separation, and redefinition stage. The cultivation stage is where the bulk of mentoring interaction occurs. During the redefinition stage the mentor and mentee decide if the relationship will progress to one based on friendship or mutual collegiality.

The Mentoring Process

During any point in the cultivation stage, the mentor and mentee maybe involved in one or more of the 10 essential elements of the mentoring process described by Dunham-Taylor *et al.* (2008) [Box 9-2]. These elements represent a continuum of developmental processes used to help the novice ANE acquire foundational knowledge, skills, values, and beliefs needed to function in academia.

Socialization represents a major element of faculty orientation. New faculty members need to be socialized to aspects of the academic and clinical settings, and to the specific courses that the mentee will be teaching. Socialization involves what Dunham-Taylor *et al.* (2008) refer to as macro and micro aspects. Macro aspects include familiarity with general teaching roles and campus-specific roles of various committees within the institution. Micro aspects involve familiarizing the mentee with program level aspects such as the nursing curriculum, policies, and individual faculty.

BOX 9-2   Elements of Effective Mentorship Programs

1. Socialization

2. Collaboration

3. Operations

4. Validation/evaluation

5. Expectations

6. Transformation

7. Reputation

8. Documentation

9. Generation

10. Perfection?

Data from Dunham-Taylor, J., Lynn, C. W., Moore, P., McDaniel, S., & Walker, J. K. (2008). What goes around comes around: Improving faculty retention through more effective mentoring. *Journal of Professional Nursing, 24*(6), 337–346.

Collaboration is another major element of faculty orientation. According to the research reviewed by Dunham-Taylor and colleagues (2008), collaboration with colleagues was found to help faculty feel more connected and less isolated. Mentors assist the new faculty in how to obtain needed information and how to work as team while also learning to function independently.

Understanding the operations of the institution and program is a common component in faculty orientation programs. Part of the mentor's task is to reinforce knowledge of policies and procedures that are essential to functioning in academia. Mentors also play a role in ensuring that new faculty know where to locate additional information and support, as needed. In addition to written policies and rules, most organizations have unwritten policies and procedures that the mentee will need to be informed of to function effectively. Therefore, the mentor plays an important role in providing knowledge related to unwritten day-to-day practices within the program.

Providing validation and feedback for new faculty is another important function of mentors. Offering timely feedback will allow new faculty to make corrective changes early in the teaching process. Feedback from the mentor about planned teaching activities can boost the new teacher's confidence in the appropriateness of the planned learning activities and may prevent mistakes, which can erode confidence.

The mentor also provides anticipatory guidance, encourages, inspires, and serves as a role model for the new faculty member. The expectation component of faculty mentoring programs involves providing anticipatory guidance. The mentor can guide new faculty in how to deal with busy times of the semester, and suggest advanced planning and organization that will help the new faculty balance the responsibilities of home and work, and avoid burnout. A related component involves providing advice concerning documentation. Teaching the mentee the importance of documenting student grades; interactions with students in clinical; and ongoing documentation of teaching, scholarship, and service activities for annual performance reviews can facilitate easy access to information when needed.

It is also beneficial for new faculty to be able to draw upon the experience of faculty members who have previously taught the same courses that the mentee is assigned to teach. The mentor can encourage sharing of teaching materials to conserve effort and provide a starting point for class preparation.

The final two components of the mentoring process—transformation and "perfection?"—are related. The transformation component of mentoring involves encouraging new faculty to use their skills and strengths and continue developing their teaching skills. It also involves monitoring for role transition from novice to expert teacher. During the orientation period for new faculty, the mentor is able to model appropriate behavior in terms of academic and community involvement. The "perfection?" component includes a question mark to emphasize the idea of continued improvement. "Perfection?" involves encouraging effective practices in teaching, scholarship, and service; and recognizing that because students, teaching practices, and health care continually change, the teacher needs to strive toward effective innovations rather than perfection.

When developing and implementing mentoring programs and serving as a mentor to novice faculty, attention to the components of a mentoring program described by Dunham-Taylor *et al* (2008) will ensure a comprehensive approach. Knowledge and information on dealing with institutional operations, generation of knowledge, and required documentation is foundational. It is also important to provide experiences to enhance role functioning through validation, feedback, and opportunities to connect, interact with, and observe other teachers. As the mentor and mentee engage in the processes of professional socialization, collaboration, and sharing expectations, the mentee is likely to acquire knowledge, confidence, and skills needed to function effectively within the academic environment. Dunham-Taylor and colleagues (2008) summed up the value of mentoring stating, "Mentorship can be the single most influential way to help in the successful development and retention of new nursing faculty" (p. 337).

Globalization and Educational Partnerships

The use of technology has affected how teachers teach, how learners acquire new knowledge and access course information. The use of technology has also enabled the ANE to more easily build educational and service partnerships with others outside the immediate local community. The enhanced ability to reach outside the classroom walls into distant communities is a result of the process of global flattening, which enables the delivery of curriculum without boundaries (Finkelman & Kenner, 2008).

In the book, *The World is Flat, A Brief History of the Twenty-First Century*, Friedman (2005), explores the concept of global flattening and identifies rules for working and flourishing in an evolving global environment (Box 9-3). Finkelman and Kenner (2008) specifically discuss how Friedman's rules are applied to nursing education and practice. The first rule reflects the need to accept rather than resist the changes in information technology and to effectively use technology. To a large extent nursing education has embraced technologically induced global flattening by expanding educational offerings using available technology and by supporting curricular changes to meet educational competencies. Several disciplines have developed competencies in the use of technology, including medicine (Committee on Educating Public Health

---

BOX 9-3   Friedman's Seven Rules for Global Working

1. When the world goes flat—and you are feeling flattened—reach for a shovel and dig inside. Don't try to build walls (p. 340).

2. The small shall act big by quickly taking advantage of tools for collaboration (p. 345).

3. The big shall act small by making the users feel connected and comfortable (p. 350).

4. The best organizations are the best collaborators (pp. 352–353).

5. The best organizations stay healthy by getting regular examinations (p. 356).

6. The best organizations outsource to win, not to shrink (p. 61).

7. Outsourcing isn't just for Benedict Arnolds. It's also for idealists (p. 61).

Data from Friedman, T. L. (2005). *The world is flat: A brief history of the twenty-first century*, NY: Farrar, Straus & Giroux.

Professionals for the 21st Century, 2003), public health (O'Carroll, 2002), and nursing (Health Resources Services Administration, 1997).

The second rule notes the ability of technology to expand collaboration and communication opportunities of individuals from smaller institutions, allowing the creation of partnerships at a distance. Rule number two encourages organizations to reach out and expand their boundaries by taking advantage of technologies that enable collaboration and partnerships. Finkelman and Kenner (2008) note that technology can equalize the playing field, allowing even smaller nursing programs to reach out and form distant educational and service partnerships.

Rule number three "And the big shall act small" is a clever way of expressing the value of the consumer and the importance of making individuals feel comfortable, connected, and in control, even in a large institution (Friedman, 2005). Business chains have learned this by offering services to individual communities through branch stores, which are directly accessible to local people. Educational institutions operating in the same fashion will be able to reach a wider market and will appeal to the consumer by reducing the feelings of distance and disconnection. For the ANE this translates into making an impersonal environment friendlier by providing direct and personalized communication, being open to inquiry, anticipating questions and individual needs, and promptly addressing questions and needs.

Friedman's (2005) fourth rule of working in a globalized environment recognizes the complexity of the environment and the processes that must be implemented to be successful. He points out that collaboration is necessary for success, in part, because of the increasing difficulty in acquiring and maintaining sufficient expertise in all required aspects of practice. In terms of collaboration, Finkelman and Kenner (2008) acknowledge that nursing practice has done a better job than education, citing administrative barriers such as determining course credit allocation, student enrollment, and headcount issues. Collaboration will allow educational institutions with a clear knowledge of their goals and strengths to be able to build relationships that will further enhance and strengthen the organization.

The fifth rule proposed by Friedman (2005) involves examining the performance of the organization and sharing the findings with the community as well as other institutions. In the age of digital technology, sharing what an institution has done in terms of processes and programs, and the results that have been achieved, can serve as exemplars to other institutions with far reaching effects. Finkelman and Kenner (2008) cite the importance of collecting data and sharing it in the form of report cards. The report card provides descriptive information about the program for the local and global community, and serves as a useful mechanism for reaching out to the community and distant populations.

According to rule number six, successful organizations will outsource not as a means to save money but because it is seen as a means for growth (Friedman, 2005). In education, outsourcing may take the form of establishing partnerships with other institutions, to sharing the teaching of a specific course, provide mentoring, and research consultation, all of which can be easily accomplished using technology.

Friedman's seventh rule involves finding solutions to existing challenges (2005). A central component of the rule involves the concept of outsourcing as a way to expand limited resources. Outsourcing involves contracting with individuals or services that are external to the institution to provide needed services. Generating "new ideas and making them work effectively by collaborating with others" is also part of the process. For example, technology can be used to provide nonlocal or retired faculty to teach specific subject matter. In summary, outsourcing may be viewed as simply finding new ways so solve old problems and enhance one's functioning in the educational environment.

Advocacy

Advocacy in nursing education is a process that requires educators to take an informed stance on an issue or concern with the goal of achieving support and affecting a desired change. Cohen, de la Vega, & Watson (2001) define advocacy as "the pursuit of influencing outcomes—including public policy and resources allocation decisions within political, economic, and social systems and institutions—that directly affect people's lives" . . . (p. 7). Advocacy is also defined as "the application of information and resources . . . to effect systematic changes" . . . (Christoffel, 2000, p. 722). When advocating for a cause, awareness of political influences that affect the institution can be extremely beneficial. Politics in this sense is understood as more than the art and science of government or using governmental procedures to affect legislative changes. Politics also refers to using influence and persuasion in relationships with others, to effect the desired change.

Often advocacy involves influencing existing proponents of policies or creating new policies that will help ensure the desired outcome is achieved. Christoffel (2000) outlined the processes in advocacy that generally occur at any level or type of advocacy (Box 9-4).

The public policy process follows a four stage model of agenda setting, adoption, implementation, and evaluation (Hall-Long, 2009). Agenda setting involves discussion and exploration of problems. Exploring the issue from the perspectives of those who will potentially be affected is a crucial part of this stage and will provide a foundation for generating a strong and well thought out policy.

The second stage, referred to as policy adoption and formulation, involves analysis of information collected, policy development, and advocacy for the proposed policy change. This stage can involve negotiation processes, developing alternative versions of a policy, and the process of developing proposals for legislative approval.

In the third stage, the policy is implemented and moves from "policy to program" (Hall-Long, 2009, p. 2). This stage involves planning, acquiring resources, develop-

---

BOX 9-4   The Advocacy Prosess

1. Identify the problem

2. Research the problem and all potential solutions

3. Select the best solution

4. Determine those who can affect desired change

5. Inform and educate others about the problem and solution

6. Assist with policy development, implementation, and monitoring as necessary

Data from Christoffel, K. K. (2000). Public health advocacy: Process and product. *American Journal of Public Health, 90*(5), 723.

ing guidelines, and developing program evaluation criteria. As with the previous stages, cultivation of relationships with community partners, stakeholders, and leaders in education and health care will smooth the implementation stage.

The final stage of the policy development process involves evaluation. However, evaluation findings hinge on the policy being properly and completely implemented. To make certain that accurate evaluation findings are obtained, it is first necessary to ensure that implementation of the policy is monitored. The evaluation criteria developed in the previous stage are used to determine if the policy is achieving the intended goals and outcomes. Based on the evaluation findings, further modifications or policy adjustments may be needed.

Leadership in Institutional Governance

One of the key aspects of functioning in an educational environment involves participating in the process of institutional governance. Each institution of higher education is comprised of a unique body of faculty, administrators, and students; therefore each has a unique organizational structure and climate. Yet there are commonalities between academic institutions in terms of organizational processes, which can be useful for faculty serving on academic committees.

In his book, *Serving on Promotion, Tenure, and Faculty Review Committees*, Diamond (2002) identifies four types of faculty review committees along with general principles that can be helpful for faculty who serve on these committees. Common academic committees include: (1) promotion, (2) tenure, (3) post-tenure, and (4) contract renewal or reappointment. Diamond notes that, "While the focus of these committees is somewhat different, the questions that are asked, much of the data that is collected, and the need for a high quality and equitable process is fairly consistent" (p. xiii).

Diamond outlines general principles and considerations that can be helpful for faculty serving on faculty review committees (Box 9-5). The first principle is concerned with the diverse perspectives of the committee members. Each of us, says Diamond, "brings to any committee on which we serve the vocabulary, traditions, and perception of our own discipline" (2002, p. 3). Our perspectives and values become especially important when serving on committees in which we are evaluating the works of faculty outside of our discipline, or even when evaluating nursing faculty who practice within a specialty different from our own. Therefore, it is important to be sensitive and aware of the perspectives of the reviewing body.

In the second principle, Diamond emphasizes that technology has a major impact on all aspects of academia including how teachers teach and how teachers engage in

---

BOX 9-5   Principles for Serving on Faculty Review Committees

1. Be sensitive to the interdisciplinary perspective of the committee members and the faculty being reviewed.

2. Be aware of the impact of technology on the roles of individual faculty.

3. Recognize the influence of common assumptions about teaching that are not supported by research.

4. Inform faculty of the review process and expectations well in advance of the review.

5. Document the processes used, the data collected, and the rationale for decisions.

Data from Diamond, R. M. (2002). *Serving on promotion, tenure, and faulty review committees: A faculty guide.* (2nd ed., pp. 3–8). Bolton, MA: Anker.

---

scholarly activities and service. Therefore it is important for the committee to know what the expectations are for individual faculty in terms of using technology and maintaining competence in the use of technology.

Third, Diamond cautions committee members to be aware of their assumptions about teaching and research, which may not be applicable across disciplines and specialties (2002). During the review process, faculty should identify the myths that commonly underlie perceptions and influence the values placed on research productivity and teaching effectiveness. One common myth reported by Terenzini and Pascarella (1994), after a review of over 2600 published manuscripts, is that "good researchers are good teachers" (p. 30). Attempts to bring such assumptions to the forefront can facilitate effective faculty review processes and enhance functioning in the academic environment.

The fourth principle involves providing clear guidelines for faculty who will be reviewed, well in advance of the review. Failure to provide the review guidelines or failure to provide a sufficient timeline for faculty to collect data to validate their performance can result in decisions being made based on insufficient or incomplete data. Because faculty welfare and livelihood can be affected by the decisions reached by the review committee, members should ensure that faculty members are informed of the process and the expectations. Diamond (2002) specifically recommends that the faculty be informed of: (1) the types of documents to be submitted, (2) the steps or processes that will be used by the committee, (3) the evaluation criteria for teaching, scholarship, and service that will be used, and (4) how the activities in these areas will be weighted. Depending upon the type of review, the faculty member may need to collect data over a sustained period of time. To ensure fairness and soundness of decisions, it is crucial to assure that decisions are based on factual evidence that has been evaluated fairly. Consideration of the first three principles will also help assure fairness and objectivity.

A final consideration is reflected in principle five, which directs the committee to document the processes used and the data analyzed (Diamond, 2002). This may be accomplished though committee minutes, written recommendations by the committee for individual faculty who have been reviewed, and through anecdotal notes by individual committee members. The documentation process helps validate that the review was conducted in an impartial and consistent manner for all faculty.

CONCLUSION

Functioning within the educational environment is the final competency, which integrates the others. Effective functioning involves understanding of educational trends such as globalization, and awareness of how these trends influence the institution and individual teaching practices. The ANE assumes accountability and works to establish effective partnerships within the community and the institution. Effective functioning is based on a foundation of adequate preparation that is enhanced by orientation and mentoring of new faculty. Experienced faculty may participate in the mentoring process as either a mentor or as a mentee, as needed for professional growth. They may also engage in leadership and advocacy processes to ensure that effective functioning is maintained.

SUMMARY

- Competency eight is delineated by eight task statements that reflect skills and processes needed to operationalize the institution's goals, mission, and philosophy.
- Competency eight requires the ANE to understand the context of the program and institution, and use teaching, technology, leadership, change, and political advocacy skills.
- Political advocacy involves influencing proponents of existing policies or creating new policies to achieve desired change.

- Understanding past and current trends in health care and education, as well as the organizational climate, institutional governance structure, processes, and policies can facilitate smooth transitioning of new faculty to the faculty role.
- Healthcare reform, changing demographics, greater emphasis on health promotion, increasing healthcare costs, and a focus on community-based care and technology are major factors influencing health care and nursing education.
- Evidence-based guidelines for faculty orientation programs include: (1) extend orientation over 1 month to 1 year; (2) integrate orientation into the faculty members development plan; (3) foster a sense of collegiality; (4) provide information on issues and expectations in teaching, scholarship, and service; and (5) provide a mentor or resource person.
- Essential elements of the mentoring process include attending to socialization, collaboration, operations, validation, expectations, transformation, reputation, documentation, generation, and perfection aspects (Dunham-Taylor and colleagues, 2008).
- Four types of faculty review committees include promotion, tenure, post-tenure, and contract renewal or reappointment.
- All faculty review committees require collection of similar types of data that document effectiveness in teaching, scholarship, and service.
- Guiding principles for serving on faculty review committees include (1) awareness of the perspectives of the review board; (2) awareness of the impact of technology on teaching; (3) awareness of discipline-specific assumptions about teaching, scholarship and service; 4) provision of clear and timely guidelines for faculty, and 5) documentation of the processes and rationale for decision making.

RECOMMENDED RESOURCES

Organizations for Educators

- The American Association of University Professors (AAUP) provides faculty support and resources on issues concerning faculty role performance, research, and research ethics. Free access to the publication *Academe Online* is available at http://www.aaup.org.
- The National League for Nursing (NLN) provides education, resources, networking, and the development of a strong work force. Visit at http://www.nln.org for more information.

Networking for Nurse Educators

- NRSINGED is a listserv for individuals involved in nursing education. This group welcomes discussion of a wide range of topics related to the role and functions of nurse educators. To join, send an e-mail message to listserv@ulkyvm.louisville.edu. Include this message in the body of your e-mail "subscribe nrsinged yourfirstname yourlastname."
- CARENETL is a discussion list for nurse faculty. To join, send an e-mail message to listserv@admin.humberc.on.ca. Include the words: "subscribe CARENETL yourfirstname yourlastname" in the body of your e-mail.

Nursing Informatics

- Nursinginformatics.com is a comprehensive resource for nurses interested in developing informatics knowledge and skills. The site features self-assessment tools to determine learning needs, extensive tutorials, and resources available at http://www.nursing-informatics.com.
- The American Nurses Informatics Association is a membership organization promoting education and networking for individuals interested in nursing informatics. The association publishes the *Computers, Informatics, and Nursing* journal, and provides extensive links to online certificate and graduate programs in informatics available at http://www.ania.org.

Political Advocacy

- The American Nurses Association offers an RN Activist Tool Kit that contains resources and information for political advocacy, available at http://nursing world.org/.
- The National League for Nursing Web site at http://www.nln.org houses a section on governmental affairs that provides guidance for nurse educators seeking to become more knowledgeable about pending educational legislation and the political advocacy process. Access to a free Nursing Education Policy Newsletter is also available.

REFERENCES

1. American Association of Colleges of Nursing. (2008). *Cultural competency in baccalaureate nursing education.* Retrieved March 30, 2009 from http://www.aacn.nche.edu/Education/pdf/competency.pdf.

2. American Association of Colleges of Nursing & The John A. Hartford Foundation Institute for Geriatric Nursing. (2005). *Older adults: Recommended baccalaureate competencies and curricular guidelines for geriatric nursing care.* Retrieved March 30, 2009 from http://www.aacn.nche.edu/ Education/gercomp.htm.

3. Christoffel, K. K. (2000). Public health advocacy: Process and product. *American Journal of Public Health, 90*(5), 722–226.

4. Cohen, D., de la Vega, R., & Watson, G. (2001). *Advocacy for social justice: A global action and reflection guide.* Sterling, VA: Kumarian Press, Inc.

5. Committee on Educating Public Health Professionals for the 21st Century. (2003). *Who will keep the public healthy: Educating public health professionals for the 21st century.* Washington, DC: The National Academies Press.

6. Diamond, R. M. (2002). *Serving on promotion, tenure, and faulty review committees: A faculty guide* (2nd ed.). Bolton, MA: Anker.

7. Dunham-Taylor, J., Lynn, C. W., Moore, P., McDaniel, S., & Walker, J. K. (2008). What goes around comes around: Improving faculty retention through more effective mentoring. *Journal of Professional Nursing, 24*(6), 337–346.

8. Finkelman, A., & Kenner, C. (2008). Educational and service partnerships: An example of global flattening. *Journal of Professional Nursing, 24*(1), 59–65.

9. Friedman, T. L. (2005). *The world is flat: A brief history of the twenty-first century,* New York: Farrar, Straus & Giroux.

10. Hall-Long, B. (2009). Nursing and public policy: A tool for excellence in education, practice, and research. *Nursing Outlook, 57,* 78–83.

11. Health Resources and Services Administration. (1997). *A national informatics agenda for nursing education and practice. Report to the secretary of the department of health and human resources.* Rockville, MD: Health Resources and Services Administration.

12. Johnson, W. B. (2007). *On being a mentor.* Mahwah, NJ: Lawrence Erlbaum Associates.

13. Morin, K. H., & Ashton, K. C. (2004). Research on faculty orientation programs: Guidelines and directions for nurse educators. *Journal of Professional Nursing, 20*(4), 239–250.

14. National Coalition for Health Professional Education in Genetics. (2007). *Core competencies in genetics for health professionals.* Retrieved March 30, 2009 from http://www.nchpeg.org.

15. National League for Nursing, Task Group on Nurse Educator Competencies. (2005). *Core competencies of nurse educators with task statements.* Retrieved September 10, 2008 from http://www.nln.org/facultydevelopment/pdf/corecompetencies.pdf.

16. O'Carroll, P. W., and the Public Health Informatics Competencies Working Group. (2002). *Informatics competencies for public health professionals.* Northwest Center for Public Health Practice. Retrieved March 26, 2009 from http://www.nwcphp.org/docs/phi/comps/phi_print.pdf.

17. Oermann, M. H. (1994). Professional nursing education in the future: Changes and challenges. *Journal of Obstetric, Gynecological, and Neonatal Nursing, 23*(2), 153–159.

18. Seok, S. (2007). Standards, accreditation, benchmarks, and guidelines in distance education. *The Quarterly Review of Distance Education, 8*(4), 387–398.

19. Staggers, N., Gassert, C. A., & Curran, C. (2001). Informatics competencies for nurses at four levels of practice. *Journal of Nursing Education, 40*(7), 303–316.

20. Terenzini, P., & Pascarella, E. (1994, January/ February). Living with myths: Undergraduate education in America. *Change,* 28–32.

INDEX

Pages followed by t or f denote tables and figures respectively.

CPSIA information can be obtained
at www.ICGtesting.com
Printed in the USA
FSHW020805040421
80075FS